Lois A. Fort Cowles, PhD

Social Work in the Health Field
A *Care Perspective*

Second Edition

*Pre-publication
REVIEWS,
COMMENTARIES,
EVALUATIONS . . .*

"This book clearly defines the knowledge, values, and skill sets necessary for social work delivery throughout the health care continuum. A strength of the book is that it begins with the historical footing and foundation of social work in health care and then delineates and elaborates on the delivery of social work services today in a wide array of settings.

This text is logical, straightforward, very readable, and helpful as a reference tool, providing a coherent view of the patchwork health care system and the social worker's varying roles. Academicians, undergraduate and graduate students, and new social work practitioners will substantially increase their understanding of the health care arena and the varying roles of social work through a careful reading of this book. This text is truly unique in its approach of combining policy, theory, and practice concepts impacting social work services in health care delivery.

I have used this book in the classroom and in workshop settings with medical social work focus groups. Repeatedly, this book has received rave reviews as being 'readable, relevant, and informative'—this from social work practitioners involved in delivering social work services within the health care arena."

Denice Goodrich Liley, PhD, ACSW
*Associate Professor,
Boise State University,
School of Social Work*

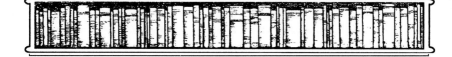

More pre-publication
REVIEWS, COMMENTARIES, EVALUATIONS . . .

"In the second edition of *Social Work in the Health Field: A Care Perspective*, Lois Cowles has produced a comprehensive and detailed portrait of social work in health care. This book is useful as a text in both practice and policy courses. Dr. Cowles does a particularly fine job identifying and explaining current policy and policy issues in each health practice setting.

Dr. Cowles documents the movement of social work and health care from the institutional, hospital setting into community-based care. Community-based care presents opportunities for social work to emphasize the public health model to primary, secondary, and tertiary prevention rather than following the 'medical repair' paradigm. Included is the strong argument for the integration of physical and mental health care in the practice of primary care. A realistic appraisal of contemporary social work practice in health care is followed by a provocative summary of future trends in health care and social work. Opportunities are seen in a future health care system more attuned to the needs of the American people.

Lois Cowles' second edition is a welcome addition to what has become a limited number of social work texts focused on health care practice."

Gary Lounsberry, PhD, MPH, LCSW
Associate Professor, Social Work,
Florida Gulf Coast University

"In her second edition of this text, Lois Cowles has given us a historical perspective and a theoretical framework with which to understand the context of social work practice in a rapidly changing health care environment. She calls for a shift from the curative medical model to a supportive and caring model and brings a public health perspective by focusing on health promotion and disease prevention.

Her integration of physical and mental health and acknowledgment of the importance of a public health approach for social work practice makes this text essential for social work health practice classes. Cowles explores social work interventions in a variety of settings, and justifies the need for evidence-based interventions. This new edition highlights recent changes in the organization and financing of health care and provides an understanding of how health policy impacts health practice. This book is a must-read for social work students planning to practice in today's ever-changing health arena. It should certainly become the text of choice for social work health practice classes."

Marjorie Sable, DrPh, MSW
Associate Professor,
School of Social Work,
University of Missouri–Columbia

THSWPP

The Haworth Social Work Practice Press
An Imprint of The Haworth Press, Inc.
New York • London • Oxford

Social Work in the Health Field

A Care Perspective

Second Edition

Social Work
in the Health Field
A Care Perspective

Second Edition

Lois A. Fort Cowles, PhD

The Haworth Social Work Practice Press
An Imprint of The Haworth Press, Inc.
New York • London • Oxford

Published by

The Haworth Social Work Practice Press, an imprint of The Haworth Press, Inc., 10 Alice Street, Binghamton, NY 13904-1580.

TR: 5.16.04

Cover design by Brooke R. Stiles.

Library of Congress Cataloging-in-Publication Data

Cowles, Lois A. Fort.
    Social work in the health field : a care perspective / Lois A. Fort Cowles.—2nd ed.
       p. cm.
    Includes bibliographical references and index.
    ISBN 0-7890-2118-8 (hc : acid-free)—ISBN 0-7890-2119-6 (pb : acid-free)
    1. Medical social work. I. Title.

HV687 .C68 2003
362.1'0425—dc21

                                 2002154815

CONTENTS

ABOUT THE AUTHOR

Lois Anne Fort Cowles, MSW, PhD, is Professor Emerita at Idaho State University in Pocatello, Idaho, where she taught both core courses and electives in aging and health care. She is also a licensed clinical social worker in Indiana and has 23 years of social work practice experience in a variety of fields, including health care, prior to shifting to university teaching in social work education programs.

Dr. Cowles is a member of the National Association of Social Workers, the Academy of Certified Social Workers, the Society for Social Work Leadership in Health Care, the Council on Social Work Education, the American Public Health Association, AGE-SW (the NASW Section on Aging), the American Society on Aging (ASA), the Idaho Women's Network, and the Honor Society of Phi Kappa Phi.

Dr. Cowles has been active in the development of an interdisciplinary gerontology education program at Idaho State and has served as a technical consultant to the SAGE-SOCIAL WORK Project of the Council on Social Work Education. She has testified in the Idaho state legislature for higher standards for social work services in nursing homes.

Foreword

Much has changed in our world and profession since the first edition of *Social Work in the Health Field: A Care Perspective* was published just three years ago. Since that time the twin towers of the World Trade Center in New York City were attacked, insidious anthrax exposures claimed lives, color-coded security alerts have become commonplace, the human genome project has increased the feasibility of mapping of inherited diseases, and epidemics such as severe acute respiratory syndrome (SARS) have spread rapidly around the globe. The gap between the wealthy and the poor has widened, the population in the United States has aged, and ethnic populations have increased. Against this dynamic backdrop, I found Dr. Lois Cowles' latest textbook to be an exciting and necessary guide for current and future health care practice.

The integrative nature of this book is perhaps its most unique quality. Building on core social work theories of human behavior and the social environment, knowledge, values, skills, and ethics, Cowles repeatedly links fundamental social work perspectives to the practice of social work in health care settings. She then locates both client difficulties and social work functions within a complex, interactive environment composed of the corporatization of health care, the shift from acute to chronic illness and disability, changing demographics in the United States, and globalization of medical issues. The meticulous interweaving of health policy, research, and practice methods into whole cloth fosters a clear understanding of the interrelationships between micro, mezzo, and macro issues.

To say that Cowles' book is extremely well researched and comprehensive is an understatement. Expanding the content of the first edition, this *Social Work in the Health Field* includes more emphasis on the impacts of ethnicity, race, culture, gender, age, education, religion and spirituality, urbanity, rurality, and poverty on health beliefs, behaviors, and status. These psychosocial impacts and the paradigm shift to caring for more persons with chronic illnesses and disabilities are addressed in new material regarding complementary and alternative medicine, wellness programs, risk factors, and the importance of interdisciplinary teams. Specific approaches to the prevention or reduction of medical problems correlated with obesity, smoking, domestic violence, dementia, and congestive heart failure are discussed.

Building upon her extensive experience as a clinical social worker, university professor, and researcher in the fields of aging and health care, Cowles combines scholarly integrity and updated, disease-specific statistics with a most enjoyable, readable writing style. Her book is well organized, and the logical format of each chapter is followed by a succinct summary. Chapters that examine various settings such as primary care, hospitals, home care, hospice, and nursing begin with rich histories of social work practice in those traditional industry segments. Informed by knowledge of the past, practitioners are encouraged to understand current and future implications for the unique client difficulties, professional roles and functions, and organizational structure of diverse settings. These writings prepare the reader for the challenging and expansive vision of social work practice in health care in the future that is offered in the final chapter.

In summary, this "must-have" textbook is a source of new knowledge for beginning and seasoned practitioners alike. Former students have exclaimed that they "loved" Cowles' first book. I have no doubt that the accolades for this second edition will greatly surpass those of the first.

Carlean Gilbert, DSW, LCSW
Assistant Professor
School of Social Work
Loyola University, Chicago

Preface

In this second edition of *Social Work in the Health Field: A Care Perspective,* the major changes include an update of research findings and statistical data on social work in health care and on the health care system in general, especially extensive material incorporated into Chapter 3 on primary care. An additional effort has been made to highlight certain important definitions and concepts through the use of "barred text."

This book is designed to provide an introduction to social work practice in the field of health care. An effort has been made to address both physical and mental health in the same text because continued separation of the two arenas makes less sense than it once did.

Traditionally, social work in mental and physical health has been practiced from the perspective of the biopsychosocial model. Now developing scientific evidence suggests that physical health problems not only can produce psychological and social environmental problems for people but also, to some extent, may be induced by them. There is also growing recognition that some mental health problems have physical manifestations, such as differences in body chemistry, and may even have a genetic component in their etiology. At the same time, both emotional and social environmental conditions continue to be seen as playing a vital role in the course and management of severe mental illness and in the etiology of less serious mental health problems.

A theme of this text is that health professionals need to expand the focus of their attention from preoccupation with repairing human problems (curing) to a more supportive approach to helping (caring) at each of three levels of health intervention: (1) health promotion and primary prevention of disease; (2) secondary prevention, or prevention of the development of existing health problems; and (3) tertiary prevention, or prevention of avoidable discomfort and disability associated with chronic or terminal health problems.

Chapter 1

- highlights the historical background and current settings of social work in health care;

- describes some basic theoretical concepts for social work in health care—such as the person-in-environment perspective, the biopsychosocial model, medical care and health care, and curing and caring—and relates them to the three basic levels of health service intervention;
- discusses the relationship between human diversity and health behavior, illness behavior, and sick-role behavior and its relevance to social work in health care;
- addresses the multidisciplinary nature of health care organizations, interdisciplinary teamwork within such settings, and the implications for social work practice in health care;
- describes other features of health care organizations of significance to social work practice in health care, such as their secondary setting nature; differences between public, voluntary, and proprietary organizations, as well as between secular and sectarian ones; organizational functions; the authority structure and the problem of authority and role definition in professional organizations; and the constraints imposed by Medicare and Medicaid on social work practice; and
- discusses the basic functions of social workers in health care settings, including presenting some common problem types faced by patients and their families that social workers address in their practice.

Chapter 2

- presents the generic and special knowledge requirements for effective social work practice in health settings;
- addresses issues of values and ethics for social work in health care and their relationship to human diversity;
- discusses the generic and special skills needed for social work practice in health care; and
- examines social work intervention in health care, with particular emphasis on the concept of "the care approach to helping," which leads to empowerment and reduction in helplessness of the patient and family through various forms of supportive assistance.

Chapters 3 through 7, respectively, address social work in primary care, hospitals, home care, nursing homes, and hospice care.

Chapter 8 overviews the strengths and shortcomings of the U.S. health care system and some alternate models for health care delivery and financing.

Chapter 9 summarizes the multiple trends in health care in the United States and their implications for the future of social work in the field. The need is highlighted for outcomes research in social work to firm up our body of knowledge of best practices, and for development of "care technology" directed to primary, secondary, and tertiary prevention.

Acknowledgments

I was remiss in the first edition of this book in not acknowledging the other people who had a clear and positive influence on my writing it. I want to make amends for this oversight now.

The person who had the most direct effect on the development of my ideas was Professor Martin B. Loeb, PhD, who was Director of the Faye McBeth Institute on Aging at the University of Wisconsin in Madison when I was a doctoral student there in the social welfare program. He hired me as a student research associate to assist him in developing the "concept of caring." He called it the "Care Project."

When Martin first described my assignment, I was speechless, and muttered something like, "Well everyone knows what caring means, don't they?" He responded, "Do they?" I then attempted to define it and found that I was not as clear about its meaning as I thought I was. Martin commented to me that it seemed to him that there surely must be something one can "do" for a person, even when you cannot "cure" him or her. He added, "We often hear people use the phrase 'curing and caring,' but what does it really mean?"

The ideas that grew from that work with Martin Loeb eventually developed into this book. Martin and I both came to realize that we had also been subconsciously influenced by the medical sociologist, David Mechanic, a friend of Martin's, who had earlier taught at the University of Wisconsin at Madison and in his textbook on medical sociology in 1978 had a section on "the technology of caring" which he referred to as " . . . a range of techniques based not only on human feeling, or even on the techniques associated with psychotherapy, but on scientific knowledge of how to provide human support" (1978:309).

I also wish to express my gratitude to the man who chaired my dissertation committee, Dr. Myron J. Lefcowitz (Jack), who was supportive and encouraging, even after I graduated and began teaching. We co-authored a couple of journal articles based on my dissertation. He was a man of principle, a kind man who liked to teach by asking you questions; the "Socratic method," he called it.

My Maryland sister, Barbara Malinowski, provided much encouragement via Saturday phone calls while I was writing this book, and my brother, Brad Fort, let me visit him at his Montana log home when I needed some "R and R."

Finally, I owe my life and everything else to my parents, Charles and Rebecca Fort, who both lived to be 94 years old, and whose last several years of life I shared as their family caregiver here in this house to which I have now returned. This is where I built a 25 x 50 foot hedge-enclosed formal flower garden when I was so confined with caregiving that I learned to find much beauty and richness where I was. The garden survives and is being revitalized. My brother, Robert Fort, who, more than anyone, taught me to believe in myself, had the stone to mark our parents' burial site engraved with the true statement: "They gave us life and taught us how to live."

Abbreviations

AAA	Area Agency on Aging
AAHSW	American Association of Hospital Social Workers
AASW	American Association of Social Workers
ADL	activity of daily living
AFDC	Aid to Families with Dependent Children
AHA	American Hospital Association
AIDS	acquired immunodeficiency syndrome
AMA	American Medical Association
APHA	American Public Health Association
BBRA	Balanced Budget Reconciliation Act
CABG	coronary artery bypass graft
CEO	chief executive officer
CHF	congestive heart failure
CHAMPUS	Civilian Health and Medical Programs of the Uniformed Services
CISD	critical incident stress debriefing
CMHC	community mental health center
CNA	certified nursing assistant
COPD	chronic obstructive pulmonary disease
CSWE	Council on Social Work Education
CVA	cerebral vascular accident
DHHS	Department of Health and Human Services
DNR	do not resuscitate
DOL	Department of Labor
DPS	disproportionate share
DRG	diagnosis-related group
DSM	*Diagnostic and Statistical Manual of Mental Disorders*
EEG	electroencephalogram
GDP	gross domestic product
GED	general equivalency diploma
HCA	Hospital Corporation of America
HCFA	Health Care Financing Administration
HHC	home health care

HIV	human immunodeficiency virus
HMO	health maintenance organization
HRQL	health-related quality of life
IADL	instrumental activities of daily living
ID	interdisciplinary
IOM	Institute of Medicine
IPA	independent practice association
JAMA	*Journal of the American Medical Association*
JCAHO	Joint Commission on the Accreditation of Healthcare Organizations
MGH	Massachusetts General Hospital
MRI	magnetic resonance imaging
NAACP	National Association for the Advancement of Colored People
NAHC	National Association for Home Care
NASW	National Association of Social Workers
NFCSP	National Family Caregiver Support Program
NHPCO	National Hospice and Palliative Care Organization
NIH	National Institutes of Health
NIMH	National Institute of Mental Health
NLN	National League of Nursing
NMA	National Medical Association
OARS	Older Americans Resources Survey
OECD	Organization for Economic Cooperation and Development
OMBRA	Omnibus Budget Reconciliation Act
PACE	Program of All-Inclusive Care for the Elderly
PCG	primary caregiver
POS	point of service
PPO	preferred provider organization
PPS	prospective payment system
PRIME-MD	Primary Care Evaluation of Mental Health Disorders
PSDA	Patient Self-Determination Act
PSO	provider service organization
QOL	quality of life
QUIG	quality indicator group
RUG	resource utilization group
SNF	skilled nursing facility
SSI	Supplemental Security Income
SSWAHC	Society for Social Work Administrators in Health Care
VA	Veterans Administration
VNA	Visiting Nurse Association
WHO	World Health Organization

SECTION I:
INTRODUCTION AND OVERVIEW

Chapter 1

Orientation to Social Work in the Health Field

HISTORICAL BACKGROUND AND DEVELOPMENT

The Birth of Social Work in Health Care

Social work in health care began in the hospital setting in 1905 when a nurse, Garnet I. Pelton, was appointed by a physician, Richard C. Cabot, to fill the first hospital social worker position at Massachusetts General Hospital (MGH) in the Internal Medicine Clinic (Cannon, 1923, cited in Cowles, 1990:2). Two years later, in 1907, social work services were placed in the Neurology Clinic of MGH, and this event is sometimes heralded as the beginning of social work in mental health (Stuart, 1997:26). However, there is little evidence that anyone at the time made a distinction between medical and psychiatric social work.

According to Ida Cannon (1923), who soon succeeded Garnet Pelton in the social worker position and became a pioneer in hospital social work, the birth of social work in hospitals was closely related to the extension of medical practice from the physician's office and home visits to the hospital as the setting for medical diagnosis and treatment. An effect of this change, which occurred around the turn of the twentieth century, was what Cannon called "a constriction of the field of vision" of the physician (1923:30). The physician was cut off from observation of patients in the context of their homes, work, and other life situations. Thus, the physician was left to focus primarily on physical factors (Cowles, 1990).

Social work in hospitals was conceptualized as a means of compensating for this deficit by having its practitioners provide reports to the medical and nursing staff describing the patient's home and work situations. According to Cannon (1923:14), Dr. Cabot saw the potential for social work in hospitals to be "a potent means for more accurate diagnosis and more effective treatment" (cited in Cowles, 1990:3). Cannon described this function of hospital social work:

It seeks to understand and to treat the social complications of disease by establishing a close relationship between the medical care of patients in hospitals or dispensaries and the services of those skilled in the profession of social work, to bring to the institutionalized care of the sick such personal knowledge of their social condition as will hasten and safeguard their recovery. (Cannon, 1923:i)

In a speech titled "Hospital and Dispensary Social Work" delivered at the International Conference of Social Work held in Paris, France, in July 1928, Dr. Cabot agreed that a primary function of hospital social work was to teach doctors and nurses about "the social and psychological aspects of disease" (Cabot, 1928:265).

The Complementary Function of Hospital Social Work

"It seeks to understand and to treat the social complications of disease by establishing a close relationship between the medical care of patients in hospitals or dispensaries and the services of those skilled in the profession of social work, to bring to the institutionalized care of the sick such personal knowledge of their social condition as will hasten and safeguard their recovery." (Cannon, 1923:i)

Early Seeds of Role Conflict

The disagreement that lingers today between physicians and social workers concerning the hospital social worker role emerged in this seminal period and is evident when Cannon's (1923) and Cabot's (1928) other expectations are compared.

The difference was that Cannon expected the social work role to include the direct treatment of the patient's social and psychological problems, which she believed were among the causes or effects of the patient's health problems or acted as barriers to cooperation with the medical treatment plan:

> The social worker seeks to remove those obstacles in the patient's surroundings, or in his mental attitude, that interfere with successful treatment, thus freeing him to aid in his own recovery. (Cannon, 1923:15)

This view of the social worker's role is also evident in Cannon's reference to

> the need for the cooperation of one skilled in understanding social problems, and equipped by training and experience to guide a patient

in solving those personal ones, that may arise from his illness or to which his illness may have been due in part. (1923:30)

In contrast, when Cabot spoke of the main functions of hospital social work, he described the social worker as a liaison or bridge between the hospital and the social environment and community resources of the patient: "For one of the chief functions of such a department [hospital social work] is to connect the hospital with all the social forces and helpful agencies outside its walls" (1928:260).

The Direct Treatment Role of Social Work in Health Care

"The social worker seeks to remove those obstacles in the patient's surroundings, or in his mental attitude, that interfere with successful treatment, thus freeing him to aid in his own recovery." (Cannon, 1923:15)

Similarly, Cabot expected the hospital social worker to help patients adjust to hospitalization (e.g., to explain the hospital system to patients and provide reassurance if they were frightened by it and to explain their health condition to them if it appeared the medical and nursing staff had not adequately done so) and to help patients adjust to returning home (e.g., help patients and their families understand the implications of the patients' health condition for the posthospital stage, such as the expected length of disability) (1928:262-263).

In short, Cabot (1928) expected the role of the social worker to revolve around bridging the gap between the hospital environment and the usual social environment of the patients in order to remove barriers to effective medical treatment, while Cannon (1923) additionally expected the hospital social work role to include efforts to modify any social, environmental, or emotional causes or effects impacting the patients' health condition.

The Biopsychosocial Perspective of Social Work in Health Care

This view of the social worker's role is also evident in Cannon's reference to "the need for the cooperation of one skilled in understanding social problems, and equipped by training and experience to guide a patient in solving those personal ones, that may arise from his illness or to which his illness may have been due in part." (Cannon, 1923:30)

Growth of Social Work in Hospital Health Care

From this beginning, with one social worker in one hospital in 1905, so-cial workers were established in 100 hospitals by 1913 and in 400 by 1923 (Cannon, 1923:vii). By 2000, 76 percent of psychiatric hospitals and 86 per-cent of general acute-care hospitals reported having social work services (American Hospital Association, 2002). Although the majority of all types of hospitals claim to have social work services, the 1995 National Associa-tion of Social Workers (NASW) membership survey results indicate that only 18.2 percent of social worker respondents name their primary practice setting as nonpsychiatric inpatient facilities and less than 1 percent (0.7 per-cent) report their primary practice setting as an inpatient mental health facil-ity (Gibelman and Schervish, 1996:94).

Overall Practice Settings and Practice Areas

A 1982 NASW membership survey found that mental health was the largest practice area of its approximately 90,000 members (26.6 percent), while the physical health field was second largest (18.1 percent), indicating that nearly 45 percent (44.7 percent) of NASW members were practicing in mental or physical health care (Gibelman and Schervish, 1996:94).

Data from the 1995 NASW membership survey indicated that mental health continues to be identified by social workers as the largest social work *practice area,* with 39 percent so naming it, and another 12.9 percent named medical health as their primary practice area (coming in third after family and children's services—24.9 percent of NASW members responding), in-dicating that 51.9 percent of NASW members then reported their primary practice area as mental or physical health care (Gibelman and Schervish, 1996:94).

However, it should be pointed out that less than 4 percent (3.2 percent) of all 1995 survey respondents classified their primary *practice setting* as either inpatient or outpatient mental health, while a total of 34.6 percent classified their primary practice setting as a medical health site. Inpatient medical facilities (i.e., hospitals), were named by 18.2 percent of respondents as their primary practice setting, second only to social services agencies, named by 20.5 percent (Gibelman and Schervish, 1996:94).

This suggests some discrepancy between what social workers consider their practice area and their practice setting. Perhaps an increasing percent-age of clinical social workers in health care settings have come to think of themselves as practicing in mental health more than in health care. In addition, many clinical social workers in private social work practice probably classify their practice area as mental health.

The 2000 NASW Practice Research Network Survey (NASW, 2000) of a sample of its members found that although 39 percent of respondents continued to classify their primary practice area as *mental* health, only 8 percent reported *medical* health as their primary practice area, down from 12.9 percent in the previous membership survey. However, an additional 14 percent of respondents named unspecified multiple practice areas, and another 14 percent were classified as "other." Thus 28 percent of the responses are uninterpretable. According to the report, a total of 47 percent of NASW members practice in the "health" area, combining mental and physical health. Again, as in the 1995 memberwide survey, a smaller percentage (20 percent) of members named mental health as their organizational practice setting than the percentage (39 percent) who named mental health as their practice area. Curiously, although only 8 percent said medical health was their primary practice *area,* 12 percent named it as their primary practice setting and an additional 5 percent named it as their secondary practice setting.

The First Specialty Area and Secondary Setting of Social Work

Social work in the health field has the distinction of being the first specialty area of social work practice, which also marked the entry of social work into *secondary settings* of practice, or settings in which the primary organizational function is not social work but another function, such as medical care, education, law enforcement, or business and industry.

In 1918, hospital social workers banded together to form the American Association of Hospital Social Workers (AAHSW), which published the journal *Hospital Social Service* from 1919 until 1933 (Bracht, 1978:11, 14). In 1955, the AAHSW merged with other specialty groups and with the American Association of Social Workers (AASW) to become the National Association of Social Workers (NASW) (Popple and Leighninger, 1993: 72).

Currently, two specialty journals of social work in health care are published: *Health and Social Work,* a publication of the NASW, and *Social Work in Health Care,* published by The Haworth Press, Inc. On their inside front covers, both journals broadly define health care to include both mental and physical health care. The major national specialty organization in health care is the Society for Social Work Leadership in Health Care, formerly known as the Society for Social Work Administrators in Health Care (SSWAHC) of the American Hospital Association (AHA), founded in 1965.

The Separation of Medical from Psychiatric Social Work

What little literature exists concerning the development of psychiatric social work suggests that prior to the 1920s, social workers employed in medical and psychiatric clinics were engaged in much the same types of roles and functions as described earlier by Cannon (1923) and Cabot (1928), that is, providing relevant social environmental information concerning patients to nurses and physicians, facilitating patient discharge and posthospital adjustment, and linking patients and families with needed community resources. This is reflected in the following commentary on early psychiatric social work:

> Before 1920 psychiatric social work was based on the assumption that a knowledge of the social environment was vital to an understanding of individual behavior. The gathering of such information by means of social casework was, in theory, the primary function of the specialty. In practice, however, social casework was fluid rather than fixed. The daily activities of social workers centered on providing assistance and aid to distressed individuals and to help them take advantage of a variety of supportive services. (Grob, 1983:250)

What began as "social work in health care" eventually divided into medical and psychiatric social work, a division stimulated by the introduction of Freudian psychoanalytic concepts around 1920. This division was further solidified by the acceleration of the mental hygiene movement following World War I, which involved the rapid expansion of psychiatric hospital and home services to returning servicemen (Lubove, 1965:76, 89). Many servicemen were suffering from what was then called "shell shock," but is now labeled post-traumatic stress disorder (PTSD).

Freudian theory became popular in America around 1920, at a time when social workers were in the throes of distress over Abraham Flexnor's 1915 address to them. Flexnor asserted that social work was not a profession because it did not have a body of knowledge rooted in science and did not focus on direct services to individuals, as much as on environmental modification and consultation and linkage of clients to other direct-service providers (Trattner, 1989:234-235). Flexnor's message stimulated a struggle within the social work profession to make the needed changes to win professional status. It also marked the beginning of a rift between practitioners who continued to see the basic mission of social work as improving environmental conditions for people and those who sought professional status through shifting to a focus on person-centered problems with a psychoanalytic theory base.

A training school for psychiatric social work was established at Smith College in 1918 (Lubove, 1965:78), and in 1922 a section on psychiatric social work was organized within the AAHSW (Lubove, 1965:127).

Following both World War I and World War II, thousands of American servicemen returned home with both psychological and physical injuries. Veterans Administration (VA) hospitals rapidly expanded after World War II and employed large numbers of both medical and psychiatric social workers.

Then, the *deinstitutionalization movement,* a push to reduce the population of mental institutions and to transfer the patients to community-based care, took off in the 1950s. A variety of events combined to provide the momentum for change, including the growing recognition that (1) America's mental hospitals were overcrowded; (2) they were warehouses more than treatment or rehabilitation centers; (3) their bureaucratic organization tended to create *secondary* disabilities (disabilities resulting from social responses to people with primary disabilities), which added to the primary mental dysfunction; and (4) their cost to taxpayers had reached alarming proportions. The movement culminated in the serendipitous discovery of *psychotropic drugs* (drugs that alter mood or mental functioning), which made it possible to consider community-based treatment as an alternative to institutionalization (Trattner, 1989:187-188).

The Community Mental Health Center (CMHC) Program accompanied the deinstitutionalization movement. The program began with the passage of the Community Mental Health Services Acts of 1963 and 1965, which provided for the nationwide development of federal and state tax-funded, community-based, comprehensive mental health service centers (Karger and Stoesz, 1998:340-341).

This development of community mental health centers, like the earlier expansion of VA hospitals, greatly increased job opportunities in social work, especially in psychiatric social work. Unfortunately, during the Reagan administration of the 1980s, the federal government's share of CMHC funding dropped from 24 percent in 1976 to 2 percent by 1984. Many states were unable to make up the difference and, as a result, the centers, whose original intent was to provide comprehensive services to everyone who needed them, with an emphasis on prevention and early intervention, had to be downsized to provide publicly funded services for only the most seriously disturbed (Karger and Stoesz, 1994:321).

Since its inception in 1905 in the general hospital setting, social work in the health field has expanded to include practice in a variety of health care settings, such as psychiatric and other specialty hospitals, public health agencies, nursing homes and rehabilitation centers, health maintenance organizations, community-based clinics, private medical practice, home care

TABLE 1.1. Practice Settings of Health Care Social Workers, 1992

Types of Practice Settings	Percent of all social workers	Number of health care social workers	Percent of health care social workers
Physician's office	1.48	7,025	6.0
Other health professional's office	1.22	5,805	5.0
Nursing/personal care facility	2.99	14,200	12.0
Hospital, public or private	14.13	67,022	54.3
Medical or dental laboratory	0.01	51	0.04
Home health care service	0.90	4,257	4.0
Allied health service	5.28	25,013	20.0
TOTAL	26.01	123,373	101.34

Source: Ginsberg, Leon (1995). *The Social Work Almanac* (Second Edition). Washington, DC: NASW Press, p. 355. Data obtained from U.S. Department of Labor, Bureau of Labor Statistics, November 1993.

agencies, and hospice programs. Whereas in 1983 about 75 percent of medical social workers were employed in hospitals (NASW, 1983) and the majority of psychiatric social workers (i.e., clinical social workers) were presumably employed in community mental health centers, by 1992 the U.S. Department of Labor reported 474,176 employed social workers in the United States, of which 26.02 percent, or 123,372, were in health services. The employment distribution across health care settings is shown in Table 1.1.

The data in Table 1.1 show that by 1992, only about 54.3 percent of health care social workers were employed in hospitals, probably reflecting the downsizing of acute inpatient hospital care as part of the nation's cost-containment efforts, combined with an overall shift of the center of health care from the acute care hospital to community settings, such as outpatient clinics, outpatient surgical centers, outpatient rehabilitation centers, formal and informal home care services, adult day care programs, nursing homes, and hospice programs.

The 2000 National Occupational Employment and Wage Estimates of the U.S. Department of Labor, Bureau of Labor Statistics, indicate that employment classification 21-1022 (Medical and Public Health Social Workers) had approximately 103,390 persons employed in that category, whose function is to

[p]rovide persons, families, or vulnerable populations with the psychosocial support needed to cope with chronic, acute, or terminal illnesses, such as Alzheimer's, cancer, or AIDS. Services include advising family caregivers, providing patient education and counseling, and making necessary referrals for other social services. (USDOL, 2000)

This employment category does not specify degree levels but appears to include the range of social work degrees, including BSW, MSW, DSW, and PhD. However, no data are provided concerning the distribution of organizational settings where these persons were employed.

THEORETICAL PERSPECTIVES

The Person-in-Environment Perspective

The unifying theoretical perspective of all current social work practice is the view that people can best be understood and helped in the context of the conditions and resources of their social environment. *Social environment* refers to the quality and characteristics of one's life situation, including interpersonal relationships, resources, and one's positions, roles, and participation in the society. More specifically, the social environment encompasses factors such as family and home life, employment and income, school situation and educational opportunities, housing and utilities, social welfare resources in the community, opportunities for political participation, access to health services, relationships with neighbors and friends, police protection and crime control, and recreational resources.

Sociologists speak of social institutions or social systems when they refer to the economy, politics, the family, education, health care, transportation, and religion. These are abstractions that characterize the mechanisms through which society provides for its members' basic needs. In a sense, describing a person's social environment means describing his or her situation in life relative to the social institutions of the society.

In real life, the nature of these social institutions is revealed in business and industry, employment opportunities, wage levels, schools, police departments, courts and correctional facilities, religious organizations, health service facilities, a variety of housing types and conditions, and families with a range of cultures, structures, compositions, and levels of functioning. Social workers refer to these real-life manifestations when speaking of the social environment.

Social workers believe that individuals, comprised of their attitudes, feelings, values, beliefs, behaviors, mental and physical health status, and their functioning in social roles in their families, workplaces, schools, neighborhoods, and so forth, can best be understood by taking into account their social environmental situation, as described in the previous paragraph. This belief is called the *person-in-environment perspective.*

The Biopsychosocial Model and the Medical Model

Beginning with the work of Ida Cannon at Massachusetts General Hospital in the early 1900s, the underlying theoretical perspective of social work in the health field has been that physical, psychological, and social environmental conditions tend to influence one another and must be taken into account in order to understand and help clients and their families in health settings. This is called the *biopsychosocial model.*

The biopsychosocial perspective is similar to the person-in-environment perspective. The person-in-environment concept claims that people both affect and reflect their social environment, and this depicts the *dual focus* of the social work profession. The biopsychosocial perspective is an elaboration of the person-in-environment view; it suggests that a person has both psychological and physical components that combine to interact with the social environment.

The biopsychosocial perspective is sometimes referred to as a *holistic* view because it seeks to encompass the "whole picture" of a person. It is often contrasted with the *medical model* that focuses on physical aspects of health problems. Another difference between the medical and biopsychosocial models is that the medical model is focused on physical or mental disease in the individual, while the biopsychosocial model is also attuned to the social environmental causes and effects of health problems.

The biopsychosocial model also is an example of *general systems theory* because it views a person's health status as reflecting the interdependency of physical, psychological, and social environmental systems. General systems theory holds that all levels of organization in nature are linked so that change in one affects change in the others (Engel, 1977).

Social workers in health care settings are concerned with the interaction of physical, psychological, and social conditions of the client, both as causes and effects. A social situation or life change event (such as marital dysfunction, social isolation, loss of one's job, or death of a loved one) can produce emotional distress that can lead to changes in physical functioning that increase vulnerability to disease. On the other hand, a physical health problem can erode self-confidence or interfere with the ability to perform customary activities, which can affect work, marriage, or other social roles and relationships and, in turn, lead to emotional distress.

Health Care and Medical Care

The distinctions between the biopsychosocial model and the medical model are related to the distinction between *health care* and *medical care*. A common failure to understand this difference is one of the problems in the U.S. health care system.

Medical care is what physicians provide in the course of monitoring patient health status and diagnosing and treating health problems. *Health care* refers to individual and societal efforts to prevent health problems from emerging and to promote an optimal level of health. Examples include individuals' efforts at proper diet and exercise, weight control, adequate rest and relaxation, safety precautions, and avoidance of hazardous chemicals. In addition, health care requires an environment that is supportive of physical needs, personal development, and social integration, as well as free of environmental pollution in all its forms.

In other words, health care requires both personal responsibility to choose a healthy lifestyle and social provision of the necessary resources and conditions to enable successful individual efforts. The World Health Organization (WHO) has taken the position that "health is a state of complete physical, mental, and social well-being and not merely the absence of disease or infirmity" (World Health Organization, 1978).

The Concept of Caring

Curing refers to efforts to correct the underlying condition. **Caring** refers to the provision of supportive assistance to: (1) promote healthy growth and development, (2) sustain function and relieve distress during a temporary problem episode, and (3) maximize comfort and function when a problem is permanent or even terminal.

Curing and Caring

Much of medical care is "repair work" for existing health problems. Unfortunately, few serious health problems can be cured (McLachlan and McKeown, 1971:48). Today, the major health problems are chronic rather than acute infectious diseases. In the early 1900s, when social work in health care began, acute infectious disease was the cause of most major health problems.

Curing refers to efforts to correct the underlying condition. *Caring* refers to the provision of supportive assistance to (1) promote healthy growth and development, (2) sustain function and relieve distress during a temporary problem episode, and (3) maximize comfort and function when a problem is permanent or even terminal. Although caring is not limited to any particular level of health service, medical care, as presently constituted, is primarily focused on the secondary level of repair of acute problems (see Chapter 4).

Levels of Health Service and Associated Practice Settings

The health care delivery system has three basic levels of services that represent stages of health status: primary, secondary, and tertiary. These stages revolve around (1) prevention, (2) repair, and (3) compensation.

Primary care, the first level of health service, focuses on primary prevention and health maintenance, that is, preventing health problems from emerging and providing very early intervention. Associated practice settings for social workers and other health professionals include public health agencies, private medical practice (general practice, family practice, internal medicine, and pediatrics), outpatient clinics, and health maintenance organizations (HMOs).

Secondary care focuses on secondary prevention, or preventing health problems that have already emerged from developing into a worsened state, that is, repair and management. Hospitals and other residential treatment centers are the main settings of secondary, or "acute," care.

Tertiary care, the last level of health service, focuses on providing supportive assistance to maximize the comfort and function of persons with well-advanced health problems that cannot be cured, being either chronic or terminal in nature. The practice settings associated with tertiary care include rehabilitation centers, nursing homes, hospice programs, home care agencies, and day care centers.

However, in recent years, it has become less clear which settings are associated with which levels of health service. Hospital emergency rooms and outpatient clinics have increasingly become centers of primary care, especially for the poor. In addition, both nursing homes and home care agencies have begun to serve an increasing number of persons whose conditions are neither chronic nor terminal, but who are recovering from an acute health problem, such as an injury or surgical procedure.

HUMAN DIVERSITY AND BEHAVIOR

Human diversity refers to the fact that people vary, one from another, in a multitude of biopsychosocial dimensions, such as age, gender, racial identity, ethnicity or culture, sexual orientation, religious beliefs and practices, and socioeconomic class (assessed by education, occupation, and income). People also vary in intelligence, talents, interests and hobbies, physical appearance and size, genetic makeup, physical and mental health status, personality traits and coping mechanisms, personal norms and values, support groups and reference groups, rural or urban background, family structure and composition, and relationships, as well as life history and experience. *Sensitivity to human diversity* means being knowledgeable about, attentive to, and respectful of differences in culture, perception, and behavioral patterns that may be associated with human variation. This sensitivity requires individualizing every person by taking into account all that makes them special.

It is important in all social work practice to be sensitive to human diversity variables, because otherwise we cannot truly understand people or their behavior, nor can we work with them effectively. Sensitivity to human diversity is important in health care settings because these variables play important roles in (1) health behavior, (2) illness behavior, and (3) sick-role behavior.

Health behavior refers to what a person does, or does not do, in an effort to take care of his or her health. *Illness behavior* involves how a person interprets and responds to signs and symptoms of health problems. *Sick-role behavior* is a person's behavior following determination of illness or injury.

Sensitivity to Human Diversity

Sensitivity to human diversity means being knowledgeable about, attentive to, and respectful of differences in culture, perception, and behavioral patterns that may be associated with human variation and individualizing every person (i.e., in working with them, take into account all that makes them special).

Relevance of Human Diversity Variables and Behaviors to Social Work Practice

Social workers who practice in health service settings provide a variety of direct services to patients and their families, which will be discussed in Chapter 2. In the course of providing these direct services, it sometimes becomes evident that the patient or family is engaging in behaviors that (1) seem to endanger the patient's health, (2) suggest a lack of attention or excessive attention to symptoms or represent unconventional methods of treatment, or (3) indicate lack of compliance with medical recommendations addressing diet, activity, medications, and stress.

Health behavior can be influenced by such variables as income, education, ethnicity, religion, occupation, intelligence, age, and sexual orientation. Illness behavior can reflect a person's gender, age, mental health status, or ethnicity. Whether a person seeks help from a neighbor, physician, chiropractor, midwife, or spiritual healer can be influenced by social class, religious beliefs, ethnicity, or rural/urban location. Finally, sick-role behavior, such as whether a person's behavior complies with medical or other health service provider recommendations, can be affected by such variables as social class, religious beliefs, ethnicity, available social supports, and gender.

Health, Illness, and Sick-Role Behavior

Health behavior refers to what a person does, or does not do, in an effort to take care of his or her health. **Illness behavior** involves how a person interprets and responds to signs and symptoms of health problems. **Sick-role behavior** is a person's behavior following determination of illness or injury.

In mental health care settings, where social workers are among the primary providers of health treatment services, these behaviors are an integral concern. In physical health care settings, health behavior, illness behavior, and sick-role behavior are primarily the concern of the medical and nursing staff. However, medical social workers may become involved with these behaviors while assisting patients and their families with such social work services as

1. preadmission planning,
2. discharge planning,
3. adjustment to the health care setting or service,
4. adjustment to the diagnosis, prognosis, or medical treatment plan, or
5. helping them to understand and make decisions concerning treatment-related issues.

It is helpful for social workers to be familiar with the literature concerning human diversity as it relates to general differences in human behavior. However, social workers must take care not to assume that because a person is of a particular racial or ethnic group, religion, gender, age, or social class he or she necessarily believes in certain things, adheres to certain customs, or behaves in a prescribed manner. Every human being is a multifaceted individual.

INTERDISCIPLINARY TEAMWORK

Multidisciplinary Organizations

All health service settings are *multidisciplinary,* except perhaps private practice involving one discipline of one professional group. A multidisciplinary setting means that more than one professional group or more than one *discipline* (specialty) within a professional group are working in the same setting.

The Interdisciplinary Concept

However, multidisciplinary settings are not necessarily *interdisciplinary;* interdisciplinary means that various professions or disciplines are working together and collaborating rather than merely working in the same place.

Models of Collaboration

Interdisciplinary teamwork is the consensus form of *collaboration.* Mailick and Jordon (1977) refer to three models of collaboration: (1) *the authoritarian model* (e.g., an operating-room team); (2) *the matrix model* (casual, informal, low-contact interaction among any number of professionals); and (3) *the consensus model* (interdisciplinary teamwork that relies heavily on joint decision making).

Characteristics of Interdisciplinary Teamwork

Theoretically, interdisciplinary teamwork is distinguished from other forms of collaboration by (1) small group size, (2) the operation of small-group dynamics (such as a sense of group bond), (3) shared decision making, and (4) more frequent, regular, and direct face-to-face communication (Mailick and Jordon, 1977).

Interdisciplinary Teams As a Form of Group Practice

Interdisciplinary teamwork is a form of group practice (Rubin and Beckhard, 1972). It revolves around services to a particular patient or client and does not include routine staff meetings (which usually concern staff business). Interdisciplinary teamwork is an alternative to one person of one professional group trying to be all things to the patient; it also is an alternative to several persons being involved without planning and intervening in a collaborative manner.

Social workers in health care settings often are asked to serve on interdisciplinary teams and sometimes to lead them (Kane, 1978, 1980). The core of such teams usually consists of all, or representatives of, the professional staff who are working with the same patient or whose expertise is considered relevant. In addition, teams may include some of the nonprofessional staff who are providing hands-on care, the patient, and some family members.

Background of Interdisciplinary Teamwork in Health Settings

Interdisciplinary health care teams first emerged in community mental health centers and expanded to general hospitals, rehabilitation centers, nursing homes, and other health service settings (Harris, Saunders, and Zasorin-Conners, 1978).

Several developments in the field of health care combined to promote the concept of interdisciplinary teamwork. One of these was the increased specialization and division of labor (Nagi, 1978). Where once there were only general practitioners, multiple medical and surgical specialties grew. Where once hospitals were staffed mostly by physicians and nurses, a variety of other professions, paraprofessions, and technician types of occupations emerged. This increased specialization and division of labor resulted in one patient sometimes having several physicians and other personnel involved in his or her care.

A second development that contributed to the idea of health care teams was the expanding scope of the concept of health (Nagi, 1978), from thinking of it as the absence of physical disease to thinking of it as including healthy environment and lifestyle, weight control, adequate exercise, satisfactory social-role functioning, a positive mental outlook, satisfying involvement in personal development, and a general sense of well-being.

A third factor was the growing recognition that human problems tend to be *complex* (multiple) rather than *simple* (singular). As a hypothetical example, a patient whose main problem seems to be a diseased gallbladder that requires surgical removal may also have a chronic obesity problem and a tendency to eat too much fat, lack regular exercise, be socially isolated, and have marriage problems. Or a person who is diagnosed with schizophrenia may also be alcoholic, homeless, and malnourished, have a venereal disease, be estranged from family or friends, and be without income, support, or occupation.

Finally, a fourth recognition that led to interdisciplinary teamwork, which is related to the third, is that clusters of problems often are interdependent and constitute a *pathology system,* so that one cannot effectively treat one problem without addressing them all (Nagi, 1978; Platt, 1994).

As Platt has noted:

> In health, the nature of problems related to the so-called new morbidity—chronic disease, emotional problems, recurrent illness—and an appreciation of the interaction among social, emotional, and biologic factors require both a new framework for problem analysis and a new way of practice. Systems theory provides the framework for analysis, and a team approach provides a method for practice. (1994:5)

Payne (2000) argues that the nature of health problems today, as well as the new health care systems which are focused on efficiency and community-centered care services, requires that health care teams not only include representatives of relevant health professions but also identify and collaborate with the patient's social network as both service extenders and sources of social support. Payne (2000) calls such teams *open teamwork,* or a combination of the concept of traditional multiprofessional teams with the concept of networking (4-5). Payne (2000:18) cites Wenger's (1994) concept of five types of networks that are important to distinguish in network analysis:

1. *Family-dependent networks*—consisting primarily of contacts with close family members
2. *Locally integrated networks*—consisting of family, neighbors, and friends, with many friends and neighbors being the same
3. *Local self-contained networks*—consisting of distant relationships and low-contact interactions with neighbors and perhaps one nearby relative
4. *Wider community-focused networks*—Active contact with family at a distance, and actively involved in community life and had many friends, but not among neighbors
5. *Private restricted networks*—usually an elderly person living alone or with a spouse, but having little interaction or relationship with anyone else (Such persons were often noted to have a personality type that was a barrier to sustained social interaction.)

By a "network" Payne refers to the patient's social support network, including individuals, organizations, and other resources with which the patient is linked and on which they depend in some way. In a sense, the person's network contains the people and organizations that would be included in what social work often refers to as an *ecomap.*

To paraphrase Briggs (1997:19), the effective interdisciplinary health team, as with all effective small groups, is synergistic in the sense that *the potential power and product of each member is enhanced by interaction and cooperation with the other members.*

Open Teamwork

"In health, the nature of problems related to the so-called new morbidity—chronic disease, emotional problems, recurrent illness—and an appreciation of the interaction among social, emotional, and biologic factors require both a new framework for problem analysis and a new way of practice. Systems theory provides the framework for analysis, and a team approach provides a method for practice." (Platt, 1994:5)

Payne advises that, rather than depend on team members simply to be gracious enough to work cooperatively within the team, it is likely to be more effective "to provide incentives to cooperation which equalize power and let negotiation take place" (2000:29) by means of building in a system of mutual exchanges or benefits. That is, what each one contributes must be shown to be beneficial to the others. In other words, as I interpret Payne's perspective: The multiprofessional team, linked with a bolstered social network (open teamwork), provides the patient with an integrated system of needed supports, which could be called a *care system.*

Rationale for Interdisciplinary Teamwork

The rationale for interdisciplinary teamwork is that multiple kinds of knowledge and skill need to be involved and coordinated to maximize efficiency and effectiveness (Jonas, 1981). *Efficiency* refers to getting the most for the buck, that is, the least waste and cost, relative to the outcome or benefit. On the other hand, *effectiveness* involves a successful outcome in terms of what one aimed to achieve. Thus, the efficiency and/or effectiveness *objectives of interdisciplinary teamwork* include comprehensive and coordinated service delivery, optimal use of staff resources, improved quality of patient care, whole-person care, and cost savings by reducing gaps and overlap in services (Friedson, 1978). As a result, "The recipient of services, the team member, the profession, and society as a whole all benefit from interprofessional collaboration" (Julia and Thompson, 1994a:53).

Functions of Interdisciplinary Teams

The functions of interdisciplinary teams include

1. shared assessment of patient problems and needs,
2. exchange of relevant information,
3. team teaching of clients/patients,
4. ethical decision making,
5. development of intervention plans,
6. delegation of tasks and responsibilities,
7. modification of plans as needed, and
8. evaluation of outcome. (Bope and Jost, 1994)

Common Problems in Interdisciplinary Team Functioning

Interdisciplinary teams may encounter at least six problems:

1. turf protection,
2. different values and perceptions of the problems and needs,
3. self-promotion,
4. prestige and status discrepancies that impair open communication,
5. lack of understanding of one another's language, skills, and knowledge areas, and
6. differences in the problem-solving process. (Julia and Thompson, 1994b)

Teamwork Requirements

Finally, in order for interdisciplinary teams to work well, a number of requirements, which have been identified in a variety of sources (Given and Simmons, 1977; Kane, 1978; French, 1979; Rubin and Beckhard, 1972; Sheps, 1974; Julia and Thompson, 1994a; Briggs, 1997), should be met, including the following:

1. Role clarity, but also role flexibility
2. Mutual respect and trust
3. Consensus on group norms, values, commitment, and purpose
4. An egalitarian attitude; a sense of equal importance
5. A sense of group bond and interdependence, not autonomy
6. Open communication and sharing
7. Flexible leadership and decision making; shared power
8. Flexible membership composition based on case needs

9. A stable core membership
10. A sense of both group identity and professional identity
11. Ability to negotiate and reach consensus
12. Goal focus and goal clarity
13. Record keeping of meetings: dates, members present, issues discussed, decisions made
14. Attention to both the task and maintenance functions of the team
15. A systems perspective

Group Decision-Making Styles

There are at least four decision-making styles in any group: (1) *default* (no decision), (2) *unilateral* (imposed from above), (3) *majority vote* (most agree), and (4) *consensus* (all agree) (Rubin and Beckhard, 1972).

Although consensus is the ideal outcome, it is important to achieve it fairly. Unfortunately, team decision making in health care settings and elsewhere is often undemocratically influenced by those with more prestige or power. In reality, we live in a society in which the medical professional is accorded a level of prestige and power far exceeding that of any other health care profession (Caputi, 1978). In addition, professional education in all fields is primarily university based, with a reward system that reinforces autonomy and competition rather than cooperation and interdisciplinary education and experience (Lodge, 1974). As a result, members of various health professions enter health care settings with little orientation to or experience with one another (Kane, 1976-1977). Furthermore, in most health care settings, the physician is ultimately responsible for patient outcomes and timely discharge. Thus, in a real sense, the call to interdisciplinary teamwork may be experienced as disorienting (Lonsdale, Webb, and Briggs, 1980:106), and those involved may encounter difficulty in achieving its theoretically ideal process and benefits.

Still, we must persist in efforts to develop professional educational preparation for interdisciplinary teamwork, both in the classroom and in practice, if we expect to make collaborative practice work (Waugaman, 1994; Casto, 1994).

Although health service settings are usually multidisciplinary and are sometimes interdisciplinary, additional features of health service organizations can influence social work practice in them. These are explored next.

OTHER ORGANIZATIONAL CONSIDERATIONS

Health service settings are secondary settings of social work practice and professional organizations that sometimes have a dual-authority system.

They may be complex organizations that also vary by whether they are public, voluntary, or proprietary and by whether they are sectarian or secular. Government efforts to control the rising cost of health services have brought major changes in professional autonomy, paperwork, and intervention criteria, time frame, and prioritization.

Secondary Settings

Health service settings are examples of *secondary settings* of social work practice because their main function is something other than social work. In this case, the primary function is health service. Thus, social work services in health settings are *auxiliary* (supplementary or supportive) and *ancillary* (subordinate) to the services of the medical and nursing care staff. The obvious exception to this is the community mental health agency, in which social workers are among the primary, rather than secondary, service providers.

This does not necessarily mean that social work services are not highly valued by the medical and nursing staff or that social workers are expected to behave subserviently to them. It simply means that the medical and nursing functions are more central than the social work functions to the operation of the organizational system. The situation would be reversed if, for example, a social work organization, such as a child welfare agency, employed one or more physicians or nurses as consultants to the social work staff or to assess and treat children with physical signs and symptoms of abuse or neglect.

What the secondary-setting nature of health service organizations does imply for social workers who practice in them is that to be accepted by the primary service providers and to be utilized fully and appropriately, social workers must (1) be considerate and respectful of the primary service providers and their work and responsibilities; (2) be mindful of the fact that medical and nursing staff view the patient as "their patient" and will appreciate the social worker keeping them informed of any developments concerning the patient or family; and (3) keep in mind the primary and priority functions of the organization, as well as the associated perspectives and concerns of the primary service providers.

Problems in cooperating with these primary providers usually arise when social workers become too preoccupied with their own work and neglect this caveat.

Professional Organizations

Another feature of health service settings is that they are professional organizations, since members of professions are the primary staff. In professional organizations, roles are not firmly defined or established by the personnel office or the professional group itself but must be "won" through a kind of political process in which *turf* (domain) is negotiated with other professionals in an ongoing fashion (Bucher and Stelling, 1978).

This means that social workers cannot expect to enter the organization and simply do their job as they envision it from their professional education. Instead, they must be aware that their role definition is dependent on the cooperation and tacit consent of other professionals in the organization, who may or may not perceive their own roles as including some of what social workers think is part of the social work domain.

For example, in most hospitals, a main function of social work is *discharge planning*. However, physicians and nurses may see some aspects of discharge planning as part of their own functions. Another example is that social workers tend to think of *psychosocial* problems as a social work arena. Yet physicians and nurses increasingly perceive psychosocial problems as appropriate to their domains (Cowles and Lefcowitz, 1995).

On the other hand, social workers may obtain information from patients or families that suggests a different diagnosis of the patient's health problem than the physician has assigned. If the social worker shares this information with the attending physician, the physician may be less than enthusiastic and view it as a turf violation.

The point is that in professional organizations, each professional is not as autonomous as he or she might be in private practice or in a predominately bureaucratic organization.

Dual-Authority System

An unusual organizational characteristic in hospitals is that two lines of authority often exist: the bureaucratic chain of command and the medical staff chain of command (Coe, 1978; Smith, 1978). Because of the unique authority, autonomy, and responsibility granted to the medical profession, its members do not always concur with, or concede to, the rules, regulations, and policies established by the board of directors or administrators. This means that social workers and other personnel who practice in such settings cannot assume that simply because they are acting in compliance with the official policy of the organization that the medical staff will not sometimes take exception to their actions and demand another course. There is no easy solution to this potential problem. It is simply important to be aware that it exists and to develop sensitivity to the types of situations that might provoke its appearance.

Complex Organizations

Complex organizations provide multiple services or functions and/or have multiple staff positions and roles. Health service organizations, especially hospitals, are referred to as complex organizations because they have a complex division of labor and several functions, which sometimes are subdivided into multiple-service units.

A *complex division of labor* means that the assignment of labor and responsibility is delegated among multiple personnel. This is not always easy to sort out. There are various positions among medical and nursing staff, and sometimes several layers of personnel in other departments, such as dietary, pharmacy, and physical therapy. Social workers need to be familiar with the division of labor among the personnel in their practice organization. If they are not clear about it, they are likely to seek information from, or report information to, inappropriate persons.

In addition, especially in hospitals, the organization often has more than one function (i.e., complex functions). Although the primary function is health care service, hospitals have multiple *units of health service,* such as the emergency room, outpatient clinics, and a variety of inpatient service units. The organization may also provide *education* or training for various types of health service professionals and other personnel. *Research* is another common function, especially of large teaching hospitals.

It is important for social workers to be familiar with the functions of the organization itself. First, to develop their own roles in an organization, social workers must know what the organization does. A setting with a professional education function may afford opportunities for social workers to teach students in the program about the social worker perspective of their role in the setting or about the biopsychosocial perspective as it relates to specific types of health problems. Similarly, settings whose functions include research may provide opportunities for social workers to collaborate on research projects. Second, a social worker employed in an organization is a representative of the organization and ought to be able to accurately describe its functions to others. Finally, organizational function is a major determinant of the social worker role in the organization. Although all health service organizations share the common and primary function of providing "health service," the form this function takes, and the function of the social worker, varies with whether the level of intervention is primary, secondary, or tertiary care.

For example, hospitals provide short-term intervention at the secondary level, which limits the length of time the social worker has to work with the patient or family. It also means that much of the time the patient is there, he or she often will be quite ill, which also limits social work intervention with the patient. Thus, for the most part, social and/or emotional problems that the social worker identifies will be referred to outside agencies for service, and the social worker will need to focus on services that support and complement the short-term care objectives of the hospital setting. On the other hand, in a hospice program the health care service is often of longer duration and focuses on supporting the function and comfort of the patient rather than on repairing the health problem. The social worker function is accordingly adapted to enhance this particular organizational function. Similar differences in the health care functions of rehabilitation centers, nursing homes, and primary care settings exist, which will be discussed further in later chapters.

Funding Sources and the Profit Motive

A variable present in health service organizations is the source of their funds and the extent to which they operate for financial profit. There are three main types of organizations with regard to funding source and profit: (1) public, (2) voluntary, and (3) proprietary.

Public organizations are owned and operated by federal, state, or local government, receive the largest share of their funds from public tax support, and are nonprofit. There are many examples of such publicly funded health service organizations, such as VA hospitals, county tax-supported hospitals, state tax-supported general medical and surgical-type hospitals, and specialty hospitals such as those for the chronically mentally ill or developmentally disabled. The VA also supports some nursing home, home care, and rehabilitation programs. Some counties also support nursing homes, drug and alcohol treatment programs, and day treatment programs for the chronically mentally ill or the impaired elderly, such as patients with Alzheimer's disease. Other examples of public organizations include federal, state, and county *public health services,* which are usually concerned with primary prevention of health problems through controlling communicable diseases, operating prenatal and well-baby clinics, providing public education, and conducting research.

Voluntary organizations are private but nonprofit and often are *sectarian* (affiliated with some religious sect). Examples of such health service organizations include Catholic, Jewish, Lutheran, and Methodist hospitals, nursing homes, and hospice programs. In addition, certain civic organizations, such as the Shriners, Masons, and American Legion, also operate hospitals and nursing home care facilities. Voluntary organizations that are not religiously affiliated are called *secular* organizations.

Finally, health service organizations increasingly are *proprietary,* which means that they are both privately owned and operated for profit. Of the three types of health service organizations, proprietary organizations are the most rapidly growing. Examples include the Columbia/HCA (Hospital Corporation of America), the largest nationwide chain of profit-making hospitals; Beverly Enterprises, the largest nationwide nursing home chain; Caremark, the largest chain of home health care agencies; and CIGNA, an insurance company and the largest chain of managed care facilities. In addition, many of the community mental health centers that were originally established as public tax-supported facilities to provide both outpatient and inpatient services for mental health problems and drug and alcohol addiction have now become private profit-making organizations, such as community psychiatric centers. The number of profit-making home care agencies also has mushroomed in recent years (Karger and Stoesz, 1998:188-191).

The funding source differences among these three types of organizations are growing increasingly difficult to distinguish. Since the Medicaid and Medicare programs were established in the mid-1960s, an increasing share of funding for all kinds of health services is coming from these tax-supported programs. Whereas Medicare is a federally funded program whose revenue is derived from payroll taxes, Medicaid is both federal and state supported, meaning its funds come from the general revenues of federal and state governments. Today, whether a health service is a public, voluntary, or proprietary facility, large parts of its funds are derived from government-financed programs.

All three types of organizations may obtain a considerable share of their funds from patient *fees for service* (charges that are based on the kind and number of provided services, in contrast to a *prepaid fee system,* whereby a set amount is paid before service, which covers whatever services are later determined to be needed). However, patient fees may be obtained *out of pocket* (fees that the individual pays because he or she lacks insurance coverage for all or part of the service), through private or public insurance programs, or from other tax-supported programs, such as Title XX, an amendment to the Social Security Act.

The issue, then, is whether any significant differences exist among the three types of organizations that are relevant to social work practice in such settings. Research has provided few answers to this question. However, there are also many other questions, largely about the quality of patient care in for-profit organizations, especially nursing homes and mental health programs. The following list presents some of those questions. Is there a tendency for proprietary health service organizations to

1. keep the direct service staff-to-patient ratio as low as possible?
2. exclude patients needing service who lack the ability to pay the established rates?

3. adapt length of service to patient ability to continue to pay?
4. rely too heavily on *psychotropic medications* in place of more time-consuming and costly interventions?
5. neglect the needs of those who are less able to advocate for themselves, such as the elderly and chronically impaired, in favor of those who are more demanding?
6. place too much emphasis on "public appearance," in terms of exterior and front entrance decor, relative to the less visible facilities, equipment, and staff needed to rehabilitate patients and support their comfort and function?
7. keep regular full-time staff to a minimum and rely on part-time or temporary staff from health personnel employment agencies?
8. generously pay certain key administrative and professional staff but require them to fulfill role expectations that serve the profit objective more than the patient care objective?
9. employ online staff who meet the minimum standards rather than optimal standards and provide compensation and benefits that are minimal?

The theme of these alleged tendencies of proprietary organizations is that they place more importance on *the bottom line* (profit) than on high quality patient care. If these allegations are true, social workers who practice in proprietary settings may experience constraints on their ability to practice in accordance with the standards, values, and ethics of their profession, in spite of appealing "perks" that may sometimes accompany positions in these organizations.

The Impact of Medicaid and Medicare

I have already alluded to the rapid growth in the Medicaid and Medicare programs in recent years and the increasing share of health care costs that these programs finance. This development has affected social work practice in health service settings, largely as a result of government efforts to control the cost of health care.

One effect of these cost-control efforts has been a general trend toward limiting social work services reimbursable by the two main government health insurance programs to those which are clearly related to the patient's current health condition and to the health care services being provided for that condition. Another effect has been an increase in organizational paperwork required to document claims for reimbursement. This has led to a corresponding increased rate of error and loss of reimbursement. This fear of not being reimbursed has led to a general tendency to limit services to those which are essential. Since the two government financing programs only reimburse services that are ordered or approved by the physician, this too has acted as a constraint on the provision of social work services.

Finally, federal government efforts to contain the rapid increase in health care costs led to passage of the Tax Equity and Fiscal Responsibility Act in 1983, which established the now familiar DRG (diagnosis-related group) system. This system limits the length of stay of hospitalized patients to a prescribed period of time, depending on the diagnosis. Overstay expenses must be absorbed by the hospital itself, not charged to the patient. Thus, the overall effect of the DRG system has been earlier release of most patients. This reduction in length of stay has further constrained what the social worker can attempt to do with inpatients and places even greater priority on the social worker function of assisting with arrangements for posthospital continuity of care in a nursing home, home care, or other plan.

Similarly, an increasing percentage of nursing home care is being reimbursed by government-funded programs, especially for Medicare-eligible persons who need a setting such as an extended care facility following a hospitalization. Often, however, the brief Medicare reimbursable period expires before the patient is ready to be released from the nursing home. This frequently requires the social worker serving the nursing home to assist in finding other sources of reimbursement or to arrange for home care.

SOCIAL WORKER FUNCTIONS
AND CLIENT PROBLEMS

Professional Standards for Social Worker Functions

The following is part of a standard set by the National Association of Social Workers regarding social work in health care settings (Standard 4):

> The functions of the social work program shall include specific services to the client population and the community in keeping with the overall mission of the organization. These shall include direct services, consultation, education, policy and program planning, quality assurance, advocacy, and liaison with the community. When the organization assumes teaching and research functions, the social work program should participate in them. Research, social work field instruction, and other teaching responsibilities are appropriate and recommended functions of all social work programs.* (NASW, 1987:6)

---

*Copyright 1987, National Association of Social Workers, Inc., NASW Standards for Social Work in Health Care Settings.

This standard (NASW, 1987:6-7) elaborates on the previous statement as follows:

> Specific services to the client population shall include but not be limited to these:
> - Assessment of the need for social work services.
> - Preadmission planning and discharge planning.
> - Direct services and treatment to individuals, families, and groups.
> - Case-finding and outreach.
> - Information and referral.
> - Client advocacy within and outside the organization, including attention to fiscal constraints.
> - Protection of clients' rights and entitlement, including the right to redress.
> - Short- and long-term planning.
> - Promotion and maintenance of health and mental health.
> - Preventive, remedial, and rehabilitative measures.
> - Provision for continuity of care, including guarantee of access and effective utilization.
>
> Services to the community shall include but not be limited to the following:
> - Identification of unmet needs and unserved groups.
> - Identification of and service to at-risk populations.
> - Consultation and collaboration with outside organizations and professionals concerning the care of populations and the promotion of health.
> - Community liaison services.
> - Community planning and coordination activities.
> - Psychosocial health education and promotion.
>
> Since the services to the client population and the community are interrelated and may overlap, the foregoing classifications of functions are not restricted to the particular areas mentioned.
>
> Consultation regarding the social, environmental, psychological, and cultural factors that affect health maintenance should be provided to those involved in the client's care. They may include the agency and its staff, the community, outside agencies and professionals, and significant others.

Four NASW expectations concerning functions of social workers in health care settings are particularly important to note: (1) both direct and indirect services should be provided; (2) social workers should reach out to clients who need their services; (3) the primary obligation of social workers is to their clients' rights and needs; and (4) services should be provided not only to individual clients but also to families, groups, and the community.

Both Direct and Indirect Services

The first paragraph in the fourth NASW standard clarifies that the core social worker functions in health care settings should include both *direct services* to clients and *indirect services* such as consultation, teaching, research, and program development. This is important to heed because social workers in health care settings, especially in hospitals, have tended to focus too heavily on direct services and too little on indirect services. Yet it is research that serves to develop the body of practice knowledge on which the claim to professionalism is primarily based, while program development is the mechanism for improving services and other resources for clients, and consultation and teaching are major instruments for promoting social work knowledge, skills, values, and influence.

A major direct-service function of social workers in health care settings is treatment of patient problems. It should be noted that social workers do not "treat" physical health problems, except insofar as modification of client attitudes, feelings, behaviors, and so forth, or modification of the environmental situation may serve to improve the client's health. However, in mental health settings, social workers with a master's or doctoral degree and a clinical social work license are often among the major providers of treatment for mental health problems.

Case Finding

The second paragraph in the NASW statement elaborates on the kinds of social work services that should be available to clients in health care settings and includes reference to "assessment of the need for social work services" and "case-finding and outreach." This is important because it underscores the need for social workers in health care settings to avoid the tendency to rely heavily on referrals from physicians and nurses, allowing these other groups to select the kinds of client problems the social workers would address.

Primacy of the Clients' Rights and Needs

The references to "client advocacy," "protection of clients' rights," and "provision of continuity of care, including provision of access and effective utilization" highlight the need for social workers to remember their primary obligation to the clients' rights and needs and to actively avoid becoming a party either to organizational or other constraints on meeting client needs or to violations of client rights.

Services to All Client Levels

Finally, the reference to "direct services and treatment to individuals, families, and groups," and to specification of "services to the community," implies that the NASW expects social workers in health care settings to work with all "client levels" and, in this sense, to function as generalists rather than specialists.

Health-Related Psychosocial Problems of Clients

The NASW standard for social worker functions in health care settings reflects the kinds of problems often addressed by social workers when working with patients and their families, including

1. barriers to admission to the service or facility;
2. problems of adjustment to the service or facility;
3. problems of adjustment to the diagnosis, prognosis, or health care plan;
4. lack of information to make informed decisions and to feel in control;
5. lack of resources to meet needs; and
6. barriers to discharge from the service or facility.

Barriers to Admission

First, patients sometimes experience *barriers to admission,* that is, conditions that prevent the person from receiving a needed health service. Such barriers may be psychological, financial, informational, or related to family care, transportation, or other concerns or resource needs.

Examples of *psychological barriers* include fear of being admitted to a hospital, nursing home, or other residential care facility, feeling embarrassed to seek help for mental or certain physical health problems, and avoiding having diagnostic tests done for fear of pain, side effects, or the findings.

Financial barriers can include lacking adequate health insurance to cover the anticipated costs of the services, fearing the loss of a job due to time off from work, and worrying about accumulating debt due to a temporary loss of income.

Informational barriers to admission tend to include both lack of mis-information and information, for example, uncertainty about what the service experience will be like or having heard rumors or read stories about "terrible things that could happen."

In addition, patients sometimes have other practical concerns such as who will take care of their family, pets, or house while they are an inpatient, not having any transportation to an outpatient service, or having their work accumulate because of missed time. Most such barriers revolve around social-environmental and/or emotional situations or concerns, so assistance with preadmission planning is an appropriate function of social workers.

Adjusting to the Setting or Service

Problems of adjustment to the service or setting are difficulties experienced by the patient or family in feeling comfortable and satisfied with the inpatient or outpatient health service or setting.

Institutional settings, such as hospitals, residential treatment centers, and nursing homes, tend to strip people of their usual supports (Goffman, 1961), that is, things on which people have come to depend. These supports may include family, friends, familiar places and furnishings, familiar location of things one relies on, freedom to make personal decisions, familiar daily routines, activities, and favorite foods. Most of us are not aware of how dependent we are on these things until we are required to be separated from them.

As a result of these and other situational changes, inpatients can experience an uncomfortable sense of loss of control over their own lives. Residents of health care facilities react in various ways to such changes; some adapt with little apparent difficulty, others withdraw (sometimes to the point of losing touch with reality) or become hostile and defiant, and some even try to leave, sometimes succeeding.

If not resolved through preadmission planning, inpatients of hospitals or nursing homes can also have realistic concerns about what may be happening to their family members, pets, homes, work situations, or unpaid bills in their absence. In addition, both inpatients and outpatients are sometimes concerned, justifiably or not, about the quality of care they receive through the health service. These and similar problems of adaption to the health service or setting are often well understood and dealt with by social workers.

Adjusting to the Diagnosis, Prognosis, or Treatment Plan

Another common problem of patients and/or their family members concerns coping with the diagnosis, prognosis, or treatment plan. Probably the most difficult adjustment is presented when the diagnosis, prognosis, or treatment plan indicates a likelihood or possibility of impending death. However, more often the diagnosis, prognosis, or treatment plan has implications for living with temporary losses of comfort and function or with *chronic* (ongoing) disabilities that may involve discomfort; functional incapacities; changes in role responsibilities and relationships; disfigurement; dependency on medications, prostheses, or machines; dietary restrictions; altering lifestyle habits such as drinking, smoking, exercise, and hobbies; or the need for significant changes in the home environment, such as ramps, grab bars, changes in floor coverings, width of doorways, or height of cabinets and light fixtures.

In short, often the diagnosis, prognosis, or treatment plan requires major changes in the lives of patients and their family members. The effects usually are both emotional and social environmental. For example, patients who learn they have a health problem that will require them to quit working or change the nature of their work may face both economic problems and emotional reactions. Patients who learn that they will require nursing home care may need to make practical decisions about their homes and families but usually experience feelings of distress about such life changes. Patients who are permanently paralyzed from the waist down face not only a multitude of practical problems concerning how they will function but also must deal with emotional issues concerning, for example, self-image, sexual relationships, and fears of dependency. Patients who have permanent and severe kidney damage that will require dialysis several hours a week on different days encounter practical problems and often experience accompanying emotional responses to dependency on machinery for survival. These are examples of psychosocial problems because they have both emotional and social environmental components. Such problems are well-suited to the competency preparation of professional social workers.

Need for Information to Make Informed Decisions and Take Control

Another common problem of patients and their family members in health care settings is a sense of diminished control. Actions are planned and sometimes carried out without adequate patient forewarning, explanation, or consent, whether by physicians, nurses, nurse aides, or other staff. The effect can be to provoke a sense of helplessness that compounds problems they may already have in adjusting to the setting or service.

This sense of loss of control is of particular significance in health care settings because, as considerable research evidence suggests, it can lead to depression and "giving up," which in turn tend to negatively impact optimal comfort, function, and even recovery (Schmale, 1972; Levy, 1974). In short, when people feel a loss of control over their life situations, they may quit trying. Although the biochemical process is not clearly understood, there is indication that such an emotional response may affect the immune system and other physiological systems that play a role in health status and life expectancy.

The social worker can play an important role by providing appropriate information to patients and their families to assist them in making informed decisions about matters that concern them. When the information they require is clearly the responsibility of the physician or nurse to provide, the social worker can act in the role of a mediator or liaison to bridge the gap between them. Social workers also assist patients and family members in thinking through their options—whether it involves a proposed medical procedure, the location and type of posthospital care, or choice of resources to assist them in dealing with the patients' health problem. Finally, social workers need to advocate for the patients' right to know the facts about their options, to assure their clients that they have this right, and to support clients in claiming it.

Lack of Resources to Meet Needs

Probably no function in health care settings is more appreciated by patients and families, as well as by physicians and nurses, than the assistance social workers provide patients and their families in obtaining resources to help meet patients' health care needs. Such resources usually fall into five categories:

1. medical aids and appliances,
2. support services,
3. income supports,
4. environmental adaptations, and
5. interpersonal supports.

Medical aids and appliances, or tools and equipment, can encompass a range of items such as wheelchairs, walkers, canes, grab bars, raised toilet seats, portable commodes, long-handled prongs for reaching, eyeglasses, hearing aids, hospital beds, geri-chairs, cardiac chairs, alternating air pressure mattresses, suction machines, blood sugar testing kits, blood pressure cuffs, incontinence pads, Hoya-lifts, gel-filled chair pads, corrective shoes, and braces. The need for such equipment is usually associated with home care situations, although there are occasions when patients in hospitals or nursing care facilities need special equipment that is not furnished by the facility.

Support services also vary widely. Those most often required in the field of health care include the following:

1. personal care services (assistance with activities of daily living, such as bathing, feeding, dressing, grooming, elimination), which may be provided by family members, home care agencies, or independent nursing assistants;
2. professional nursing services (for example, wound care, monitoring vital signs, catheter changes, and IV regulation, often provided by visiting nurse services associated with or independent of a home care agency);
3. physical therapy;
4. housekeeping services;
5. transportation services for the elderly and handicapped;
6. home-delivered meal services;
7. family counseling services;
8. drug and alcohol treatment services;
9. hospice care programs;
10. telephone reassurance services;
11. lifeline services;
12. adult or child protection services;
13. respite care services;
14. day care;
15. foreign language interpreter services; and
16. vocational retraining.

Income support is a major area of resources often needed by patients and their families. Frequently, the need for income assistance is associated with paying for the health care service agency itself, whether outpatient care, hospitalization, nursing home care, home care, day care agency services, or hospice program services. In addition, income assistance is often needed to pay for medical aids and appliances and many of the various services previously listed. Furthermore, patients in health care settings sometimes lack resources to support basic living needs, such as adequate housing and food, without which their health is further threatened.

Income supports generally come in two main forms: cash or in kind. *Cash income supports* are economic assistance received in the form of cash/checks to be used as needed. Examples of cash income assistance include Social Security, Supplemental Security Income, Temporary Assistance to Needy Families, Veterans' pensions, unemployment compensation, worker compensation, and general assistance (which in some states is provided through the township trustees). On the other hand, *in-kind income supports* are economic assistance that is received not in cash but in the form of the service or resource needed (e.g., food, clothing, housing, medical care). Examples of in-kind income support programs include Medicare, Medicaid, public housing, subsidized private housing, food stamps, food and clothing bank programs, and shelters for the homeless.

Environmental adaptations are important resources for persons who have mental or physical disabilities that require certain changes in the setting around them in order to be able to function as well as possible. For the physically impaired, these may include ramps, wider doorways to accommodate wheelchairs, rearrangement of furnishings to make them reachable, nonskid floors, or low-pile carpets. Depending on the type of mental impairment, helpful environmental adaptations could include a fenced-in yard (to prevent wandering), low-level sounds, avoidance of interpersonal conflicts, simplicity and continuity of furnishings, or strategically placed labels to help locate vital areas.

Interpersonal supports are needed by most people. These involve having ready access to other people who provide human relationships and social interactions that are experienced as emotionally supportive, including feeling cared about and valued. Having such interpersonal support is a fundamental human need and plays a vital role at all levels of health care service.

Barriers to Discharge

Patient and family *barriers to discharge* are factors that prevent patients from terminating their inpatient or outpatient services once they are ready for release. Such barriers are similar to barriers to admission to health care services; they may be psychological, financial, informational, or related to family care, transportation, or other concerns or resource needs.

A psychological barrier to discharge could be that the patient has grown emotionally dependent on the service and fears being separated from it. A financial barrier to discharge could be that the patient has no income and no place to go after discharge. An informational barrier to discharge could be that the patient does not know enough about nursing homes or home care agencies to make arrangements for such services. An example of a family care barrier to discharge is that a patient may need extended care in another facility but does not know how his or her family would manage during such a prolonged absence by the patient. Finally, the patient may simply have no way to travel from the inpatient location to the next service location and may require assistance in arranging for transportation and/or paying for it.

In many instances, hospitalized patients and/or their family members are fully able to handle the release and aftercare without professional assistance. However, this is not always the case.

Patients usually need assistance with discharge planning when (1) their health condition at the expected time of release is such that they will require some kind of assistance afterward; (2) it is not clear to the medical or nursing staff what resources patients have at home to manage their aftercare; (3) the patients or families need information about and assistance in making arrangements for nursing homes, home care, or hospice care programs; and (4) the patients or families need assistance in identifying their options and making decisions concerning their choice of aftercare.

It is important to understand that when social workers help with these various types of problems, services are often, but not always, directed to individual patients and individual family members. Social workers also sometimes relate to all or several members of a family together, or to a group of patients or families with similar problems or needs—whether to provide information, orientation, instruction, or some sort of counseling or problem solving.

In addition, in the course of serving clients in these direct ways, social workers sometimes identify gaps in community resources for certain types of client needs, or they may identify some unhealthy condition in a community that needs to be corrected to reduce the future incidence of problems such as those faced by their clients. Thus, social workers may need to become involved in what is variously called community organization, social action, and policy/program planning and development. Such community-directed services, along with teaching, research, and consultation, are termed *indirect services* because they are not provided to clients but on behalf of clients.

It should also be remembered that the need for improved resources or environmental changes, calling for policy/program planning and development, may be within the health service itself. Social workers are often in a unique position to learn from clients what is problematic about the service or facility itself, as clients often more readily share such information with social workers than with physicians or nurses. Social workers have a responsibility to try to help improve the quality and delivery of services in the setting where they practice.

The next chapter discusses the knowledge, values and ethics, skills, and interventions of social workers in health service settings.

SUMMARY

Since the beginning of social work in health care in the general hospital setting in 1905, its practitioners have seen their role as complementing the functions of the medical and nursing staff by addressing the problematic social, environmental, and psychological experiences of the patient and family that affect the patient's health condition and its treatment. Currently, about 47 percent of NASW members practice in the health field, in mental and physical health areas combined, while about 32 percent of NASW members are located primarily in mental or physical health organizational settings, predominately medical facilities.

The underlying theoretical perspective of social work in the health field is that biological, psychological, and social systems reciprocally influence one another as causes and effects of health problems. Although "medical care" is what physicians provide in their efforts to monitor patient health and to treat health problems, social work practice in the health field addresses the individual attitudes, behaviors, and social environmental resources of people—factors vital to "health care" at the three levels of prevention, remediation, and compensation.

What people do, or do not do, to take care of their own health, how people interpret and respond to what could be symptoms of health problems, and how people behave after they are determined to be ill or injured are complex phenomena that reflect multiple human diversity variables. There is a body of knowledge about broad differences in human behavior associated with gender, ethnicity, socioeconomic class, and age. However, such knowledge cannot predict how particular individuals will behave given their combined characteristics.

Most health service settings employ a multidisciplinary staff. Sometimes such settings utilize interdisciplinary teams to assess and intervene in health care. The mission of these teams is to coordinate comprehensive services addressed to the often multiple and interdependent problems of the whole patient in an effort to enhance the success of services and to reduce gaps and overlap in services. Although information is available regarding the functions, requirements, and problems of interdisciplinary teams, unfortunately most professional education does not adequately prepare workers for this type of group practice.

Health service organizations are secondary settings of social work, and they are professional rather than typical bureaucratic organizations. In those settings with physician-dominated health services, such as hospitals, there may be a dual-authority system, that is, both a bureaucratic and a physician chain of command that run parallel to each other. In addition, health service organizations such as hospitals, community mental health centers, and public health agencies often have a complex division of labor and/or complex functions, and thus are called complex organizations.

Health service organizations also vary by whether they are public, voluntary, or proprietary and by whether they are sectarian or secular. Proprietary health service organizations are the most rapidly growing type, and considerable concern has been expressed about the alleged impact of a financial profit incentive on the quality of health services and on the concept of a "profession."

Finally, as the increased cost of health services has become recognized as one of our nation's most serious social problems, cost-containment efforts of government health care financing programs have intensified in ways that include effects on social work in health services.

Thus, a variety of characteristics of health service organizations tends to constrain the role and function of the social workers who practice in them. The challenge for social workers is to find ways to adapt that will maximize their own efficiency and effectiveness for the sake of all concerned—patient and family, organization, and funding source.

The basic and essential functions of social workers in health service settings include direct services to patients and families, individually or in small groups, as well as the functions of consultation, education, policy and program planning, quality assurance, advocacy, *and* liaison with the community. Recommended functions of social workers in the health field include research, social work field instruction, and other teaching experiences.

Chapter 2

Fundamentals of Health Care Social Work Practice

KNOWLEDGE REQUIREMENTS

The Knowledge Base of Professionalism

The basic characteristic that distinguishes a profession from an occupation is that a profession lays claim to or "professes" to have a body of knowledge on which its members base their practice of service to others. The specialized nature of this knowledge leads people outside the profession to view a member of the profession as "an authority" in the knowledge area and to grant the profession "the authority" to practice with little interference from outsiders, that is, autonomy of practice (Greenwood, 1957). This body of professional knowledge is expected to be sufficiently extensive and complex that preparation for entrance to the profession requires a lengthy educational process, which is usually university based.

Definition of the Social Work Profession

Social work has been defined as the *professional* activity of helping individuals, families, groups, or communities to enhance or restore their capacity for social functioning and of creating societal conditions favorable to this goal (NASW, 1991). Thus, as a profession, social work claims to have special knowledge and skills that better qualify its members, as opposed to nonmembers, to provide such helping services.

The Meaning of Knowledge

For centuries, philosophers, theologians, scientists, and members of other disciplines have debated about what constitutes "knowledge." Much of their debate revolves around the issue of the *process* through which knowledge is obtained. Philosophy and theology are prescientific or extrascientific fields because they predate science and adhere to processes of

41

"knowing," such as logical deduction and religious experience, which are outside the process of modern science. For the most part, professions, including social work, uphold the *scientific* process of developing knowledge, which emphasizes the importance of *unbiased observation* (objectivity) and theory building.

Knowledge As Theory

In the realm of science, knowledge is not mere fact finding, such as might be performed through a population census, an opinion poll, or other modes of observing phenomena. Instead, gathered facts or pieces of information need to be related to explanations of what the facts mean, of how they are related to one another or to other facts (Wing, 1978). Preliminary or tentative explanations are called *hypotheses*. As hypotheses are tested and found to be supported or not, a body of *theory* (explanation) is developed; this is called knowledge. Knowledge and theory are never final or complete, but instead are always open to modification as additional research gathers new evidence.

One concession that science owes to other more intuitive approaches to knowledge is that much of scientific development begins with *casual observations,* or hunches, about some aspect of reality. That is, before people formulate a hypothesis about something, they usually "happened to notice . . ." or "got an idea that . . ." Often this occurs in the course of everyday experience, or, in professions, in the course of practice experience. In the latter case, we call these *practice hunches,* or pieces of practice wisdom. Often, such hunches are the seeds of knowledge development in that they may be used to formulate a research question, which is the first step in the scientific process.

The Scientific Process

In all science, a particular process is required. Although the initial stimulus may be only a hunch about some aspect of reality, the scientific process involves a series of particular steps (Neuman, 1994:11):

1. Formulate a research question.
2. Review the literature.
3. Refine the research question.
4. Design a plan for researching that question, including
   a. sampling,
   b. data collection, and
   c. data analysis.
5. Conduct the study.
6. Analyze the data to draw conclusions regarding the research question.
7. Disseminate the findings to others.

As noted earlier, a hunch, or *piece of practice wisdom,* is often the basis for formulating a research question, such as "Is the poverty rate correlated with the reported child abuse rate?" or "Does the level of patient participation in discharge planning affect patients' likelihood of relapse?" Research questions are then explored by reading previous studies of the issue to determine what their findings and conclusions have been. Based on these, the research question is refined and/or translated into a hypothesis, such as "As the poverty rate increases in a population, the reported child abuse rate increases," or "The less patient involvement in discharge planning, the earlier patients relapse." The hypothesis is then tested through the research process, and the findings are disseminated through professional journals, adding to the cumulative *body of knowledge* (theory) on the subject.

In summary, a profession must have a body of knowledge that justifies its authority to practice. Scientific knowledge is theory building through a specific process that helps to (1) ensure that each new study builds on previous ones and (2) force researchers to think through how they will address the particular research question beforehand to determine whether the issue can be researched.

Generic Social Work Knowledge Areas

Social work education programs revolve around four core knowledge areas that are considered essential for all social work, regardless of client population, field of practice, or setting. These generic areas of social work knowledge are as follows:

1. *Human behavior and the social environment:* an integration of scientific theory about the role of biological, psychological, and sociocultural factors in human behavior and development.
2. *Social welfare policy and programs:* knowledge of the historical development and current features of social welfare programs and policies in society to address social problems—including community resources available to help people, gaps in resources, the process of policy/program development in society, and how social workers can influence such development.
3. *Social work practice:* theory concerning the social work helping process, methods of social work practice, skills, techniques, and intervention modalities, as well as the values and ethics of professional social work practice.
4. *Research methods:* knowledge of the scientific research process, both quantitative and qualitative, principles and methods of sampling, data collection, and data analysis that are suited to social work practice.

Of these four knowledge areas, number 3 is uniquely social work knowledge—social work practice knowledge. It is this knowledge that needs ongoing development so that social work can maintain its status as a profession.

Because social workers address such a broad range of human problems and often practice in a variety of fields and practice settings in the course of their careers, the additional knowledge needed for effective practice with particular client populations, fields, and settings is acquired largely through continuing education, both formal and informal, often while working in the setting.

Health Field–Specific Knowledge Areas

Social work practice within the health field varies somewhat with the particular client population, problem area, organizational setting, and community context of practice; it is therefore helpful if the social worker has the following additional knowledge:

1. *Client population and problem area:* the characteristics of the client population, the nature of the health problem(s) dealt with in the setting, and the common path, treatment, or management of the disorder(s); the biopsychosocial perspective of these disorders; the role of human diversity in the onset and course of the disorders and its influence on (a) health behavior, (b) illness behavior, and (c) sick-role behavior. Inevitably, this type of knowledge involves acquiring some additional vocabulary, often medical and psychiatric terms.
2. *Organizational setting:* the characteristics of the organizational setting and their implications for social work, such as whether it is for-profit or nonprofit and secular or sectarian; its mission and function(s); its level of health service intervention; its authority structure; the types of health professions and occupations in the setting and their roles and role expectations of social work; organizational policy, rules, and regulations; and interdisciplinary teamwork principles and practice problems.
3. *Community characteristics and resources:* the characteristics of the surrounding community, such as rural, urban, or suburban, population demographics, political attitudes, major business and industry, and the resources of that community, including general resources and those of special relevance to the needs of the client population and problem area served by the practice setting.
4. *Specific intervention modalities:* approaches tailored to the needs of the particular client population, problem area, and organizational

characteristics, such as crisis intervention, grief counseling, behavioral modification, or case management.

5. *Research, evaluation, and documentation:* the findings and methods of research, evaluation, and documentation that are appropriate to and/or required by the practice setting.

The Relationship Between Generic and Specific Knowledge

The special knowledge required for practice in the health field is not different from generic social work knowledge; it is a more in-depth development or specialized understanding of certain aspects of it.

Knowledge of the *particular client population and problem area* in the context of the biopsychosocial model and human diversity and knowledge of community characteristics are in-depth developments of generic knowledge of human behavior and the social environment. Knowledge of the *organizational setting and community resources* is a development of general knowledge of social welfare policy and programs. Although all social workers gain some introduction to and overview of a range of *intervention modalities* in social work practice during their basic professional education, practice in a specific setting usually requires development of knowledge of particular interventions that are most appropriate in that setting. Finally, knowledge of appropriate *research, evaluation, and documentation* useful to and/or required in the setting is a development of basic social work research methods.

In short, generic social work knowledge is the foundation upon which all social work practice is based. Social work practice in the health field, or in any other field, simply requires further development of this basic knowledge in ways that are specific to the clientele, problems, organization, and community of the particular practice setting.

VALUES AND ETHICS CONSIDERATIONS

The Values Base of Professionalism

In addition to a knowledge base, a profession must have a code of ethics that reflects the underlying values of the profession and delineates its standards for the professional behavior of its members. The rationale for this is that since a profession is granted relative autonomy from outside supervision, it must assume responsibility for regulating its own members.

The Meaning of and Relationship Between Values and Ethics

Values are what one regards as important or worthwhile. *Ethics* are behavioral norms that usually reflect our underlying values. What we consider *appropriate behavior* (proper to the situation) tends to reflect what we view to be important or worthwhile. A *code of ethics* is a set of these behavioral expectations or norms.

The Basic Values and Practice Principles of the Social Work Profession

Ethical Principles*

The following broad ethical principles are based on social work's core values of service, social justice, dignity and worth of the person, importance of human relationships, integrity, and competence. These principles set forth ideals to which all social workers should aspire.

Value: *Service*

Ethical Principle: *Social workers' primary goal is to help people in need and to address social problems.*

Social workers elevate service to others above self-interest. Social workers draw on their knowledge, values, and skills to help people in need and to address social problems. Social workers are encouraged to volunteer some portion of their professional skills with no expectation of significant financial return (pro bono service).

Value: *Social Justice*

Ethical Principle: *Social workers challenge social injustice.*

Social workers pursue social change, particularly with and on behalf of vulnerable and oppressed individuals and groups of people. Social workers' social change efforts are focused primarily on issues of poverty, unemployment, discrimination, and other forms of social injustice. These activities seek to promote sensitivity to and knowledge about oppression and cultural and ethnic diversity. Social workers strive to ensure access to needed information, services, and resources; equality of opportunity; and meaningful participation in decision making for all people.

---

*Copyright 1996, National Association of Social Workers, Inc., Code of Ethics.

3 — **Value:** *Dignity and Worth of the Person*

Ethical Principle: *Social workers respect the inherent dignity and worth of the person.*

Social workers treat each person in a caring and respectful fashion, mindful of individual differences and cultural and ethnic diversity. Social workers promote clients' socially responsible self-determination. Social workers seek to enhance clients' capacity and opportunity to change and to address their own needs. Social workers are cognizant of their dual responsibility to clients and to the broader society. They seek to resolve conflicts between clients' interests and the broader society's interests in a socially responsible manner consistent with the values, ethical principles, and ethical standards of the profession.

4 **Value:** *Importance of Human Relationships*

Ethical Principle: *Social workers recognize the central importance of human relationships.*

Social workers understand that relationships between and among people are an important vehicle for change. Social workers engage people as partners in the helping process. Social workers seek to strengthen relationships among people in a purposeful effort to promote, restore, maintain, and enhance the well-being of individuals, families, social groups, organizations, and communities.

5 **Value:** *Integrity*

Ethical Principle: *Social workers behave in a trustworthy manner.*

Social workers are continually aware of the profession's mission, values, ethical principles, and ethical standards and practice in a manner consistent with them. Social workers act honestly and responsibly and promote ethical practices on the part of the organizations with which they are affiliated.

6 **Value:** *Competence*

Ethical Principle: *Social workers practice within their areas of competence and develop and enhance their professional expertise.*

Social workers continually strive to increase their professional knowledge and skills and to apply them in practice. Social workers should aspire to contribute to the knowledge base of the profession. (NASW, 1996:5-6)

Ethical Standards of Professional Social Work Practice

Ethical Standards

1.   SOCIAL WORKERS' ETHICAL RESPONSIBILITIES TO CLIENTS

1.01 Commitment to Clients

Social workers' primary responsibility is to promote the well-being of clients. In general, clients' interests are primary. However, social workers' responsibility to the larger society or specific legal obligations may on limited occasions supersede the loyalty owed clients, and clients should be so advised. (Examples include when a social worker is required by law to report that a client has abused a child or has threatened to harm self or others.)

1.02 Self-Determination

Social workers respect and promote the right of clients to self-determination and assist clients in their efforts to identify and clarify their goals. Social workers may limit clients' right to self-determination when, in the social workers' professional judgment, clients' actions or potential actions pose a serious, foreseeable, and imminent risk to themselves or others.

1.03 Informed Consent

(a) Social workers should provide services to clients only in the context of a professional relationship based, when appropriate, on valid informed consent. Social workers should use clear and understandable language to inform clients of the purpose of the services, risks related to the services, limits to services because of the requirements of a third-party payer, relevant costs, reasonable alternatives, clients' right to refuse or withdraw consent, and the time frame covered by the consent. Social workers should provide clients with an opportunity to ask questions.

(b) In instances when clients are not literate or have difficulty understanding the primary language used in the practice setting, social workers should take steps to ensure clients' comprehension. This may include providing clients with a detailed verbal explanation or arranging for a qualified interpreter or translator whenever possible.

(c) In instances when clients lack the capacity to provide informed consent, social workers should protect clients' interests by seeking permission from an appropriate third party, informing clients consistent with the clients' level of understanding. In such instances social workers should seek to ensure that the third party acts in a manner consistent with clients' wishes and interests. Social workers should take reasonable steps to enhance such clients' ability to give informed consent.

(d) In instances when clients are receiving services involuntarily, social workers should provide information about the nature and extent of services and about the extent of clients' right to refuse service.

(e) Social workers who provide services via electronic media (such as computer, telephone, radio, and television) should inform recipients of the limitations and risks associated with such services.

(f) Social workers should obtain clients' informed consent before audiotaping or videotaping clients or permitting observation of services to clients by a third party.

1.04 Competence

(a) Social workers should provide services and represent themselves as competent only within the boundaries of their education, training, license, certification, consultation received, supervised experience, or other relevant professional experience.

(b) Social workers should provide services in substantive areas or use intervention techniques or approaches that are new to them only after engaging in appropriate study, training, consultation, and supervision from people who are competent in those interventions or techniques.

(c) When generally recognized standards do not exist with respect to an emerging area of practice, social workers should exercise careful judgment and take responsible steps (including appropriate education, research, training, consultation, and supervision) to ensure the competence of their work and to protect clients from harm.

1.05 Cultural Competence and Social Diversity

(a) Social workers should understand culture and its function in human behavior and society, recognizing the strengths that exist in all cultures.

(b) Social workers should have a knowledge base of their clients' cultures and be able to demonstrate competence in the provision of services that are sensitive to clients' cultures and to differences among people and cultural groups.

(c) Social workers should obtain education about and seek to understand the nature of social diversity and oppression with respect to race, ethnicity, national origin, color, sex, sexual orientation, age, marital status, political belief, religion, and mental or physical disability.

1.06 Conflicts of Interest

(a) Social workers should be alert to and avoid conflicts of interest that interfere with the exercise of professional discretion and impartial judgment. Social workers should inform clients when a real or potential conflict of interest arises and take reasonable steps to resolve the issue in a manner that makes the clients' interests primary and protects clients' interests to the greatest extent possible. In some cases, protecting clients' interests may require termination of the professional relationship with proper referral of the client.

(b) Social workers should not take unfair advantage of any professional relationship or exploit others to further their personal, religious, political, or business interests.

(c) Social workers should not engage in dual or multiple relationships with clients or former clients in which there is a risk of exploitation or potential harm to the client. In instances when dual or multiple relationships are unavoidable, social workers should take steps to protect clients and are responsible for setting clear, appropriate, and culturally sensitive boundaries. (Dual or multiple relationships occur when social workers relate to clients in more than one relationship, whether professional, social, or business. Dual or multiple relationships can occur simultaneously or consecutively.)

(d) When social workers provide services to two or more people who have a relationship with each other (for example, couples, family members), social workers should clarify with all parties which individuals will be considered clients and the nature of social workers' professional obligations to the various individuals who are receiving services. Social workers who anticipate a conflict of interest among the individuals receiving services or who anticipate having to perform in potentially conflicting roles (for example, when a social worker is asked to testify in a child custody dispute or divorce proceedings involving clients) should clarify their role with the parties involved and take appropriate action to minimize any conflict of interest.

1.07 Privacy and Confidentiality

(a) Social workers should respect clients' right to privacy. Social workers should not solicit private information from clients unless it is essential to providing services or conducting social work evaluation or research. Once private information is shared, standards of confidentiality apply.

(b) Social workers may disclose confidential information when appropriate with valid consent from a client or a person legally authorized to consent on behalf of a client.

(c) Social workers should protect the confidentiality of all information obtained in the course of professional service, except for compelling professional reasons. The general expectation that social workers will keep information confidential does not apply when disclosure is necessary to prevent serious, foreseeable, and imminent harm to a client or other identifiable person or when laws or regulations require disclosure without a client's consent. In all instances, social workers should disclose the least amount of confidential information necessary to achieve the desired purpose; only information that is directly relevant to the purpose for which the disclosure is made should be revealed.

(d) Social workers should inform clients, to the extent possible, about the disclosure of confidential information and the potential consequences, when feasible before the disclosure is made. This applies whether social workers disclose confidential information on the basis of a legal requirement or client consent.

(e) Social workers should discuss with clients and other interested parties the nature of confidentiality and limitations of clients' right to confidentiality. Social workers should review with clients circumstances where confidential information may be requested and where disclosure of confidential information may be legally required. This discussion should occur as soon as possible in the social worker-client relationship and as needed throughout the course of the relationship.

(f) When social workers provide counseling services to families, couples, or groups, social workers should seek agreement among the parties involved concerning each individual's right to confidentiality and obligation to preserve the confidentiality of information shared by others. Social workers should inform participants in family, couples, or group counseling that social workers cannot guarantee that all participants will honor such agreements.

(g) Social workers should inform clients involved in family, couples, marital, or group counseling of the social worker's, employer's, and agency's policy concerning the social worker's disclosure of confidential information among the parties involved in the counseling.

(h) Social workers should not disclose confidential information to third-party payers unless clients have authorized such disclosure.

(i) Social workers should not discuss confidential information in any setting unless privacy can be ensured. Social workers should not discuss confidential information in public or semipublic areas such as hallways, waiting rooms, elevators, and restaurants.

(j) Social workers should protect the confidentiality of clients during legal proceedings to the extent permitted by law. When a court of law or other legally authorized body orders social workers to disclose confidential or privileged information without a client's consent and such disclosure could cause harm to the client, social workers should request that the court withdraw the order or limit the order as narrowly as possible or maintain the records under seal, unavailable for public inspection.

(k) Social workers should protect the confidentiality of clients when responding to requests from members of the media.

(l) Social workers should protect the confidentiality of clients' written and electronic records and other sensitive information. Social workers should take reasonable steps to ensure that clients' records are stored in a secure location and that clients' records are not available to others who are not authorized to have access.

(m) Social workers should take precautions to ensure and maintain the confidentiality of information transmitted to other parties through the use of computers, electronic mail, facsimile machines, telephones and telephone answering machines, and other electronic or computer technology. Disclosure of identifying information should be avoided whenever possible.

(n) Social workers should transfer or dispose of clients' records in a manner that protects clients' confidentiality and is consistent with state statutes governing records and social work licensure.

(o) Social workers should take reasonable precautions to protect client confidentiality in the event of the social worker's termination of practice, incapacitation, or death.

(p) Social workers should not disclose identifying information when discussing clients for teaching or training purposes unless the client has consented to disclosure of confidential information.

(q) Social workers should not disclose identifying information when discussing clients with consultants unless the client has consented to disclosure of confidential information or there is a compelling need for such disclosure.

(r) Social workers should protect the confidentiality of deceased clients consistent with the preceding standards.

1.08 Access to Records

(a) Social workers should provide clients with reasonable access to records concerning the clients. Social workers who are concerned that clients' access to their records could cause serious misunderstanding or harm to the client should provide assistance in interpreting the records and consultation with the client regarding the records. Social workers should limit clients' access to their records, or portions of their records, only in exceptional circumstances when there is compelling evidence that such access would cause serious harm to the client. Both clients' requests and the rationale for withholding some or all of the record should be documented in clients' files.

(b) When providing clients with access to their records, social workers should take steps to protect the confidentiality of other individuals identified or discussed in such records.

1.09 Sexual Relationships

(a) Social workers should under no circumstances engage in sexual activities or sexual contact with current clients, whether such contact is consensual or forced.

(b) Social workers should not engage in sexual activities or sexual contact with clients' relatives or other individuals with whom clients maintain a close personal relationship when there is a risk of exploitation or potential harm to the client. Sexual activity or sexual contact with clients' relatives or other individuals with whom clients maintain a personal relationship has the potential to be harmful to the client and may make it difficult for the social worker and client to maintain appropriate professional boundaries. Social workers—not their clients, their clients' relatives, or other individuals with whom the client maintains a personal relationship—assume the full burden for setting clear, appropriate, and culturally sensitive boundaries.

(c) Social workers should not engage in sexual activities or sexual contact with former clients because of the potential for harm to the client. If social workers engage in conduct contrary to this prohibition or claim that an exception to this prohibition is warranted because of extraordinary circumstances, it is social workers—not their clients—who assume the full burden of demonstrating that the former client has not been exploited, coerced, or manipulated, intentionally or unintentionally.

(d) Social workers should not provide clinical services to individuals with whom they have had a prior sexual relationship. Providing clinical services to a former sexual partner has the potential to be harmful to the individual and is likely to make it difficult for the social worker and individual to maintain appropriate professional boundaries.

1.10 Physical Contact

Social workers should not engage in physical contact with clients when there is a possibility of psychological harm to the client as a result of the contact (such as cradling or caressing clients). Social workers who engage in appropriate physical contact with clients are responsible for setting clear, appropriate, and culturally sensitive boundaries that govern such physical contact.

1.11 Sexual Harassment

Social workers should not sexually harass clients. Sexual harassment includes sexual advances, sexual solicitation, requests for sexual favors, and other verbal or physical conduct of a sexual nature.

1.12 Derogatory Language

Social workers should not use derogatory language in their written or verbal communications to or about clients. Social workers should use accurate and respectful language in all communications to and about clients.

1.13 Payment for Services

(a) When setting fees, social workers should ensure that the fees are fair, reasonable, and commensurate with the services performed. Consideration should be given to clients' ability to pay.

(b) Social workers should avoid accepting goods or services from clients as payment for professional services. Bartering arrangements, particularly involving services, create the potential for conflicts of interest, exploitation, and inappropriate boundaries in social workers' relationships with clients. Social workers should explore and may participate in bartering only in very limited circumstances when it can be demonstrated that such arrangements are an accepted practice among professionals in the local community, considered to be essential for the provision of services, negotiated without coercion, and entered into at the client's initiative and with the client's informed consent. Social workers who accept goods or services from clients as payment for professional services assume the full burden of demonstrating that this arrangement will not be detrimental to the client or the professional relationship.

(c) Social workers should not solicit a private fee or other remuneration for providing services to clients who are entitled to such available services through the social workers' employer or agency.

1.14 Clients Who Lack Decision-Making Capacity

When social workers act on behalf of clients who lack the capacity to make informed decisions, social workers should take reasonable steps to safeguard the interests and rights of those clients.

1.15 Interruption of Services

Social workers should make reasonable efforts to ensure continuity of services in the event that services are interrupted by factors such as unavailability, relocation, illness, disability, or death.

1.16 Termination of Services

(a) Social workers should terminate services to clients and professional relationships with them when such services and relationships are no longer required or no longer serve the clients' needs or interests.

(b) Social workers should take reasonable steps to avoid abandoning clients who are still in need of services. Social workers should withdraw services precipitously only under unusual circumstances, giving careful consideration to all factors in the situation and taking care to minimize possible adverse effects. Social workers should assist in making appropriate arrangements for continuation of services when necessary.

(c) Social workers in fee-for-service settings may terminate services to clients who are not paying an overdue balance if the financial contractual arrangements have been made clear to the client, if the client does not pose an imminent danger to self or others, and if the clinical and other consequences of the current nonpayment have been addressed and discussed with the client.

(d) Social workers should not terminate services to pursue a social, financial, or sexual relationship with a client.

(e) Social workers who anticipate the termination or interruption of services to clients should notify clients promptly and seek the transfer, referral, or continuation of services in relation to the clients' needs and preferences.

(f) Social workers who are leaving an employment setting should inform clients of appropriate options for the continuation of services and of the benefits and risks of the options. (NASW, 1996:7-15)

Values and Ethics Considerations in Health Care Settings

The following client-related social work values, principles, and ethical standards have particular significance in health care settings.

The Value of the Dignity and Worth of the Person

The dignity and worth of the person takes on special significance in health care settings where we sometimes work with persons who are severely deteriorated, deformed, demented, deranged, or dying.

In addition, the client population of health care settings sometimes resembles a *microcosm* of society, in that it may include rich and poor, young and old, "saints and sinners," geniuses and mentally retarded persons, people of a variety of races, subcultures, religions, both males and females—some of whom are heterosexual and some homosexual—corporation heads, laborers, rock stars, athletes, and politicians.

As professional social workers, we are challenged to remember that every individual is of value. We accept each person regardless of his or her behavior. Each person has a right to fulfill his or her potential. We individualize people and address our approach and services to *their* needs. We reach out to vulnerable people and advocate for them, and we avoid imposing our values and norms on them, but instead seek out and respect theirs and work within the framework of who *they* are.

The Ethical Standard of Client Confidentiality

The word *confidentiality* literally means "with faith" or "with trust." In health care settings, clients are highly vulnerable. Not only will they be physically exposed in their bedclothes or even naked, but they are also "stripped of their customary supports" (Goffman, 1961) when in institutional settings such as hospitals and nursing homes. This vulnerability can cause clients to share things about themselves they might not ordinarily discuss, which later can add to their feelings of vulnerability. In addition, you will have access to their medical records, which often detail much personal information. Finally, you may encounter someone you know, or know of, among clients and their families—whether a former lover, a member of the clergy, a former teacher, or some public figure.

It is essential that you keep what you know about clients to yourself. Never gossip, even to your family, friends, or colleagues. Record only what you would be willing for them to read, and keep confidential files locked.

Trust is the sine qua non (prerequisite) of effective social work practice. Violation of this trust will tend to diminish your credibility as a professional in the eyes of anyone who witnesses it.

Exceptions to the confidentiality standard include cases of public health dangers, threatened suicide or homicide, or other criminal behavior. In these instances, social workers simply inform clients that they cannot promise confidentiality.

The Ethical Standard of Client Self-Determination

Health care settings often pose important questions for patients and their families that cover a wide range of topics, such as the following:

- Whether to initiate or continue life support
- Whether to have a recommended medical or surgical procedure
- Whether to accept the treatment that will reduce the symptoms or even extend life, but will cause unpleasant side effects
- Which treatment option to select
- Whether to tell significant others about their health condition
- What to do about their lives in the future
- Whether to go home or to a nursing home after discharge from the hospital

In addition, the self-determination standard takes on special significance in health care settings because there is some evidence that when people experience a strong sense of loss of control over their lives, they tend to give up the struggle, which can negatively affect their recovery (Schmale, 1972; Seligman, 1975; Levy, 1974).

Thus, it is very important for the social worker to (1) assist the client and/or family to gain access to needed information on which to base *informed decisions;* (2) assist them in identifying and assessing their options to make an appropriate selection; and (3) support their preferences and assist them in realizing their goals.

The Value of Social Justice

It is our obligation to support and actively promote equal opportunity and equitable treatment for all people—regardless of our personal feelings about them, their health condition, or their behavior. In spite of our own views about politics, morality, religion, and so forth, as professionals, we must realize that social justice exists for everyone or it may not exist for anyone.

Values and Ethics Conflicts

From time to time, practice situations arise that cause professionals some sense of uncertainty, strain, or temptation concerning their professional values and ethics. These are known as *values and ethics conflicts*. Such conflicts tend to be related to (1) client health conditions, personal characteristics, or behavior; (2) organizational situations or practices; or (3) community resource provider promotional efforts.

Client-Related Conflicts

Values and ethics conflicts in health settings can be stimulated by subjective reactions of social workers to clients' health conditions or their behavior. Such conflicts can impair social workers' ability to uphold their professional values and ethics, as depicted in the following examples:

- The patient's health condition is so deteriorated or impaired that the social worker may privately question whether he or she is worth the costly care being supplied.
- The patient has a health problem that arouses emotion-laden memories of some personal family situation.
- The patient's personal characteristics are so like those of the social worker that the social worker fears that the problem could happen to him or her, creating distress.

- The patient has health problems that are the result of behaviors such as physical or sexual abuse, drug or alcohol dependency, homosexuality, or induced abortion, about which the social worker may have some value-laden feelings.
- The patient is determined to go home following release, or the family is determined to take him or her home, when the social worker strongly believes that even with all available resources, the patient will be unable to manage the needed care for his or her health condition.

Organization-Related Conflicts

Values and ethics conflicts may also arise from situations involving the organizational setting itself, as in the following examples:

- An administrator in the setting asks the social worker to talk with members of the patient's family, who have been complaining about the patient's care, in order to "get them off our backs."
- An administrator in the setting asks the social worker to lead a series of group meetings for family members of recently admitted patients, using a manual prepared by the corporation headquarters that does not provide for the relatives to freely talk about their feelings and concerns, but rather is designed to persuade them to disengage from monitoring their loved one's care and simply entrust the care to the facility.
- It is evident that the health care facility is seriously understaffed, and numerous incidents of patient neglect and overuse of physical and chemical restraints have occurred.
- When the social worker has tried to identify and reach out to patients who are "at risk," sometimes the patients' private physicians resent what they see as interference with "their patient."
- "Patient rights," outlined in writing by the organization, are sometimes violated.
- The for-profit organization appears to be basing its decisions regarding intake and discharge more on the adequacy of the insurance coverage than on the person's need for treatment.
- The physician insists that the social worker is to arrange for the patient's discharge before it is possible to do so without compromising the client's or family's well-being in the social worker's opinion.
- One or more patients complain to the social worker that another professional in the setting has been physically, emotionally, or sexually abusive to them.

Community Liaison-Related Conflicts

Values and ethics conflicts also can arise in the course of linking clients with community resources. In their role as *brokers* (people who know the resource options and help clients to link up with the ones best suited to their needs), social workers are in a position of influence by having personal preferences regarding community resources. This has become especially true in recent years as for-profit organizations have proliferated in the health sector of the economy, often creating a tight marketplace. Examples include community mental health centers, nursing homes, home care agencies, and medical equipment suppliers.

As a result of this increase in business-oriented service suppliers, social workers in health care settings may become the target of a sometimes bewildering bombardment of promotional materials, gifts, invitations to expensive lunches, and offers of special favors, all designed to induce social workers to steer clients to a particular service. There is probably nothing inherently wrong with social workers accepting these things, as long as it does not interfere with ongoing objective assessment of the comparative quality of clients' available resource options.

Coping with Values and Ethics Conflicts

There is no easy answer for dealing with these types of conflicts that social workers sometimes face in their practice in health care settings. In coping with those conflicts which are stimulated by subjective responses to *client* characteristics, social workers simply need to recall the admonition to "keep personal needs and feelings separate from the professional relationship." To deal with those conflicts raised by situations involving the *organizational setting,* social workers may be aided by remembering to "keep your commitments to your employing organization" but also respect "the primacy of the client's interests and well-being." Finally, when faced with conflicts that arise from promotional efforts of some business-oriented *community resource agency,* it is best to remember that "professional behavior should be characterized by honesty and integrity."

As social workers mature in their professionalism, they generally realize that the values and ethics of their profession can help them resolve the temptations that inevitably arise. The nurturance of professional knowledge, blended with and tempered by professional values and ethics, cultivates social worker skills, which are addressed next.

SKILL REQUIREMENTS

The Meaning of Skill

In everyday life, we think of skill as the ability to do something well, whether riding a bike, laying bricks, or performing brain surgery. One thing that distinguishes the skill of a professional from that of a bike rider or bricklayer is the level of knowledge required to perform the activity well. The level of required knowledge reflects the level of *complexity* and *stability* of the phenomenon involved. Complexity refers to the multiplicity of factors. Level of stability involves the extent to which these factors are constant or changing, that is, dynamic. In other words, if every human being and human problem were identical and singular, and every client responded the same during the helping process, social work practice would be more like laying bricks.

Another distinguishing characteristic of professional skill is that it is constrained by professional values and ethics. That is, there are things we *could* but would not do because we believe them to be a violation of what our profession upholds as important, worthwhile, or appropriate behavior.

Thus, *professional skill* is not mechanical, but involves the ability to act appropriately by drawing upon a body of knowledge and a set of values and ethics while interacting with a complex set of often-changing conditions. Likewise, professional social work skills are not learned simply by observing others performing them, nor only from practicing them, but are rooted in (1) knowledge of human behavior and the social environment, social welfare policy and programs, methods of social work practice, and research and evaluation methods and in (2) the values and ethics of social work.

Four Characteristics of Professional Skill

As a result of this relationship between practice activity and the knowledge, values, and ethics of one's profession, the practice activity of a professional is expected to exhibit the following characteristics:

1. *Conscious*—performed with awareness of what is being done
2. *Purposeful*—performed with an objective
3. *Disciplined*—performed not impulsively but with control
4. *Responsible*—performed with mindfulness of obligations to the values and ethics of the profession

The Meaning of Social Work Skills

Thus, we can define *social work skills* as the application of social work knowledge, values, and ethics to the performance of social work practice activity. Actually, any or all activities of social workers in the course of their practice, whether in direct services to clients, consultation, community liaison work, policy/program planning and development, teaching, or research and evaluation, are "skills"—that is, skilled activities, if they are rooted in social work knowledge, values, and ethics and, as a result, are conscious, purposeful, disciplined, and responsible.

Generic Social Work Skills

Generic social work skills are those which are common to all social work practice and which largely revolve around direct services to clients. The various approaches to categorizing social work skills reflect the basic steps and associated activities in the helping process of social work (DiNitto and McNeece, 1997; Morales and Sheafor, 1989).

Skilled Activities in Helping	Stages of Helping Process
Engagement	Engagement
Observation	Data collection
Assessment	Assessment
Cooperative planning	Contracted intervention planning
Intervention modality	Plan implementation
Research/evaluation	Evaluation of progress/effect
Termination/closure	Termination
Communication	(Throughout the helping process)
Empathy	(Throughout the helping process)

In addition to these skills associated with the helping process, basic social work education helps develop a broad range of research skills, as well as skills that are specific to group and community intervention.

The Difference Between Skills and Techniques

A skill is broader than a technique. A skill is a category of performance ability that identifies *what* is being done, whereas a technique is a specific behavior or set of behaviors used in skill performance that identifies *how* it is being done. For example, active listening is a communication skills technique. For each of the previous skill areas, or categories of performance ability, there is a set of associated techniques or behaviors used in skill performance (Morales and Sheafor, 1989).

Special Skills Required in Social Work in the Health Field

Earlier, I described the special knowledge areas required for social work in health care settings. The special skills for social work practice in health care settings are associated with these special knowledge areas:

1. the client population and problem area;
2. the organizational setting;
3. the community characteristics and resources;
4. the specific intervention modalities; and ·
5. the methods of research, program evaluation, and documentation appropriate to the particular setting.

Delineation of these relationships follows.

Client Population and Problem Area

Knowledge of the client population and problem area served by the health care setting will enhance the social worker's skill in the following practice activities:

1. Engagement, observation, assessment, cooperative planning, intervention, evaluation, termination, and overall communication and empathy associated with the process of helping patients and their families
2. Communicating with members of other health professions in the setting (because you "speak their language" and they are impressed with your insight and sensitivity to the client population and problem area)

Organizational Setting

Knowledge of the characteristics of the organizational setting will enable the social worker to develop skill in the following practice activities:

1. Developing the social work role in the organizational system so that it becomes a valued, complementary, integrated, and efficient component of that system, one that is well adapted to organizational constraints, priorities, and expectations
2. Facilitating interdisciplinary teamwork
3. Engaging in informal client advocacy with other staff in the setting

Community Characteristics and Resources

Knowledge of the characteristics, resources, and resource needs of the particular community will likely enhance the social worker's skill in these practice activities:

1. Interagency communication
2. Linking clients to resources
3. Community program/policy planning and development
4. Liaison work between the practice setting and community

Specific Intervention Modalities

Social worker knowledge of intervention methods and approaches that are particularly well suited to the needs of the particular client population, problem area, and organization will enable the social worker to develop skill in effectively helping clients to resolve their problems.

Research, Program Evaluation, and Documentation Needs

Social worker knowledge of methods of research, program evaluation, and documentation that are appropriate to and/or required by the organization setting and its funding sources will serve the social worker well in developing skill in the following areas:

1. Designing and conducting research that will help develop the practice knowledge base of social work in health care
2. Evaluating the effectiveness of the social work program in the setting as a basis for further development of that program
3. Documenting what is required for maximizing funding reimbursement to the setting
4. Encouraging interprofessional coordination by documenting case activity in medical records to inform other professional staff of it

In the next section, I explore some dimensions of service interventions in social work in health care settings.

DIMENSIONS OF HELPING

The Mission of Social Work

Preamble*

The primary mission of the social work profession is to enhance human well-being and help meet the basic human needs of all people, with particular attention to the needs and empowerment of people who are vulnerable, oppressed, and living in poverty. A historic and defining feature of social work is the profession's focus on individual well-being in a social context and the well-being of society. Fundamental to social work is attention to the environmental forces that create, contribute to, and address problems in living.

Social workers promote social justice and social change with and on behalf of clients. "Clients" is used inclusively to refer to individuals, families, groups, organizations, and communities. Social workers are sensitive to cultural and ethnic diversity and strive to end discrimination, oppression, poverty, and other forms of social injustice. These activities may be in the form of direct practice, community organizing, supervision, consultation, administration, advocacy, social and political action, policy development and implementation, education, and research and evaluation. Social workers seek to enhance the capacity of people to address their own needs. Social workers also seek to promote the responsiveness of organizations, communities, and other social institutions to individuals' needs and social problems.

The mission of the social work profession is rooted in a set of core values. These core values, embraced by social workers throughout the profession's history, are the foundation of social work's unique purpose and perspective:

- Service
- Social justice
- Dignity and worth of the person
- Importance of human relationships
- Integrity
- Competence

This constellation of core values reflects what is unique to the social work profession. Core values, and the principles that flow from them, must be balanced within the context and complexity of the human experience. (NASW, 1996:1)

---

*Copyright 1996, National Association of Social Workers, Inc., Code of Ethics.

Toward this end, professional social workers *serve* clients, through direct or indirect interventions, with the goal of restoring or enhancing their social functioning, that is, person-in-environment fit.

Direct and Indirect Social Work Services in Health Care

The basic social worker functions in health settings (NASW, 1987) identify areas of service activity and can be grouped by *direct* services, provided directly to or for the client, and *indirect* services, which are performed on behalf of or to benefit some population of potential clients.

Direct service functions include

- case finding and outreach,
- assessment of need for social work services,
- intervention planning,
- intervention (treatment),
- preadmission planning,
- discharge planning,
- information and referral,
- advocacy for a client,
- protection of rights or entitlement of a client,
- health promotion and maintenance,
- preventive, remedial, and rehabilitative measures, and
- provision of continuity of care—including guaranteed access and effective utilization.

Indirect service functions include

- advocacy for a population,
- consultation,
- liaison with the community,
- policy and program planning and development,
- quality assurance,
- research,
- social work field instruction, and
- teaching (other than field instruction).

Social Worker Roles

Roles are labels for actors that identify the function or part they are performing. Depending on which function a social worker is performing at any given time, his or her role in intervention may include that of

- an *advocate* who fights for or defends client rights;
- a *broker* who knows all of the relevant resources and links the client with the most appropriate ones;
- a *case manager* who assesses a client's needs, links that client with needed resources, and coordinates and oversees resource delivery;
- a *consultant* who provides expert opinions to others, when asked;
- a *counselor* who engages in personalized interpersonal interaction with a client, which involves the client's feelings, attitudes, perceptions, or behaviors;
- a *liaison* who acts as a go-between, link, or bridge between two or more people or organizations;
- a *mediator* who facilitates conflict resolution between parties;
- a *researcher* who develops new knowledge;
- a *planner* who prepares a design for a course of action; and/or
- a *teacher* who transmits knowledge to others.

The Social Work Helping Process

The social work profession conceives of a particular helping process, or series of steps or stages, in service intervention with clients. This conceptualized process serves to remind practitioners that professional social work intervention is disciplined and orderly; it requires client involvement, systematic gathering and interpretation of relevant information, and planning with the client before intervention itself is initiated, followed by ongoing monitoring and final evaluation of the intervention progress, effectiveness, and outcome, and ultimately concludes with closure or termination of the intervention process (DiNitto and McNeece, 1997).

The Meaning of Intervention

This helping process is the conceptualized series of steps that precedes, includes, and follows the intervention itself. Theoretically, the intervention, or what is sometimes called the treatment or treatment modality, is what is actually done in an effort to address the client's problem(s). In practice, it is difficult to separate the steps that precede and follow the intervention from the intervention itself because all social worker interaction with the client throughout the process has therapeutic potential.

Four Client Levels of Intervention

The *client* of social work services, or interventions, in the health field may be an individual patient (one on one), all or part of a patient's family, any other small group of people, or another larger sector of the community or society—such as the people in a neighborhood, a population of people concerned with a particular health problem, all residents of a treatment center, rehabilitation center, or halfway house, or all patients in a day treatment, day care, or other outpatient program. The client is the person or group that requests and/or will benefit from the social work intervention.

Intervention Objectives

Although the overall goal of social work is to restore or enhance the social functioning of clients, the more immediate *objectives* of intervention may be to

- modify attitudes, perceptions, feelings, or behaviors;
- improve interpersonal relationships or communication;
- facilitate decision making and self-determination;
- enhance adaptation and coping capacity; and
- sustain or enhance mental or physical comfort and functioning.

Intervention Approaches

In addressing these objectives, a variety of approaches may be considered, the selection of which depends on assessment of the client's needs and capacities. Essentially, there are six approaches:

1. Counseling in some form
2. Education or skill training
3. Resource information and resource linkage assistance
4. Advocacy to help the client obtain what he or she needs and is entitled to have
5. Modification of the environment to adapt it to client needs
6. Community resource development

Affective-Expressive and Concrete-Instrumental Interventions

Historically, social workers have tended to categorize their interventions in health care settings as either (1) affective-expressive or (2) concrete-instrumental.

Affective-expressive interventions are the various forms of counseling that involve a process of personalized interpersonal interaction between the social worker and client in which the focus is on attitudes, feelings, perceptions, decisions, or behaviors of the client. Frequently, such services target client problems that are related to *adjustment* to the health service or facility or to the diagnosis, prognosis, or medical treatment plan. However, in mental health settings, affective-expressive interventions are also often directed toward treating the health problem itself. Such interventions are termed affective-expressive because they focus on "affect," that is, feelings/moods, and "expression," or behavior.

Concrete-instrumental interventions, on the other hand, are those which revolve around resource information and referral activity, that is, linking the client with needed resources—such as assisting with arrangements for admission and aftercare, the care of the patient's family during his or her absence or disability, assistance with transportation to health services, helping to obtain medical aids and appliances, or assisting with financial arrangements for the patient's care. In other words, concrete-instrumental interventions are usually tangible services in which the social worker acts as an agent for the client; they focus on social environmental problems, needs, and resources and often are associated with patient problems relating to admission and aftercare.

More recently, however, social workers are realizing that this traditional distinction between affective-expressive and concrete-instrumental social work interventions is somewhat artificial (Blazyk and Canavan, 1985). This is because preadmission and discharge planning often need to involve the attitudes, feelings, perceptions, decisions, or behaviors of patients and/or their family members; conversely, patients with problems of adjustment to the health care service or facility or to the diagnosis, prognosis, or treatment plan, or patients whose primary health problem is mental rather than physical, often have a variety of concrete concerns and needs.

The Concept of Psychosocial Problems

Psychosocial problems are problems with both psychological and social environmental components, which reflects the inevitable influence each arena has on the other.

Fundamental to social work in health care is the perspective that the social functioning of people reflects what is variously termed the interaction, intersection, interface, or transactions between the *person* with attitudes, feelings, perceptions, and behavior patterns and the *environment,* with its presenting situation, resources, and supports (Germain and Gitterman, 1980). Thus, a person's social functioning reflects both his or her interpretation of a situation and the actual situation. For this reason, the interventions of the social worker address psychosocial problems that impair optimal social functioning.

Intervention Methods

Intervention methods, sometimes called treatment modalities, are more or less specific techniques or models for intervention, each with a premise concerning how or why it ought to help solve the problem.

There are many intervention or treatment approaches that the social worker may view as a repertoire of options, the choice of which depends on the nature of the client's problem, needs, and capacities. In one text (Kerson, 1989), the combined social workers who contributed case studies to that anthology of readings identified more than twenty treatment modalities or types of interventions that they have used in their practice in health care settings: crisis intervention, problem solving, education and information, task-oriented counseling, ego-oriented casework, confrontation, peer group therapy, assertiveness training, group work, case management, family therapy, behavior modification, entitlement and advocacy, concrete services, milieu therapy, skill training, psychoanalysis, cognitive therapy, relaxation therapy, modeling, supportive counseling, reminiscence therapy, and nondirective client-centered counseling.

The second edition of Kerson's text *Social Work in Health Settings: Practice in Context* (1997) follows the same format, including identification of the social worker's intervention(s) in each case study—that range includes many of the same interventions as well as a few new ones, including community organization, supportive environment development, critical incident stress debriefing, and anticipatory and postdeath grief counseling.

Although many of the same interventions are named in the second edition as in the first edition, the most striking difference is the more frequent use of crisis intervention and case management in the 1997 edition. The inevitable question is whether this apparent change may be the result of the increase in managed care and short-term, solution-focused approaches. In any case, the Kerson works indicate that social workers, in both mental and physical health settings, call upon a wide range of approaches, interventions, techniques, and roles in their efforts to help clients with problems of social functioning that are related to their health problems.

Premises of Alternate Interventions

The use of these interventions for various client needs in the health field suggests the following premises of their selection. People may benefit from

- *education and information* to make informed decisions and take charge of their lives and health;
- outreach coupled with caring *confrontation* to get the client to address his or her health behavior or health problem;
- rehearsing those behaviors which are required to change a problem situation *(task-oriented counseling);*
- social interaction (discussion, recreational activity, shared task activity) with a group of other people the client respects and can identify with in order to change attitudes, feelings, perceptions, or behaviors *(group therapy/peer group therapy);*
- learning new skills in order to change problem situations or develop adaptive behaviors *(skill training);*
- direct, focused, practical, supportive assistance when in a crisis *(crisis intervention);*
- learning *problem-solving skills,* such as partializing and focusing;
- learning to interpret events as less threatening and to recognize positive rather than self-defeating messages *(cognitive therapy);*
- a supportive environment or milieu *(milieu therapy);*
- counseling with family groups to identify and eliminate dysfunctional patterns of communication within them *(family therapy);*
- ego building to cope with stress *(ego-oriented casework);*
- developing insight into past experience to help cope with the present *(psychoanalysis);*
- having a professional who is designated to coordinate service delivery when the client requires services from a variety of agencies or specialists *(case management);*
- positive reinforcement of progress in the client's efforts to make behavioral changes *(behavior modification);*
- having someone to fight for the client's rights *(advocacy);*
- *concrete services* and resources to meet basic material needs instead of, or before, services to address emotional or behavioral problems;
- learning how to assert one's position on issues without attacking or provoking others *(assertiveness training);*
- learning how to induce a period of relaxation to avert unhealthy behavioral responses *(relaxation therapy);*
- observing other people demonstrate appropriate behaviors in order to learn them *(modeling);*
- recollecting and reminiscing about good times in the past to help restore the client's sense of ego integrity when overwhelmed by life change events *(reminiscence therapy);* and
- having someone listen and provide *support* while the client thinks through problems and restores ego functioning *(supportive counseling).*

DeCoster conducted a content analysis of social work journal articles published between 1977 and 1999 concerning social worker interventions in health care social work practice across the range of health care settings and populations. The purpose of the study was to identify the types of interventions used by the social workers to address particular forms of emotional distress of patients, and to develop a classification of specific interventions for specific forms of emotional distress. DeCoster reported that the forty-five mutually exclusive strategies or interventions utilized fell into two broad categories: cognitive (69 percent) and behavioral (31 percent). The most frequently reported social work emotion-treatment strategies were

1. *to reassure*—talk to instill confidence for present situation, being optimistic
2. *to educate*—provide accurate information on the present or upcoming situation (procedure, event) and ensure that it is comprehended
3. *to express*—active cathartic expression of emotion
4. *to verbalize*—discuss the client's experienced or expressed emotions (2000:14-15)

DeCoster (2000) also points out that health care social workers often utilize a combination of such strategies as they "listen, normalize, empower, and identify needs" (19).

The Meaning of Counseling in Social Work

With the exceptions of education and information, milieu therapy, problem solving, skill training, case management, advocacy, community organization, information and referral, and concrete services, the treatment modalities or interventions identified in the Kerson (1997) text fall primarily under the category of *counseling*. Counseling is a broad term that refers to a personalized interpersonal process of helping which relies heavily on verbal and nonverbal communication between the social worker and client(s). Counseling may be provided to an individual, family, or other small group.

Counseling in social work is generally thought of as the medium through which social workers attempt to treat problems in social functioning that require a focus on the client's attitudes, feelings, perceptions, or behaviors. Because counseling involves emotional and behavioral functioning, it is sometimes called an affective-expressive activity. The objective of counseling may be to

1. change a person's attitudes, feelings, perceptions, or behaviors;
2. change interpersonal relationships and communication patterns;

3. help the client to think through and make some needed decisions; and/or
4. sustain or enhance a person's coping capacity.

Although counseling can, and often does, include teaching new skills, providing needed information, education, or advocacy, or linking clients with needed concrete resources, these activities must be coupled with a personalized interpersonal process and linked with one or more of the previous four objectives to be considered counseling.

Social work is distinguished from other helping professions by its dual focus on *the person and the environment*. Therefore, if social workers who do counseling wish to retain their identity as social workers, they need to sustain this dual focus. In theory, social workers who disregard the social-environmental context of the client as a person and address only the client's intrapsychic functioning are not practicing social work.

The Theoretical Perspective of Care or Caring

Once established, few of the major mental or physical health problems today are amenable to complete cure. Earlier in this century when social work in health care began, the major health problems in the United States were acute *infectious* diseases (those caused by bacteria or viruses), such as typhoid, typhus, pneumonia, and tuberculosis. As a result of their prevalence, life expectancy was about 60 percent of what it is today. However, as public health measures and medical technology developed, these diseases were brought under control and more people began to live longer.

One result of longer life expectancy is that *chronic* health problems (permanent and incurable ones) have now emerged as the major health problems. This is because chronic disorders, such as heart disease, hypertension, cancer, type II diabetes, strokes, and arthritis, tend to emerge with advancing age. In addition, younger people with chronic diseases and disabilities, such as epilepsy, type I diabetes, severe mental illness, mental retardation, and other developmental disabilities, also live longer now because of the development of anticonvulsive drugs, insulin, and antipsychotic drugs, as well as antibiotics that help control the infectious diseases that once tended to shorten people's lives.

Although heart disease, hypertension, strokes, and cancer are the major causes of death and disability, certain psychosocial problems are also gaining prominence, sometimes as contributing causes of chronic disease. Examples of such *psychosocial problems* include alcoholism and other drug abuse, cigarette smoking, eating disorders, domestic violence, rape and other forms of sexual abuse, homicide, suicide, and motor vehicle accidents.

Neither the chronic health problems nor the psychosocial or behavioral ones are curable in the same sense that infectious diseases often are. For this reason, the focus must be on *care interventions* (supportive forms of assistance) to: (1) promote health and prevent disease from emerging, (2) prevent the development of health problems that have already emerged, and (3) prevent secondary disabilities, or avoidable impairment of function and comfort associated with chronic or terminal problems, once they reach that stage:

> Since most serious diseases and disabilities are likely to prove relatively intractable if they cannot be prevented, the role of therapeutic medicine should be modified to include as the major commitment the *concept of care*. Such a change would carry major implications for medical science and service and should affect the content and orientation of medical education. (McLachlan and McKeown, 1971:48) (emphasis added)

Since the terms *care* and *caring* are so commonly but variously used, it is important to clarify what they mean. I agree with David Mechanic, who wrote:

> It is unfortunately common for many physicians to conceive of the caring functions of medical care as simply the expression of kindness and acceptance of the patient. While this is no trivial aspect, *caring constitutes* a much wider *range of techniques based* not only on human feeling, or even on the techniques usually associated with psychotherapy, but *on scientific knowledge of how to provide human support. . . . In short, caring is a technology, the dimensions of which can be concretely identified, studied, manipulated and transmitted to practitioners who apply the technology in concrete situations.* Caring is thus much more than a communication of feeling. (1978:309) (emphasis added)

Rationale for the Concept of Care

"Since most serious diseases and disabilities are likely to prove relatively intractable if they cannot be prevented, the role of therapeutic medicine should be modified to include as the major commitment the concept of care. Such a change would carry major implications for medical science and service and should affect the content and orientation of medical education." (McLachlan and McKeown, 1971:48)

The Purpose of Caring

Often, people need extensive supportive types of assistance to
1. help prevent the onset of health problems;
2. enhance the cure process and keep health and other human problems from compounding or developing into a worsened state once emerged; and
3. maximize comfort and function once health problems have become chronic and/or terminal and to prevent secondary disabilities.

The Concept of Caring

"It is unfortunately common for many physicians to conceive of the caring functions of medical care as simply the expression of kindness and acceptance of the patient. While this is no trivial aspect, caring constitutes a much wider range of techniques based not only on human feeling, or even on the techniques usually associated with psychotherapy, but on scientific knowledge of how to provide human support. . . . In short, caring is a technology, the dimensions of which can be concretely identified, studied, manipulated and transmitted to practitioners who apply the technology in concrete situations. Caring is thus much more than a communication of feeling." (Mechanic, 1978:309)

"Health is a complete state of biological, psychological, and social well-being, not simply the absence of disease" (WHO, 1978). Care interventions, or supportive kinds of assistance, are directed toward a combination of biological (physical), psychological (mental and emotional), and social well-being. For this reason, caring is an interdisciplinary and biopsychosocial approach to helping.

An underlying premise of the care approach to helping is that service providers must cooperate *with*, not operate *on*, the patient and family to

1. empower them and engage them in efforts to achieve the goal appropriate to the patient's health status level (prevention, repair, compensation), and
2. promote their self-determination and the sense of control and mastery needed to ward off feelings of helplessness, powerlessness, and giving up.

The Rationale for Care Interventions

The *rationale* for providing supportive assistance, that is, care interventions, at all three levels of health service intervention is as follows:

1. At the *primary level,* initially, some health problems emerge, in part, because of one or more of the following:
   a. People engage in self-destructive or high-risk behavior.
   b. People fall prey to environmental dangers.
   c. People have stressful life experiences that erode their coping capacity and their resistance to health problems.
2. At the *secondary level,* when people are ill or injured with acute health problems that could be cured or repaired, or whose development could be slowed or stopped, the following problems arise:
   a. People do not always recognize that they are ill or injured or need help.
   b. People do not always know where to go to seek appropriate help.
   c. People sometimes are afraid to seek such help.
   d. People sometimes feel they cannot afford to accept the help, for financial reasons or due to other responsibilities.
   e. People sometimes have other barriers to getting the needed help, for example, transportation, discrimination, or cultural beliefs.
   f. People with acute health conditions, once they gain access to the needed treatment service, often experience impairment of their functional capacity and/or mental, physical, or social comfort, which, if not supported for them, can act as a barrier to attaining their level of potential recovery.
   g. People who are ready for release but still need some special care are more likely to relapse if supportive assistance is not provided to help ensure continuity of care.
3. At the *tertiary level,* when people have chronic and/or terminal health conditions that cannot be cured, the following issues must be considered:
   a. People often experience considerable impairment of comfort and functioning, whether mental, physical, or social.
   b. People require extensive supportive forms of assistance to help them compensate for such impairment (Morris and Anderson, 1975)

When I say that neither the chronic health problems (e.g., heart disease, hypertension, strokes, and cancer) nor the psychosocial or behavioral problems (e.g., alcoholism and other drug abuse, cigarette smoking, eating disorders, domestic violence, rape and other forms of sexual abuse, homicide, suicide, and motor vehicle accidents) are curable in the same sense that infectious diseases often are, I mean that psychosocial and behavioral health problems are not ones that we know how to repair through surgical procedures or medications. Instead, *they are adaptations to social and emotional experiences in life.* The problem is that when we allow behavioral and psychosocial problems to develop, when we ignore people's excesses until some crisis occurs, when we allow people to remain in situations in which they are being mistreated physically, emotionally, educationally, and sexually, scars are formed and tend to remain. Brain function may become altered and may never be restored to its original normal state.

We must instead try to prevent people from habitually engaging in health behaviors that tend to contribute to chronic diseases. A high percentage of the U.S. population is currently classified as overweight or obese—both of which are correlates of the four major causes of death today. Thus, the primary form of caring is primary prevention. This is likely to require interventions directed at both individuals and communities. Caring consists of supportive forms of assistance. Supports can be thought of as pillars that are necessary, but not sufficient, to hold something up. In the case of human beings, I believe that, at the primary level, caring is health promotion and disease prevention at both personal and community levels.

Primary prevention requires a society that promotes health

- through the foods it allows to be sold;
- through the advertisements it allows to be distributed;
- through the standards it sets and enforces for the physical environment (air, water, soil);
- through the quality of the schools it provides for all of its citizens;
- through the preventive and early intervention services it guarantees its citizens for mental and physical health problems, for interpersonal behavior problems, for child-rearing problems, such as supportive human relationships (social support), behavior modification, education and information, empowerment, and facilitation of access to the development of Abraham Maslow's hierarchy of human needs, which are, in ascending order, fundamental needs such as food, clothing, shelter, safety, and security, belonging, self-esteem, and self-actualization (Maslow, 1968).

In short, primary prevention implies the elimination of the sources of distress and "*dis*ease" in our social structures, such as poverty, racism, pollution, poor education, and the general lack of a nurturing environment.

Examples of Primary Care Interventions

In an ideal society, primary care interventions would include the following: *Help prevent child maltreatment by requiring people to be licensed to raise children.* This would require people who wish to parent children to take and pass written and oral exams dealing with child care and child development, proper nutrition, appropriate behavioral management and discipline, and so on. Although failure to pass such an exam could not prevent people from giving birth to children, it could establish the idea that child rearing is a serious business for which society has certain expectations and standards, and it could determine whether community services may need to be provided early on—such as public health nursing and social work team visits to educate, support, and monitor, like the system that exists in Sweden. Although people have the right to have children, they do not have the right to mistreat them. Child maltreatment is a fundamental and widespread cause of multiple social problems, such as delinquency and crime, mental health problems, learning problems, domestic violence, drug and alcohol abuse, and economic dependency. In short, if a person's behavior negatively affects others, then it is no longer simply a personal problem but a social problem, a public issue. We require people to have a license to drive a car, to hunt, to fish, to operate a boat, and so forth, but for some reason we have no requirements for people to produce and rear totally vulnerable children.

Require that every community have sufficient numbers of qualified professionals to provide early identification and intervention in situations of child maltreatment. The focus should be on helping families to become able to provide good care, and to provide substitute care when the child's safety is in jeopardy.

Make it illegal to sell food products that are determined by qualified nutrition experts to be detrimental to human health (e.g., foods that have a high content of fat, cholesterol, sugar, etc.).

Make it illegal to advertise products that are determined to be hazardous to human health (e.g., cigarettes).

Provide affordable public services to all citizens. These should include early identification and intervention for mental and physical health problems, interpersonal behavior problems, child-rearing problems, and chemical dependency problems. In other words, I am suggesting a return to public comprehensive community mental health centers.

Of course, primary preventive interventions would also include a living wage, inclusive communities, quality education for all, and so on.

Examples of Secondary Care Interventions

Secondary care interventions are appropriate when the functioning of a person is compromised due to an acute health or other human problem, that is, when the person suffers from extreme grief, feels threatened, has an illness that prevents normal physical function and responsibilities, or experiences another crisis. Examples of care interventions at this level might include these:

- *Have a social worker and nurse team reach out to assess the person's status, needs, and wishes, and to offer a care plan of appropriate intervention.* This could include homemaker services, nurse aid services, clinical crisis intervention services, provision of a volunteer visitor who shares or has shared this type of problem situation to provide ongoing support, on-site physical therapy, occupational therapy, and nutrition services.

- *Keep in touch with the needy person and address the person's specific immediate needs as they arise, with his or her permission and partnership.* Offer whatever is needed to help the person to compensate for temporary impairments so that he or she feels empowered rather than compromised.

Examples of Tertiary Care Interventions

Following are some suggested examples of supportive interventions, or care interventions. I encourage readers to think about these and other types of interventions in terms of their potential effects in addressing the purposes and rationale for caring at the three levels of health services.

Tools and equipment. This refers to all types of medical aids and appliances, such as walkers, wheelchairs, grab bars, raised toilets, handheld showers, hand-operated automobiles, TENS machines for pain relief, and blood sugar monitoring kits. This form of caring is often referred to as assistive technology.

Support services. These include a wide range of services, such as identification of and outreach to members of high-risk groups; personal care services; counseling; support groups; education, information, and skills training; meals on wheels; home care; hospice care; day care; respite care; home-repair and maintenance services; telephone reassurance service; lifeline service; visiting podiatry and hairdressing services; and social action to eliminate high-risk economic, political, physical, and social environmental conditions.

Income supports. These include both cash supports, such as Social Security, SSI, VA pensions, and other benefits paid in or convertible to cash, as well as in-kind income supports, such as food stamps, Medicare and Medicaid, subsidized housing, public housing, shelters, nutrition centers, and food pantries.

Environmental adaptations. These include ramps, kitchen and light fixtures designed for wheelchair access, amplifiers and magnified dials on telephones, low-pile carpet, nonskid floors, low-glare lighting, remote control appliances, temperature controls on water taps, and so forth.

Interpersonal supports. These are interactions, communications, and relationships with other people that are experienced as emotionally supportive, that is, as indications to patients that someone cares about them. Examples might include reaching out to people in need, calling them by the name they prefer, respecting their cultural diversity, showing interest in and attending to their thoughts and feelings, being available when needed, showing prompt attention and responsiveness to their needs, encouraging their ability to make their own decisions and do for themselves when able, facilitating their having and doing what they find enjoyable, being accepting of them as individuals, and assisting them to obtain what they need and are willing to receive.

In fact, the theoretical perspective I call caring is rooted in the principle that the supportive interventions required for health maintenance, repair, and compensation *must* include interpersonal interactions, communications, and relationships that are experienced by the client as "feeling cared about." The belief that one is of value is the source of personal motivation and empowerment, which is the sine qua non of health maintenance, recovery, and coping.

Limitations of Social Work Intervention in Health Care Settings

Social work intervention in health care settings is often constrained by a variety of conditions, usually relating to the client, setting, or community.

Client-Related Constraints

In both mental and physical health settings, the patients themselves are sometimes unable to participate fully in any type of social work intervention, either because they are children or because they are too ill or handicapped to communicate, express preferences, make decisions, or provide needed information. As a result, the social worker may need to work with family members, a legal guardian, or others with legal authority to act on the client's behalf. In lieu of the availability of such a person, the social worker may be required to initiate the legal process to appoint a guardian for the client.

Organization-Related Constraints

Depending on the characteristics of the organizational setting of practice, there may be constraints on social work intervention in terms of the following: (1) available time to work with clients when they are not engaged in other program activities or before they are discharged; (2) which kinds of services are reimbursable; (3) which kinds of services are acceptable to organizational policy (for example, Catholic organizations are unlikely to allow social worker interventions that facilitate access to abortion or artificial methods of contraception); and (4) which staff members are allocated responsibility for which types of services. For example, in some health settings, persons other than social workers may be assigned responsibility for preadmission and/or discharge planning or counseling. In addition, often an interdisciplinary team of health professionals, rather than an individual, jointly decides upon appropriate interventions.

Community-Related Constraints

Finally, the options for social work intervention are sometimes limited by community-related conditions. For example, the community simply may not have certain resources that the client needs, in which case the social worker needs to be as creative as possible to find alternate solutions. These may include seeking private or little-known benefactors to purchase something, or they may require the social worker to help develop a resource, such as a support group; it may also be helpful to consult with a professional who has expertise in that resource area (such as a particular type of medical equipment) regarding possible substitutes or alternatives.

Another common situation is that the patient may not be from the local community or is being released to a facility or family member in some other, often distant, community. In these cases, considerable exploration is usually required to determine what resources are available in that other community. A common, and particularly challenging, community-related situation for social workers occurs when the patient is being released to a very rural and remote area in another state where community resources are practically nonexistent. In such situations, it can be productive to telephone one or more large agencies in the local community that provide that type of service to ask if they know the location and phone number of a comparable service in the urban area closest to where the patient is going. By making contact with the latter organizations, the social worker can often gain considerable assistance in working out a plan for continuity of the patient care, including access to the available local resources.

SUMMARY

At the base of every profession is the claim that it has a special body of knowledge that enables its members to understand and address the phenomena encompassed by their arena of practice.

All social work practice requires knowledge of

1. human behavior and the social environment,
2. social welfare policy and programs,
3. social work practice, and
4. social work research methods.

Only social work practice knowledge is unique to the social work profession and must be continually developed through ongoing research within the profession.

In addition, social work practice in a health care setting requires some specialized knowledge of

1. the client population and problem area,
2. the particular organizational setting,
3. the community and its resources,
4. specific intervention modalities, and
5. research, evaluation, and documentation suited to the setting.

Besides having a body of knowledge, a profession must have a set of values and ethics to guide members' practice of that profession. The new code of ethics of the NASW lays out some core values, principles, and standards of the social work profession that are of special relevance to practice in health care. Challenges that sometimes confront social workers concerning their professional values and ethics often arise in relation to client, organizational, or community liaison situations. However, the resolution of these conflicts is also often aided by reviewing and reflecting on this code of ethics.

Social worker skills for practice in health care settings are cultivated through specialized knowledge and are both inspired and constrained by the guiding values and ethics of the profession—resulting in practice activity that is conscious, purposeful, disciplined, and responsible. From professional knowledge comes *conscious* practice activity—knowing what is being done. From knowledge also comes *purposeful* practice activity—knowing what the objective is. From the values and ethics of the profession comes *disciplined* activity—control of impulses, as well as *responsible* behavior—activity that is mindful of social workers' obligations to clients, colleagues, employing organizations, professions, and society at large.

Finally, professional values and ethics inspire social workers with the reminder that professionals *serve* others, and it is through our combined knowledge, values, ethics, and skills that we are able to effectively intervene in our service mission. This mission is to help sustain, enhance, or restore social functioning, that is, person-in-environment fit. Social worker functions include both direct and indirect services toward this goal. Social workers play a variety of roles, reflecting shifts in functions.

Social work intervention or treatment to help the client is part of a systematic process or series of steps that has a beginning and an end. The social work client may be an individual, family, group, or larger sector of the community. Social worker efforts to sustain or enhance social functioning may have as objectives modifying attitudes, feelings, perceptions, or behaviors; improving interpersonal relationships or communication; facilitating decision making; enhancing adaptation and coping capacity; or sustaining or enhancing mental or physical comfort and functioning.

There are a multitude of intervention methods, but they reflect six broad approaches: counseling, education or skill training, resource information and resource linkage assistance, advocacy, environmental modification, and community resource development.

In addition to the health problem itself, clients commonly experience six health-related psychosocial problems, including barriers to admission to the health service or facility; problems of adjustment to the health service or facility; problems of adjustment to the diagnosis, prognosis, or health treatment plan; lack of needed information to make informed decisions and take control; lack of resources to meet needs; and barriers to discharge. Social workers in both mental and physical health service settings address these types of psychosocial problems.

Social workers do not directly treat physical health problems, but social workers with a master's degree in social work (MSW) or doctoral degree who practice in a mental health setting often do directly treat certain types of mental health problems.

In social work practice, counseling is one intervention approach that can take many forms, but it is always a personalized interpersonal process of helping that relies heavily on verbal and nonverbal communication with the client in which the focus is on attitudes, feelings, perceptions, decisions, or behaviors of the client in the context of his or her social environmental situation.

Today's major health problems require a broad supportive approach to help more effectively prevent them, to enhance what recovery is possible once they emerge, and to prevent and compensate for impairments of comfort and function associated with having health disorders that are chronic or terminal. This requires an approach that is both biopsychosocial and interdisciplinary. This approach is what I call caring and is a developing intervention perspective in social work and other professions in health care.

Finally, social work intervention in health service settings is sometimes constrained by conditions related to the client, setting, or community.

The next five chapters further explore the opportunities and limitations of social work intervention in specific health service settings.

SECTION II:
SETTINGS AT THE THREE LEVELS
OF INTERVENTION

Chapter 3

Social Work in Primary Care Settings

HISTORICAL BACKGROUND

The early work of social workers in settlement houses during the last quarter of the nineteenth century involved engaging the community in social action efforts to modify social and physical environmental conditions seen as detrimental to public health, including those related to housing, workplaces, sewage and water, and lack of education:

> . . . their goal was to bridge the gap between the classes and races, to eliminate the sources of distress, and to improve urban living and working conditions. Like the public health reformers, with whom they frequently cooperated, theirs was the preventive approach. (Trattner, 1989:147)

In 1905, Dr. Richard C. Cabot hired social workers to work in his medicine clinic at Massachusetts General Hospital. These workers were to make home visits (Oktay, 1995:1891) to bring back to the medical and nursing staff an understanding of the conditions in the patient's home, work, and community that were relevant to the patient's health problem (Cabot, 1928: 28); they also were to address those conditions whenever possible (Cannon, 1923:15, 30).

Social work in primary health care developed further during the Great Depression when the Social Security Act was passed in 1935, which called for social workers to be employed in the Maternal and Child Health Program and the Crippled Children's Program (Oktay, 1995).

Before World War II, most Americans obtained medical care services through their family physician, primarily general practitioners and some internists and pediatricians. However, it was not until the 1960s when medical specialization was sufficiently widespread that concern began to emerge about the decline in what was termed primary care. This marked the beginning of multiple efforts by the U.S. government to promote a return to primary care, efforts that continue today (Donaldson et al., 1996:19-20).

Beginning in the 1960s, the federal government funded primary health care settings such as migrant health centers, neighborhood health centers, and homeless health care programs staffed by physicians who were repaying educational loans under the National Health Services Act (Oktay, 1995). Social workers were written into these federally funded neighborhood health centers as part of the federal antipoverty program and included as mandated staff in the first federally funded HMOs. Social workers have been widely employed in hospital outpatient clinics, as the DRG system has reduced inpatient care and hospitals have sought alternative forms of service opportunities (Oktay, 1995:1891).

In the late 1980s, the U.S. Department of Health and Human Services (DHHS), Division of Maternal and Child Health, began to support social worker training in public health concepts (Henk, 1989). Currently, the NASW and the Council on Social Work Education (CSWE)-sponsored Institute for the Advancement of Social Work Research has been cooperating with the National Institute of Mental Health (NIMH) to support research on social work in primary health care to help prevent and provide early intervention in mental disorders (Oktay, 1995:1891).

In 1990, 547 community, migrant, and homeless health centers were serving six million people, or about one-fourth of the nation's medically indigent (National Association of Community Health Centers, 1993). In addition, government funds support Maternal and Child Health Block Grant programs, public health department primary care programs, such as well-baby clinics, prenatal care, immunization and screening programs, and child development programs for prevention of and early intervention in child developmental problems (Oktay, 1995:1889).

However, during the conservative backlash of the 1980s, federal funding to train primary care physicians and to support primary care services for underserved people dropped significantly, and few health care settings in the United States now provide true primary care, although many use the term to describe their services. That is, few first-contact settings provide health service that is comprehensive, coordinated, and continuous, although HMOs may come closest to providing primary care, since they have an incentive to keep people healthy and to avoid high-cost services (Oktay, 1995:1888).

To date, social work in public health is better established than social work in primary medical care settings, reflecting, perhaps, the reluctance of physicians in private practice to collaborate with professional groups that they fear the public may associate with "welfare" and child welfare. In addition, private physicians generally have been reluctant to acknowledge the skills of other professional groups in mental health because physicians traditionally have perceived mental health as a subspecialty of medicine, i.e., psychiatry. Public health, on the other hand, became a separate discipline from medical practice in the early 1900s, about the time that medicine transitioned from social medicine with a care orientation to a medical model with a cure orientation to disease caused by bacteria and viruses, rather than social environs, and located in the individual. About the same time, social work began to transition from a focus on social-environmental causes of human problems to a person-centered, mental health focus.

The history of public health itself is one that most of the public probably took for granted until the recent publication of the seminal work by Laurie Garrett (2000), which unveiled the historical rise and fall of the public health infrastructure. It is truly a tale of clashes between public interests and a range of private interests—political and economic, including the economic interests of physicians in private practice. Following is a prophetic passage from Garrett's book, published the year before the September 11, 2001, terrorist attacks on the World Trade Center in New York City and on the Pentagon in Washington, DC, and the subsequent bioterrorist attacks involving anthrax spores delivered through the mail system to unsuspecting American citizens:

> Public health in the twenty-first century will rise or fall, then, with the ultimate course of globalization. If the passage of time finds ever-widening wealth gaps, disappearing middle classes, international financial lawlessness, and still-rising individualism, the essential elements of public health will be imperiled, perhaps nonexistent, all over the world. Capital will be skewed away from social service infrastructures in such a scenario, particularly those that meet the needs of the poor. Few public health barriers will be in place to prevent global spread of disease, and ever more drugs will be rendered useless by microbial resistence. United Nations agencies, including the World Health Organization, will witness further deterioration in their funding and influence. And political instability will foster increasingly irrational nation-state and rogue activities including, perhaps, bioterrorism. (Garrett, 2000:588)

Stephen H. Gorin (2001) laid out some of the history of the public health system in the United States, describing how recent findings about the role of socioeconomic inequality as a major determinant of population health have revitalized the validity of public health, and how those findings imply that social work ought to be at the heart of addressing the problem of social inequality.

Settings of Social Work in Primary Health Care

Primary Medical Care

Social workers in *primary care* may be found in hospital outpatient clinics, HMOs, neighborhood health center clinics, and group medical practices (Miller, 1987:323). In addition, social workers are firmly entrenched in many of the family practice residency training centers throughout the United States, functioning in accordance with the American Academy of Family Physicians (Hess, 1985:57; Zayas and Dyche, 1992). Other sites of social work in primary care include hospital emergency rooms, free clinics, public health departments (Ell and Morrison, 1981:35S), and family planning clinics (Kerson and Peachey, 1989).

The Specter of Rising Social Inequality

"Public health in the twenty-first century will rise or fall, then, with the ultimate course of globalization. If the passage of time finds ever-widening wealth gaps, disappearing middle classes, international financial lawlessness, and still-rising individualism, the essential elements of public health will be imperiled, perhaps nonexistent, all over the world. Capital will be skewed away from social service infrastructures in such a scenario, particularly those that meet the needs of the poor. Few public health barriers will be in place to prevent global spread of disease, and ever more drugs will be rendered useless by microbial resistance." (Garrett, 2000:588)

The idea of integrating social work services into primary care practice has long received conceptual support both from the medical and social work communities. In the Health Maintenance Organization Act of 1973, the federal government mandated that social work services be integrated into health maintenance organizations as an essential profession to achieve the objectives of health promotion and early intervention (Badger et al., 1997:22).

Primary Prevention

According to Bloom (1995:1898), major settings of social work in *primary prevention* include public schools; workplaces (e.g., employee assistance programs, accident prevention programs); recreational settings; social agencies that provide social support and skills training and education, such as self-help groups, and social and coping skills training (e.g., family life education, parenting training, assertiveness training, caregiver support, suicide prevention, grief support); and health settings, such as HMOs with prevention-oriented services.

For example, by the 1999-2000 school year, the number of school-based health centers increased sevenfold to a total of 1,380, according to a nationwide survey conducted by the Center for Health and Health Care in Schools at George Washington University. These school-based centers are usually operated by a local hospital or health center and provide early care to prevent or treat common health problems of children and teens, as well as chronic health conditions. Staffed by teams of nurses, physicians, and mental health professionals, they typically provide annual physical exams, offer family counseling, and work with school staff to intervene with student problems (American Public Health Association, 2001b).

Health Promotion

A recent text (Poland, Green, and Rootman, 2000) addresses the following settings of *health promotion:* home and family, school, workplace, health care institutions, clinical practice, the community, and the state. The rationale for the settings approach to health promotion reflects an ecological perspective, which recognizes that health is a product of the person-in-environment or reciprocal interaction of the two spheres:

> The ecological perspective presents health as a product of the interdependence between the individual and subsystems of the ecosystem. Subsystems for health promotion may include family, peer groups, organizations, community, culture, and physical and social environment. (McLeroy et al., 1988:16, cited in Poland, Green, and Rootman, 2000)

Primary Health Care Concepts

In the literature, the fields of primary medical care, public health, preventive medicine, and health promotion are sometimes discussed as separate disciplines, sometimes as overlapping, and sometimes as parts of a common whole. They are presented here as parts of a conceptual whole that includes the following:

1. *Professions providing primary medical care,* such as family practice, internal medicine, pediatrics, physician assistants, and nurse practitioners
2. *Settings of primary medical care practice,* including individual and group practices of any of the previous professions, outpatient clinics

located in hospitals, neighborhood health centers, freestanding clinics, and HMOs
3. *The field of public health*
4. *Primary prevention,* that is, efforts to prevent the occurrence of health problems
5. *Health promotion programs*

Primary Care

Technically, the term *primary care* refers to the emphasis on the patient's first entry into the health care system. The HMO Act of 1973 endorsed support for primary health care in the United States (Miller, 1987:321). In 1978, the World Health Organization named primary health care as the key to attaining health care for all people by the year 2000 (Oktay, 1995:1887) and identified its key concepts as including the terms *practical, affordable, acceptable to the community, accessible and community based,* and *the gateway to continuity of the health care system* (WHO, 1978:25). The 1978 Assembly of the World Health Organization on Primary Care "emphasized the promotion of health, the prevention of disease, and the integration of mental and physical health services; and advocated a holistic approach that includes the physical, mental, and social aspects of health" (Oktay, 1995: 1887).

Although the WHO concept of primary health care encompasses public health objectives of community-based health promotion and primary prevention of disease, American medical practice tends to reserve the concept of primary health care for personal health care services, excluding public health work. According to the Institute of Medicine (IOM) Committee on the Future of Primary Care:

> Primary care is the provision of *integrated, accessible* health care services by clinicians who are *accountable* for *addressing a large majority of personal health care needs,* developing a *sustained* partnership with patients, and practicing in the context of family and community. (Donaldson et al., 1996:31) (emphasis added)

Miller (1987:321) referred to these five characteristics of primary care as coordinated, accessible, comprehensive, continuous, and accountable.

The IOM refers to the need for partnership with patients and practice in the context of family and community, suggesting a developing recognition by the medical profession that effective primary care must be a cooperative venture rather than an authoritative one and that people are influenced by interaction with other social system levels, such as family and community. The IOM also acknowledges the limitation of primary medical care without public health:

> [Primary care] will have a limited impact on health status until or unless the determinants of public and social health are addressed. . . . The aggregate benefits in health status to be gained from increasing income or education greatly outweigh the gains from medical intervention. . . Similarly, preventing injuries from violence, child neglect, or motor vehicle crashes and deterring the adverse effects of teenage pregnancy, substance abuse, and sexually transmitted diseases are critical to the health of the community. (Donaldson et al., 1996:71)

The IOM acknowledges that *access* is a key requirement of primary care. If people do not have the financial and geographic ability to obtain primary health care when it is needed, there is no way to fulfill the objectives of prevention and early intervention, both of which are related to improved population health as well as to health care cost control. Thus, universal health insurance or some other form of universal access to primary health care is a necessity (Donaldson et al., 1996:113).

The Concept of Primary Care

"Primary care is the provision of integrated, accessible health care services by clinicians who are accountable for addressing a large majority of personal health care needs, developing a sustained partnership with patients, and practicing in the context of family and community." (Donaldson et al., 1996:31)

The five main attributes of high-quality primary care are as follows:

1. Primary care is grounded in both the biomedical and social sciences.
2. Primary care acknowledges the necessity of occasional diagnostic ambiguity, given the complexity of interacting environmental factors.
3. Primary care considers physical and mental health together.
4. Primary care intrinsically provides opportunities to promote health and prevent disease.
5. Primary health will increasingly utilize computerized information systems to facilitate quality practice in multiple ways. (Donaldson et al., 1996:80-81, 88)

The Limitation of Primary Medical Care

"[Primary care] will have a limited impact on health status until or unless the determinants of public and social health are addressed. . . . The aggregate benefits in health status to be gained from increasing income or education greatly outweigh the gains from medical intervention. . . . Similarly, preventing injuries from violence, child neglect, or motor vehicle crashes and deterring the adverse effects of teenage pregnancy, substance abuse, and sexually transmitted diseases are critical to the health of the community." (Donaldson et al., 1996:71)

Primary health care recognizes the interaction of physical, mental, emotional, and social functioning of a person. *Social functioning* is the ability to perform social roles, such as being a student, parent, or worker (Donaldson et al., 1996:37-38). The primary health care provider is also viewed as a gatekeeper to additional services (Donaldson et al., 1996:39).

The five main values of primary health care are that it

1. provides a one-stop service;
2. aids patient and family in navigating the health care system;
3. provides continuity of care;
4. offers prevention, early intervention, and health promotion; and
5. helps to link patient, family, and community. (Donaldson et al., 1996:53)

Attributes of High-Quality Primary Care

1. Primary care is grounded in both the biomedical and social sciences.
2. Primary care acknowledges the necessity sometimes of diagnostic ambiguity, given the complexity of interacting environmental factors.
3. Primary care considers physical and mental health together.
4. Primary care intrinsically provides opportunities to promote health and prevent disease.
5. Primary health will increasingly utilize computerized information systems to facilitate quality practice in multiple ways. (Donaldson et al., 1996:80-81, 88)

Public Health

An early pioneer in public health, C.-E. A. Winslow, in 1920, defined the field as follows:

Public Health is the science and art of: (1) preventing diseases, (2) prolonging life, and (3) promoting health and efficiency through organized community effort for:

(a) the sanitation of the environment
(b) the control of communicable infections
(c) the education of the individual in personal hygiene
(d) the organization of medical and nursing services for the prevention and treatment of diseases
(e) the development of social machinery to insure everyone a standard of living adequate for the maintenance of health . . .

so organizing these benefits as to enable every citizen to realize his birthright of health and longevity. (Winslow, 1920)

It may be noted that Winslow's inclusion of "the development of social machinery to insure everyone a standard of living adequate for the maintenance of health" indicates that he had an early recognition that if public health is to prevent disease and promote health effectively, it must address socioeconomic conditions in the community.

Primary Prevention

In public health, *primary prevention* refers to efforts to prevent the occurrence of health problems as well as very early identification and intervention. This is in contrast to *secondary prevention* aimed at the control and prevention of developing into a more serious state or level (e.g., the spread of cancer or the development of liver damage due to alcoholism) and to *tertiary prevention*, or prevention of secondary disabilities associated with chronic and/or terminal health problems.

Martin Bloom (1987:305-306) described several emerging themes of primary prevention:

1. a systems orientation, recognizing the multiple interacting causes of most health problems;
2. a proactive approach rather than a reactive one;
3. recognition of the need to teach coping skills, reduce environmental stress, and increase environmental supports;
4. an awareness that preventive interventions can be introduced at different stages in a process with varying implications;
5. a sense that it is preferable, ethically, to involve individuals in promoting their own health and preventing health problems than to instigate mass actions that affect everyone, with or without their consent.

The mixture of biological, psychological, social, and cultural factors in determining health is reflected in the five main technologies of primary prevention:

1. Education
2. Social change in the community or society
3. Promotion of competency
4. Promotion of natural caregiving
5. Consultation and collaboration (Gullotta, 1987)

According to Bloom, there is a need to design effective primary prevention strategies that are coordinated and integrated:

> Not only must problematic factors be prevented, but promotive factors must be substituted in the system of events in their place. Furthermore, gains at one system level must not be undertaken at the expense of negative changes or losses at other system levels. (1995:1896)

Green (1995) cites Levy and Kunitz (1987:938) in arguing for the need for a "strengths perspective" in disease prevention. To paraphrase, effective disease prevention programs must identify and draw upon cultural and community *strengths* rather than deficits or weaknesses.

Health Promotion   *diff % health promotion & disease prevention*

Goel and McIsaac (2000) claim that the tendency is for health professionals and laypersons alike to confound the concepts of *health promotion* and *disease prevention,* but explain that *health promotion* is directed more toward the community-based and nonmedical determinants of health—such as social status, social support, empowerment, and education/information—while *disease prevention* is directed more toward lowering the risks of particular diseases through, for example, efforts to induce individual behavioral changes, utilize biomedical screening tests, and develop and prescribe drugs to modify existing biomedical risk factors.

Health promotion facilitates the *active* participation of people, in their families, schools, workplaces, and other community settings, to identify and take action to modify conditions that affect their health rather than "doing things" to people as passive recipients of professional interventions to compensate for unhealthy social, economic, and political conditions. Thus, health promotion activity tends to demedicalize health and shifts the focus of intervention from a paternalistic to an empowerment approach. In a sense, health promotion program descriptions are reminiscent of the War on

Poverty programs of the 1960s, such as model cities and Vista. In fact, Maurice Mittelmark (1999) appears to *equate* the terms *health promotion* and *community development:*

> These [health promotion] programs focus on building community ca-
> pacities to mount and manage many different kinds of health promo-
> tion programs or to improve the basic foundations for a thriving
> community, such as equitable access to education and economic secu-
> rity, social connectedness of the citizenry, and public policy that sup-
> ports agreed-on health objectives. Such programs may have a specific
> health or human development issue as their raison d'etre, such as pro-
> moting a healthy social and physical environment in which to raise
> children. . . . In its ideal form, community development arises from the
> grass roots of the community itself. (Mittelmark, 1999:5-6)

Mittelmark describes the Ottawa Charter for Health Promotion (WHO, 1986) as a political document that "defines *health promotion* as the process of enabling people to take over, and to improve, their health" (Mittelmark, 1999:6). The World Health Organization's "Healthy Cities Project," involv-ing more than 1,000 cities worldwide, is the best known communitywide project aimed at shaping healthier public policy (Ashton, 1992, cited in Middlemark, 1999, p. 6). The Ottawa Charter for Health Promotion was ini-tiated at the First International Conference on Health Promotion held in Ottawa, Canada, November 17-21, 1986. The charter explains that "health promotion action" should:

1. Build healthy public policy
2. Create supportive environments
3. Strengthen community action
4. Develop personal skills
5. Reorient health services (WHO, 1986)

The Social Health of the Nation

The federal government has a tendency to assess how well the country is doing in terms of economic indicators such as the gross domestic product, the unemployment rate, stock market indicators, and the index of leading economic indicators (Miringoff and Miringoff, 1999). Most European coun-tries, however, make assessments of their nations' health by also examining certain indicators of social health, such as wage rates, economic inequality trends, suicide rates, life expectancy, and levels of substandard housing. This type of assessment is now done in the United States through Fordham University's Institute for Innovation in Social Policy, of which the School of

Social Service is a part, and some recent results are presented in the book *The Social Health of the Nation: How America Is Really Doing* (Miringoff and Miringoff, 1999). The data are presented with comparisons across states within the United States and between the United States and selected foreign countries.

Although the following indicators have improved in the United States over recent years, still there is

- a relatively high infant mortality rate, especially among black Americans (ranked twenty-first among developed nations);
- high rates of low birthweight infants, especially in the southern states;
- a ranking of seventeenth for high school graduation rates among developed nations (77 percent in United States compared to 99 percent in Japan and 98 percent in Finland);
- despite reduction in the poverty rate among the sixty-five and over population, an increasing percentage of the people ages eighteen through sixty-four living in poverty (reflecting low wage rates); and
- increasing life expectancy, but still ranked seventeenth among developed nations.

The following indicators have worsened over recent years:

- The rate of reported child maltreatment (all forms of abuse and neglect) has increased.
- The percentage of children under age eighteen living in poverty has increased.
- Internationally, among industrialized nations, sixteen nations have lower child poverty rates than the United States. The child poverty rate in the United States is about three times higher than in any of the Scandinavian countries (Finland, Sweden, Norway, and Denmark) or Belgium.
- Internationally, among industrialized countries, the youth suicide rate in the United States is seventh from the highest.
- The percentage of the population without health insurance coverage has increased by 43 percent since 1976 (presumably due to declining coverage through employment, combined with gaps in the covered low-income population through Medicaid).
- The hourly rate of compensation costs, or wages plus benefits, received by workers in manufacturing in the United States has declined relative to that of many other industrial nations, so that, by 1996, the United States ranked thirteenth from the highest.
- The United States has the largest gap between rich and poor among all industrialized nations.

- The United States has one of the highest incarceration rates among industrialized nations and one of the highest rates of violent crimes among youth.
- The youth homicide rate in the United States is the highest among twenty-two industrialized nations.
- The teenage birth rate in 1995 was 9 percent in the United States, 6 percent in Great Britain, 2 percent in France, and 1 percent in Poland, Germany, and Japan (percentage of women ages twenty through twenty-four who had given birth by age eighteen).

Although most of these social indicators are also direct health indicators, the rest are clearly associated with health status and therefore ought to be among the objects of health promotion efforts.

The Prerequisites of Health

"The fundamental conditions and resources for health are peace, shelter, education, food, income, a stable ecosystem, sustainable resources, social justice and equity. Improvement in health requires a secure foundation in these basic prerequisites." (WHO, 1986:1)

Macrina (1999) traces the historical development of the concept of *health promotion* and points out the persistent dual perspectives of personal responsibility and social responsibility, or what Macrina calls "market justice" and "social justice." The former, *market justice,* holds that individuals are ultimately responsible for their own health and that it is not the responsibility of the economic or political systems to take actions to regulate the marketplace or other areas of society to promote the health of its citizenry. On the other hand, the *social justice* perspective offers that it *is* the obligation of society to act to promote a socioeconomic, political, and physical environment that is as conducive to or enabling of good health as possible. In short, *health promotion* programs are distinguished by their adherence to the social justice perspective.

The Interacting Determinants of Health Behavior

"Health-related behavior is influenced both by individual characteristics such as personality type, beliefs, knowledge, and attitudes and by the external physical and sociological environments within which the behavior occurs." (Gilliland and Taylor, 1999:428)

The Ottawa Charter, which subsequently influenced WHO policy, identified the prerequisites to health as follows:

> The fundamental conditions and resources for health are peace, shelter, education, food, income, a stable ecosystem, sustainable resources, social justice and equity. Improvement in health requires a secure foundation in these basic prerequisites. (WHO, 1986:1)

However, it seems reasonable to assume that both approaches, *market justice* and *social justice,* may be required to maximize health potential i.e., to continue both *disease prevention* efforts and community-based *health promotion* efforts. In a sense, they respectively address the micro and macro levels of health status determinants, or individual behavior and environmental conditions, whether physical, social, or psychological. As Gilliland and Taylor (1999) have noted:

> Health-related behavior is influenced both by individual characteristics such as personality type, beliefs, knowledge, and attitudes and by the external physical and sociological environments within which the behavior occurs. (428)

Furthermore, the *health promotion* perspective claims that interventions designed to modify individual health behavior are simply insufficient to have enough impact on widespread chronic diseases that are nearly endemic in a population:

> With the increasing attention given to chronic disease, such as cancer and heart disease, it has become obvious that traditional interventions designed to change the behavior of high-risk individuals have too little impact to lower chronic disease rates. Community intervention is one strategy that emerged in response to that recognition in the early 1970's. Based on the idea that behavior is heavily influenced by environment, this approach seeks to change community norms and values regarding behaviors that contribute to chronic diseases. Over the past fifteen years, community health promotion has proven to be one of the most exciting and promising newer approaches. (Thompson and Kinne, 1999:45-46)

THEORETICAL PERSPECTIVES

In spite of the varying concepts, both primary health care and public health have a perspective that is biopsychosocial, holistic, sensitive to human diversity, and client empowerment oriented and is rooted in epidemiology, the primary prevention of disease and disability, and health promotion.

Epidemiology

Primary prevention, health promotion, public health, and primary health care are based on an epidemiological perspective that seeks to trace the etiology of health problems by investigating the incidence distribution of specific health problems. Epidemiology is the study of the distribution of the occurrence of health problems by such external variables as geographical location, climate, and time of year—as well as individual factors including age, sex, ethnicity, income, educational level, and occupation. These last six variables are indicators of social status, and their relationship to disease, disability, and death is the subject of *social epidemiology* (Engel, 1977). In epidemiology, the victim is termed the *host,* the causal factor becomes the *agent,* and the context in which the two encounter each other is referred to as the *environment.* Modern epidemiology is not as linked as it once was to the medical model of disease, which traditionally conceived of each health problem as having more or less a single cause, such as a bacterium or virus. Today, epidemiology more often recognizes a complexity of interacting causes (Bloom, 1995:1896).

Community Intervention As Health Promotion

"[T]raditional interventions designed to change the behavior of high-risk individuals have too little impact to lower chronic disease rates. Community intervention is one strategy that . . . seeks to change community norms and values regarding behaviors that contribute to chronic diseases. . . . community health promotion has proven to be one of the most exciting and promising newer approaches." (Thompson and Kinne, 1999:45-46)

Friis and Sellers (1996:376) present what they term "a guide to psychosocial epidemiology" that serves to identify some of the major independent variables, moderator variables, and dependent variables in a theoretical model of chronic disease etiology (see Table 3.1).

The Biopsychosocial Model

The biopsychosocial model of health and disease is usually attributed to George Engel (1977), whose seminal article, which appeared over twenty

TABLE 3.1. The Psychosocial Epidemiology of Chronic Disease

Independent Variables (Predictors)	Moderator Variables (Mediators)	Dependent Variables (Outcomes)
Stress	Personality factors, e.g., type A personality	Life and job satisfaction
Status incongruity	Culture	Mental health, e.g., affective states/depression
Person-in-environment fit	Social support	Chronic disease
Life events	Lifestyle behavior	

Source: Friis, Robert H. and Sellers, Thomas A. (1996). *Epidemiology for Public Health Practice.* Gaithersburg, MD: Aspen Publishers, 376.

years ago in the journal *Science,* is probably among the most renowned ever written. Primary health care is rooted in the belief that health status is the result of a complex interaction of biological, psychological, social, cultural, and physical environmental factors. Consequently, good health will never result from simply seeking medical intervention from any one of an array of specialist physicians, depending on the particular health problem one has already developed. Rather, the biopsychosocial model holds that health status is the result of genetic inheritance, learned behavior, cultural influences, the quality of the physical environment, socioeconomic status, one's age and sex, the amount and kind of stress experienced, coping mechanisms, diet, exercise, avoidance of intake of dangerous drugs, social supports, sense of empowerment, and access to medical care, especially at the primary level.

An example of the biopsychosocial model is the placebo effect. It has long been documented in medical research that in experiments in which patients with a particular health problem are randomly assigned to experimental and control groups a certain percentage of those in the control group who receive only inert ingredients in their medication will report improvement in symptoms and often demonstrate improved functioning and reduction in symptoms. The placebo effect seems to be evidence that cognitive perception/mental attitude or belief can influence the body in ways that can either improve or worsen physical signs of health problems. Clearly, this is support for the biopsychosocial model—the interaction of psyche and soma—and the psyche frequently is affected by social situations. According to Hafen and colleagues (1996), Albert Schweitzer, humanitarian and physician with years of experience as a physician in Africa, once was asked to explain the secret of African witch doctors, to which he replied: "The witch doctor succeeds for the same reason all the rest of us succeed. Each patient carries his own doctor inside him. We are at our best when we give the doctor within each patient a chance to go to work" (440).

In response to the widespread use of alternative medicine in the United States, the National Institutes of Health (NIH) established the Office of Alternative Medicine in 1992. Such interventions range from therapeutic touch and aromatherapy to herbal remedies, meditation, and acupuncture (Cook, Becvar, and Pontious, 2000). Furthermore, during the fall of 2001, the placebo effect was on the NIH e-mail listing of research priorities for which the institute was seeking research applications and funding. These actions of the NIH suggest a recognition of the possibility that social and psychological factors are significant variables influencing health outcomes.

It appears that mental, physical, and social health affect one another; that is, social-environmental conditions can induce a sense of helplessness and depression, which in turn may induce biochemical changes that impair the immune system and increase susceptibility to disease. In addition, socially induced depression can increase vulnerability to accidents and injuries, whether from impaired concentration and inattentiveness or high-risk behavior in search of a sense of power. On the other hand, having a disease or disability can itself produce adverse emotions due to the actual, expected, or perceived impact of the physical health problem on normal social-role functioning.

After reviewing the "inequality and health" literature, Gorin (2000:273) concluded:

> The inequality and health literature reveals that health is essentially a biopsychosocial phenomenon, and social work researchers can add to this literature. In addition, as the largest group of mental health providers, social workers can provide insight into the role of psychosocial factors in the relationship between inequality and health. Finally, social justice and advocacy have long been central to social work's mission, and in a sense, we are obligated to become involved in efforts to reverse the trend toward growing inequality.

The Interaction of Physical and Mental Health

People with mental health problems tend to seek attention for somatic complaints from primary care physicians more than from mental health specialists (Shannon, 1989:35). In much of America, especially among rural people, elderly people, Asian Americans, those of lower socioeconomic status, and certain conservative religious groups, it is often socially unacceptable to seek help for psychological distress from a mental health professional. As a result, primary care physicians may be sought instead, with patients presenting vague or confusing complaints with unclear meaning. However, most primary care physicians are not trained or motivated to provide direct counseling or psychotherapeutic services and instead tend to rely on pharmaceutical interventions, which often bring short-term symptom relief without problem relief. Cassell, a famous physician, presents his vision for medical education that would produce doctors who can competently and confidently address the psychosocial problems of primary care patients, claiming such changes in medical education are necessary because "[i]t is not uncommon to find graduating medical students who have had no training in normal or abnormal psychology, no experience with nondrug treatment of emotional illness, and no instruction in the psychology of physical illness" (1995:385).

Some evidence suggests that mental and physical health interact. Patients with chronic illness tend to become depressed (Hill, Kelleher, and Shumaker, 1992). Of patients in primary care settings, 5 to 10 percent have been diagnosed with major depression, and two to three times that number have symptoms of mild depression (Katon and Schulberg, 1992). In addition, depressed patients tend to use health services more (Katon, 1987). According to Davis (1996:83), at least thirteen studies have confirmed that individuals with various forms of mental illness have rates of physical illness far in excess of the expected frequency of illness in the general population. There is widespread concern that chronically mentally ill people receive a gross lack of medical care for physical health problems (Davis, 1996).

Mechanic (1994) has made a strong case for integrating mental health care into primary medical care. A special version of the DSM-IV has now been adapted for primary care (American Psychiatric Association, 1995) and provides a kind of algorithm or path system for simplifying the diagnosis and treatment identification of various sets of symptoms of apparent mental health problems.

Clare (1982) found that half of the patients with a mental health problem in a primary care setting also had some type of social problem, such as with family, housing, or employment. At the same time, people exposed to prolonged stress tend to have impaired immune systems (Pert et al., 1985:820s-826s; Evans, Barer, and Marmor, 1994:13). In an editorial about World Health Day, Neugebauer (2001) wrote:

> Social stress and interpersonal relations are key elements in the onset, course, and treatment of mental disorders. Exposure to physical and

sexual abuse in childhood, bereavement, acutely traumatic events, and chronic forms of adversity across the life span instigate some disorders while activating preexisting vulnerabilities or compromising prognoses for others. . . . World Health Day highlights several disorders: schizophrenia, depressive disorders, Alzheimer disease, epilepsy, mental retardation, and alcohol dependence. Additionally, emphasis is placed on reorienting mental health services to protect patients from neglect and violence, integrating mental health services into the general health system, increasing family involvement in the rehabilitation process, and shoring up social bonds in transitional economies where rapid changes in social structure place vulnerable people at extreme risk for mental disorders. (551-552)

The urgency of integrating mental health services into primary health care is underscored by the tragic status of public mental health services today in much of the United States. As Keigher (1999) noted:

The traditional state infrastructure of services for the care and maintenance of people with severe and persistent mental illness is largely gone. . . . The criminalization of mental illness has come to replace a significant share of a care and treatment system now dysfunctionally incomplete. . . . Jails and prisons are increasingly the *de facto* alternative to a functioning system of mental health care. . . . In the San Diego County Jail, 14 percent of men and 25 percent of women inmates are on psychiatric medication. The Los Angeles County jail system, where more than 3,000 of the more than 20,000 inmates were receiving psychiatric services, is now said to be the largest mental institution in the United States—not to mention, according to some accounts, the largest homeless shelter. (Currie, 1998, cited in Keigher, 1999:88-89)

The inequity in mental health services is further elaborated in a report of the surgeon general:

Even more than other areas of health and medicine, the mental health field is plagued by disparities in the availability of and access to its services. These disparities are viewed readily through the lenses of racial and cultural diversity, age, and gender. (U.S. DHHS, 1999:vi)

Another example of a biopsychosocial health problem may be physical abuse. A psychological vulnerability of both abuser and victim may be normalized by a pattern of exposure to this form of social interaction in the childhood home. Monahan and O'Leary (1999) pointed out that one of the serious results of physical domestic violence can be head injury. In their own study of women in a domestic violence shelter, 35 percent reported a history of such head injury, with associated symptoms including headaches, memory loss, dizziness, and seizures.

A Holistic Perspective

Because of the interaction of biopsychosocial factors, true primary health care requires simultaneous examination and treatment of the whole person, including physical symptoms, emotional states, social and physical environmental conditions, cultural influences, and cognitive interpretations. Many years ago, the World Health Organization defined health as "a complete state of physical, psychological, and social well-being" (WHO, 1978) and not merely the absence of disease. The WHO definition recognizes that health status is related to an individual's ability to function physically, emotionally, and socially, and to the person's subjective sense of well-being.

Sensitivity to Human Diversity

Since social, cultural, and psychological variables are now widely recognized as playing a major role in health status by interacting with biological variables, primary health care has come to realize that variation in these variables across age, gender, ethnicity, socioeconomic class, and sexual orientation is essential information to ascertain and truly understand—the result of profound empathy. My conceptualization of the meaning of "sensitivity to human diversity" includes these steps:

1. Understanding the other person's ethnicity, gender, age, socioeconomic class, sexual orientation, and so on, and what they *mean* to that person
2. Respecting their human diversity characteristics
3. Taking these characteristics into account in working with them, adapting one's interactions respectfully

There is a large body of literature on the relationships between health status and such human diversity variables as age, gender, ethnicity, and social class. This literature is central to a variety of fields, such as epidemiology, medical sociology, behavioral medicine, human development, social psychology, and medical anthropology.

It is essential that social workers in the health care field sincerely commit themselves to developing an understanding of human diversity variables as they relate to health. An excellent reference pertaining to cultural diversity for social workers and others in the helping professions is by James W.

Green, who wrote, "Ethnic competence means moving beyond the job description and learning about clients through direct observation and participation in their everyday routines in naturalistic settings" (1995:97).

Green's (1995) text is useful in understanding how to explore with a client/patient his or her health complaints and understanding of their meaning. It is clear that such an approach is a vital part of developing a strategy for effective health promotion and disease prevention with an individual, family, group, organization, or community.

Green stresses the need for social workers in health care to understand the ethnicity of their clients, while also individualizing them. He wrote, "to perceive the client's individuality as something beyond or behind, or irrelevant to these ethnographic features leaves only an insubstantial ephemera of what the individual must really be like" (1995:71-72). According to Green, in order for social workers to individualize clients within their cultural context, they must know the clients' cultural resources, including "the institutions, individuals, and customs for resolving problems that are indigenous to the client's own community" (1995:95).

Sensitivity to human diversity means

1. understanding the other person's ethnicity, gender, age, socioeconomic class, sexual orientation, and so on, and what they mean to that person;
2. respecting their human diversity characteristics; and
3. taking these characteristics into account in working with them, adapting one's interactions respectfully.

The meaning of a health behavior, such as drinking, smoking, diet, or physical activity, may be quite different from one culture to another. Behaviors that are unhealthy may have quite a different etiology, role, function, and effective prevention and treatment (Green, 1995). For example, while drinking alcohol is a problem in many Native American communities, it cannot be successfully managed without first understanding its meaning for the particular culture. For some, it is a means to spiritual visions and dreams. For others, it may contribute to a sense of solidarity in the community. For others, it may constitute a tool for ventilation of feelings.

There is no doubt from the mounting evidence that human diversity variables are associated with *morbidity* (disease) and *mortality* (death) rates worldwide. These variables are expressed through health behavior and illness behavior, which are, in turn, heavily influenced by *values and beliefs* (culture) and by an individual's sense of locus of control and *personal efficacy* (power).

Angel and Williams (2000) have advised that we remain alert to the awareness that culture, such as values, beliefs, norms, tools, and language, is generally confounded with social stratification variables, such as race, age, class, and gender:

> [W]hat we think of as culture, the purely cognitive set of symbols, rules, values, norms, and linguistic tropes that are informed by the internalized frames or schemas with which we interpret that world, is confounded with structured systems of social differentiation. This fact brings what is purely cultural into direct contact with the political and the economic. An understanding of culture, and especially its role in health and illness, must deal with all of these complex interconnections and immediately come to terms with the reality of power differentials between groups, including those based on race, and ethnicity, gender, and age. (Angel and Williams, 2000:29)

Marsella and Yamada (2000) point out that an emerging trend in the mental health field, as in the physical health field, is the recognition that biological factors are but one of a multitude of socioeconomic and cultural variables that interact in determining health status, leading to an increased focus on qualitative research. They contrast this emerging trend with

> two basic cultural assumptions of Western mental health professionals and scientists: (a) problems reside in individual minds and brains, and thus, individual brains and minds should be the locus of treatment and prevention; (b) the world in which we live can be understood objectively through the use of quantitative and empirical data. Both of these assumptions stand in direct opposition to the postmodernist views that currently characterize and inform the study of culture and mental health relationships. These views emphasize the importance of the social context of psychological problems, i.e., powerlessness, poverty, marginalization, inequality, in understanding the etiology and expression of psychopathology. They point out that the individual psyche comes to represent and reflect the struggles and conflicts in our cultural environment and the subjective nature of our knowledge about the world in which we live. This has led to increased emphasis on qualitative research. (8-9)

An important implication of this trend for social work is that qualitative research, which many social workers find more comfortable and familiar, is the preferred approach to development of knowledge concerning the person's perceptions and cognitions that have influenced his or her health status. As Marsella and Yamada noted, "Culture is the template we use in constructing, defining, and interpreting reality" (12).

The Confounding of Culture and Social Stratification

"[W]hat we think of as culture, the purely cognitive set of symbols, rules, values, norms, and linguistic tropes that are informed by the internalized frames or schemas with which we interpret that world, is confounded with structured systems of social differentiation. An understanding of culture, and especially its role in health and illness, must deal with all of these complex interconnections and immediately come to terms with the reality of power differentials between groups, including those based on race, and ethnicity, gender, and age." (Angel and Williams, 2000:29)

The Ecology of Mental Health

- The "new" mental health professional and researcher believes [that] individual and societal mental health are inextricably linked—that we must understand the ecology of mental health. Thus, mental health is not only about biology and psychology, but also about education, economics, social structure, religion, and politics.
- There can be no mental health where there is powerlessness, because powerlessness breeds despair.
- There can be no mental health where there is poverty, because poverty breeds hopelessness.
- There can be no mental health where there is inequality, because inequality breeds anger and resentment.
- There can be no mental health where there is racism, because racism breeds low self-esteem and self-denigration.
- There can be no mental health where there is cultural disintegration and destruction, because cultural disintegration and destruction breed confusion and conflict. (Marsella and Yamada, 2000:10)

Poland, Green, and Rootman (2000), citing Poland (1992), discuss the settings approach to health promotion and conclude that because health promotion is rooted in a holistic understanding of the determinants of health it will require a research shift to more "interpretive (qualitative and historical) methods as a basis for understanding the complexities and intricacies of settings, and the impact of health promotion interventions and initiatives within these contexts" (350). Again, social workers are likely to find these methods to be similar to case history taking and to exploring with clients the onset and development of a behavior or problem situation.

Finally, Paniagua (2000) lists and describes nineteen syndromes (140-141) with a mix of physical and mental symptoms that are indigenous to specific cultures throughout the world and reflect culturally determined experiences. Clearly, if a clinician did not understand the cultural context of these manifestations, inappropriate treatment responses would be probable. For example, one of these culture-bound syndromes is labeled *pibloktoq*, which is native to Arctic and subarctic Eskimos. The symptoms of this illness include "excitement, coma, and convulsive seizures resembling an abrupt dissociative episode, often associated with amnesia, withdrawal, irritability, and irrational behaviors such as breaking furniture, eating feces, and verbalization of obscenities" (Paniagua, 2000:141).

Health Behavior

The individual and family must assume primary responsibility for living in a way that encourages and promotes good health. Such *health behavior* (Cockerham, 1992:81-95) pertains to, for example, diet, exercise, abstinence from tobacco and other drugs, moderation in alcohol use, and stress management. The challenge, of course, is to find effective ways to help people to avoid behavior that is high risk for disease or disability. However, it is important to avoid the pitfall of blaming the victim, especially when commercial advertising rampantly promotes human consumption of products that are potentially lethal. Advertisers appeal to deep-seated needs, such as feeling relaxed, free, attractive, loved, and fulfilled. Sadly, much high-risk behavior may be engaged in *because* people feel unwell and are seeking some sort of relief.

Some recent community health promotion programs have been based on the premise that it is likely to be more effective to modify health behavior in a community than in the individuals within it, since individual behavior tends to reflect cultural values and norms (Thompson and Kinne, 1999). Nonetheless, individual-level disease prevention and health promotion programs are widespread, and a body of theory to guide such interventions has developed to a fairly sophisticated level.

Significance of Culture to Illness Behavior

"[A] symptom is not simply a symptom, but a valuable opportunity for understanding the myriad ways in which culture impacts health and illness. A symptom is a sign and expression of illness, but it is also an insight into the nature of health. A symptom is a communication, an interpretation, and an experience. It is also a signal from patient to self and to others of a changing relationship, a changing role, and a changing set of expectations and demands. In all these instances, whether it is expressed idiomatically or within conventional Western medical terms and contexts, a symptom reveals culture and its influences." (Marsella and Yamada, 2000:19)

Four Health Behavior Models

Kohler, Grimley, and Reynolds (1999) outline four major theories of change in individual health behavior:

1. The health belief model (Rosenstock, 1974)
2. The theory of reasoned action (Ajzen and Fishbein, 1980)
3. The social cognitive model (Bandura, 1986, 1997)
4. The transtheoretical model of change (Prochaska and DiClemente, 1983, 1984, 1986)

The health belief model (Rosenstock, 1974). The five main components of this model are

1. perceived severity of and susceptibility to a disease,
2. perceived threat level of a disease,
3. perceived benefits of an advocated health action,
4. perceived barriers to the completion of that action, and
5. cues to action.

Human diversity variables are acknowledged to impact all four perceptions, while cues to action (such as education, illness symptoms, and media information) affect the perception of threat to oneself, which in turn affects the likelihood of behavioral change.

The theory of reasoned action (Ajzen and Fishbein, 1980). This theory holds that

1. the closest determinant of a health behavior is intention;
2. intention reflects both an attitude (tendency to act) and a subjective norm (a belief that a behavior will have a desired outcome that is socially valued by one's reference group); and

3. these are influenced by one's socioeconomic status, age, gender, and so on; attitudes toward social expectations and toward the individuals involved in the situation; and individual personality traits.

The social cognitive model (Bandura, 1986, 1997). Referred to as "social learning theory," this model holds to a reciprocal determinism consisting of three elements that may be depicted as three sides of a triangle with arrows running in both directions parallel to each of the three sides: (1) person, (2) environment, and (3) behavior.

For example, a person's environment, such as a noisy party with a lot of strangers, may trigger his or her (person) urge to engage in tension-relieving behavior, such as drinking several martinis. However, some of the people nearby who are sipping light beer (environment) may soon move away from the martini drinker and make scornful comments. This may prompt the person to trade the martini for a cup of coffee (behavior).

According to Bandura, people can anticipate certain outcomes from certain actions and act accordingly. Outcomes may be predicted based on (1) past experience, (2) vicarious experience (models), (3) views of others whose opinions one values, and (4) inferences derived from other knowledge.

Furthermore, a person's behavior also is influenced by his or her self-assessment of his or her power to engage in the behaviors the person believes are conducive to good health. This is called *perceived self-efficacy* and is derived from (1) past experience, (2) the vicarious experience from observing one's model's behavior, (3) the encouragement and support of others one values, and (4) interpretations of physiological sensations. A person may perceive that the outcome of certain health behavior would be very positive and yet lack confidence in his or her efficacy to conform to that behavior. Thus, changing health behavior to more positive activities must persuade the person not only of the value of the outcome but also of his or her strength or power to do so.

According to Bandura (1986), changing individual health behavior requires (1) motivation to change, (2) the self-regulation skills to change (e.g., monitoring behavior, setting goals, establishing incentives), (3) the belief in one's ability to persevere to the extent necessary, and (4) the knowledge, skills, and resources required to adapt the desired health behavior.

The transtheoretical model of change (TMC model) (Prochaska and DiClemente, 1983, 1984, 1986). This model holds that behavioral change is a *process,* with various stages or levels of motivation to change, each of which requires different intervention strategies. The five stages of the transtheoretical model of change include

1. precontemplation—not ready to change;
2. contemplation—thinking about change;
3. preparation—ready to change;
4. action—initiating change; and
5. maintenance—continuing change.

This theory posits ten processes of change or strategies of intervention (the first five are cognitive-affective, the second five, behavioral):

1. *Consciousness-raising*—Increasing information about the healthy behavior change and awareness of one's risks: media campaigns, feedback, confrontations
2. *Dramatic relief*—Experiencing and expressing emotions associated with engaging in unhealthy behaviors: role-plays, psychodrama, personal testimonies
3. *Self-reevaluation*—Realizing how one thinks and feels about oneself (i.e., self-image) with regard to engaging in an unhealthy behavior and how this self-image might change if the behavior were to be changed: values clarification, imagery, exposure to healthy role models
4. *Environmental reevaluation*—Assessing how one's behavior may negatively impact others in the personal-social environment or the physical environment: empathy training, documentaries, couple-family system interventions
5. *Self-liberation*—Choosing and firmly committing to change: "go public" with one's decision to change, set a "quit" or "start" date, empowerment
6. *Helping relationships*—Having someone to talk to, share feelings with, and get feedback from regarding the healthy behavior change: increasing social support, rapport building, therapeutic alliances
7. *Counterconditioning*—Learning new healthy behaviors to substitute for old unhealthy ones: relaxation exercises, assertiveness training, positive "self-talk"
8. *Contingency management*—Rewarding oneself or being rewarded by others for making a healthy change: contingency contracts, overt and covert reinforcements.
9. *Stimulus control*—Avoiding people, places, or situations that might trigger unhealthy behavior and adding cues to trigger healthy behavior: avoidance techniques, restructuring one's environment (e.g., removing alcohol or fatty foods, carrying condoms), posting reminders to engage in healthy behaviors (e.g., taking prescribed medications)

10. *Social liberation*—Realizing changes in social norms with regard to certain health behaviors: advocacy, public policy changes (e.g., smoke-free malls and restaurants)

In general, the first five processes tend to be utilized in the early stages of health behavior change, and the last five processes tend to be utilized in the later stages of health behavior change and maintenance in the TMC model (Kohler, Grimley, and Reynolds, 1999).

Socioeconomic Status and Health Behavior;
Inequality and Health Status

Research indicates that people of higher socioeconomic status are more likely to engage in positive health behavior. The current preeminent theory about this phenomenon is that:

> [t]he sense of personal efficacy associated with higher social position encourages beliefs both in one's ability to break addictions and in the positive consequences of doing so. Beliefs in the effectiveness (or lack of it) of one's actions are both learned and reinforced by one's social position. (Evans, Barer, and Marmor, 1994:50)

"The issue, it seems, is not poverty. . . but inequality" (Gorin, 2000:270). There is rapidly growing evidence that social inequality, measured in part by the Gini coefficient indicator of relative poverty, is a major determinant of health status. The evidence suggests that it is not simply the inability to afford what one needs (such as proper food, shelter, clothing) to promote health, but rather the negative psychological impact of social inequality on biochemical functioning, via erosion of self-confidence and sense of empowerment, that is damaging.

Most fascinating of all is the compilation of evidence presented by Evans, Barer, and Marmor (1994) that a demonstrable direct relationship exists worldwide between social status and health status. This appears to be a reflection more of an individual's sense of power, control, competency, self-esteem, resources to combat stressors, self-actualization, and general well-being *associated* with social status rather than income. Social class is probably one of the most useful shorthand indicators of a person's power (Freund and McGuire, 1991:31). Unemployed people, across two European countries and the United States, who received entitlement benefits, reported better health than those who received means-tested benefits, suggesting that self-image and self-respect may play a significant role in health status (Rodriguez, 2001).

However, it is a mistake to reduce social inequality to social economic class because ethnicity is another variable that is not entirely a function of class, but sometimes also reflects racism in the social environment (Smith, 2000). As W. E. B. DuBois once said: "To be a poor man is hard, but to be a poor race in a land of dollars is the very bottom of hardship" (cited in Oliver and Shapiro, 1995:91).

If the issue is inequality, rather than income alone, and race/ethnicity is one social status variable, gender may well be another. The majority of the 43 million Americans who are medically underserved (who lack both adequate access to primary health care services and have poor health status) are poor, female, young, and uninsured. Gaston and colleagues note:

> Most notable among the factors that determined both limited access to health care and poor health status were low income, the maldistribution of health services in the community, absence of culturally competent service providers, and the unavailability of health insurance. The report noted that the uninsured tend to be young, low-income African American and Hispanic women and their children. (Center for Health Economics Research, 1993, cited in Gaston et al., 1998:91)

A must-read book is *The Society and Population Health Reader: Income Inequality and Health,* edited by Kawachi, Kennedy, and Wilkinson (1999). Their statistical and interpretive analysis of the relationship between social inequality and health status provides powerful evidence of the validity of the biopsychosocial perspective, and of the ultimate need to examine and address the entire social system—economic, political, educational, religious—in health promotion efforts to maximize a community's or nation's health potential.

It has been documented that increased perceptions of social inequality are associated with increased levels of violence and other health and social problems. An article that appeared a few months before the September 2001 terrorist attack on America warned: "The only effective way to reduce individual-sponsored and group-sponsored bioterrorism, we believe, is to reduce state-sponsored terrorism and to work for a world characterized by social justice and peace" (Sidel, Cohen, and Gould, 2001:717). Given the current global economy and increased interdependence between nations of the world, social inequality between *countries* may be found to contribute to the erosion of health potential among those who are relatively less advantaged. Most fascinating from a social work perspective is that the impact of social status discrepancy appears to be a negative one because of the perceived implication of inferiority, injustice, exclusion, and exploitation, which tends to erode one's sense of competency, efficacy, social belonging, and pride. Thus, one issue that arises is whether the real determinants of health are socioeconomic, or psychosocial, such as a sense of empowerment and social cohesion, or both.

For example, Japan, which has the longest life expectancy and lowest infant mortality rate in the world, also has a low level of income inequality, yet Japan expends one of the lowest percentages of its gross domestic product and least amount per capita on health care of any country in the world.

In any case, the president of the American Public Health Association, a social worker with both MSW and MPH degrees and a Native American, has commented on the disparities in access to health services and to health status among Americans: "We cannot be united as a nation until all people have the ability and opportunity to share a comparable level of health and well-being" (Bird, 2001:3).

Illness Behavior

Cultural differences, reflected in variation in values and the interpretation of symbols and events, play a key role in the impact of life events on health status (Corin, 1994).

> The meaning that illness has for the individual, and his or her response to it, are based both on individual psychological factors and the socially based cognitive models concerning pain and suffering, as well as their causes and consequences, that are part of one's cultural tradition. One experiences illness alone, but one does so using cognitive schemas and language that are part of one's culture that one inherits from ones progenitors. (Angel and Williams, 2000:25)

Illness behavior, or responses to what could be the signs and symptoms of a health problem, plays a role in determining how quickly early health problems are addressed and the effect of such interventions. Well-known variations exist between men and women, between young and old people, across ethnic groups, and across socioeconomic status groups in such illness behavior (Cockerham, 1992:97-120; Weiss and Lonnquist, 1994:143-144, 221-244).

A major problem in medical practice is lack of patient compliance with the recommended medical care plan. Noncompliance probably reflects differences in values, beliefs, and cognitive interpretations of the meaning and implications of symptoms, all of which are related to human diversity variables. As Corin noted,

> illness experience is not a simple mirror of the disease process. Rather it reflects personal and collective expectations and values; and social

and psychological components of that experience can be more powerful determinants of help-seeking behavior, and of actual disability, than biological abnormalities. (1994:113)

The essence of the significance of culture to illness behavior is captured in the following quotation:

[A] symptom is not simply a symptom, but a valuable opportunity for understanding the myriad ways in which culture impacts health and illness. A symptom is a sign and expression of illness, but it is also an insight into the nature of health. A symptom is a communication, an interpretation, and an experience. It is also a signal from patient to self and to others of a changing relationship, a changing role, and a changing set of expectations and demands. In all these instances, whether it is expressed idiomatically or within conventional Western medical terms and contexts, a symptom reveals culture and its influences. (Marsella and Yamada, 2000:19)

Marsella and Yamada (2000) end with this statement:

It seems there are many reasons to conclude that within the various mental health professions and sciences, a commitment to a bio-psychosocial approach that firmly incorporates cultural considerations and materials is the only basis for accurate and meaningful practice and research. (22)

Client Empowerment and Social Support

Client empowerment is key to health promotion and disease prevention, both to engage individuals in developing healthier lifestyles and to inspire them to become active members of the body politic, infused with confidence and competence to impact the development of policies and programs of the society to ensure that all its citizens enjoy the social supports they require to realize their full potential.

The major causes of death and disability in America today are chronic diseases, for example, heart disease, high blood pressure, cancer, chronic obstructive pulmonary disease (COPD), and diabetes. This is due, in large part, to adverse health behavior, such as smoking; excessive alcohol consumption; too much cholesterol, fat, salt, and sugar in the diet; too few fresh vegetables, fruits, whole grain breads, and cereals, or "roughage"; a lack of physical exercise; and too much stress.

Main Theories of Change in Individual Health Behavior

1. The health belief model (Rosenstock, 1974)
2. The theory of reasoned action (Ajzen and Fishbein, 1980)
3. The social cognitive model (Bandura, 1986, 1997)
4. The transtheoretical model of change (Prochaska and DiClemente, 1983, 1984, 1986)

There is considerable evidence that social supports play a major role in the mitigation of stress, although valued *sources* of social support vary across cultures and need not refer to family and friends (Corin, 1994:125). Perhaps the strongest argument for professional social workers playing a major role in health care in the future is the evidence that *mediating structures, such as social supports, are the most powerful determinant of health,* and the key role of community support in promoting a healthy society cannot be overemphasized (Kelner, 1985).

Kawachi, Kennedy, and Wilkinson (1999) point to the large volume of both qualitative and quantitative research that provides evidence of a clear link between the quantity and quality of social relationships and health outcomes. That is, what is termed *social integration,* or feeling a secure part of a supportive social network, appears to be directly associated with better health. They note:

> Just as a wide range of ecological measures of social relations are closely related to health, so also are a wide range of individual measures, including number of friends, people's involvement in community life, and whether or not they have a "confiding" relationship. Yet why social contact should have such a profound impact on health remains unclear. (Kawachi, Kennedy, and Wilkinson, 1999:xxv)

Without question, genetic inheritance also plays a fundamental role in determining health status. Causes of death and length of life tend to run in families. Of course, part of the reason for this may be that younger family members tend to learn the behavior patterns of older family members, including health and illness behavior patterns, work habits, mechanisms for coping with stress, and even mental attitudes toward locus of control (Wheaton, 1980). Although a genetic influence is clear, its impact can be significantly mitigated by a supportive social environment (Evans, Barer, and Marmor, 1994).

Social support plays one of the most important roles in mediating or moderating the impact of stressful life experience on negative health outcomes. For example, Blair (2000) conducted a secondary analysis of data from a study of 124 Cambodian refugees in the United States and found that those who had been able to live with family members in refugee camps outside of Cambodia after the end of the Khmer Rouge regime were significantly less likely to later develop post-traumatic stress disorder.

However, what is perceived as social support varies across and within human diversity variables. For example, if persons with a homosexual orientation are rejected by family and community of origin, they may join a gay community that functions as a surrogate family. African Americans, whose sense of well-being is sometimes under attack from the external world, may employ their church and extended family, including family of choice, to effectively counteract any harmful impact. This may explain why African Americans have a suicide rate half that of white Americans. However, not all African Americans find church to be a source of social support, and not all gays or lesbians are rejected by their families or find support in a gay community.

Hispanic teenage girls have a suicide attempt rate that is twice that of either white or African-American adolescent girls (Zayas et al., 2000). Zayas and colleagues attribute this phenomenon to a combination of factors, including lower socioeconomic status, rigid authoritarian parenting, lack of extended family supports, discrepancies between parents' and daughters' acculturation, mothers' overdependence on the daughters in the absence of the fathers, and mothers' reluctance to seek adult social support outside the family unit. In any case, the pattern suggests a loss of traditional social supports in this ethnic group as a result of immigration to a foreign environment.

Fitzpatrick and Bosse (2000:54) found that "[b]eing employed is an important source of support for bereaved older men especially on physical health measures." Paster (2001:34) argues that one's social milieu is as important as physical exercise and eating right to achieve good health and a long life, and in the social sphere, he prescribes, "Have a good marriage or its equivalent, build a strong social network, engage in good relationships with family and friends, and foster mutual support." In a study of HIV-infected women, scores on a depression screening scale were higher when scores on both tangible support and emotional support were lower, and depression scores were particularly higher when the women did not have family members who listened to their concerns (Richardson et al., 2001:103).

Lisa Berkman (2000), of the Harvard School of Public Health, reported on a longitudinal study of 211 people age sixty-five or older living in the community outside of institutions who were followed from 1982 through 1996 to track their health status and level of social support. The researchers found that the death rate was more than twice as high among those with no social support compared to those who reported having someone they could count on for emotional support. In fact, when the researchers controlled for a variety of physical variables correlated with likelihood of dying, the strength of the relationship between having significant social support (versus no social support) and the death rate increased further.

Berkman reviewed other findings concerning the relevance of social support to health status and mortality rates that are remarkably similar to her own findings. In addition, Berkman reported additional findings of a colleague concerning the importance of conditions within a community or group, such as trust between citizens and levels of reciprocity—referred to as social capital indicators—which are seen as indicators of working together for mutual benefit (in contrast to community conditions of intergroup indifference, conflict, and competition). The level of such social capital has been found strongly and inversely correlated with the death rates in those states. Dr. Berkman discusses the social policy implications of these kinds of findings, suggesting that social workers and other health care professionals could do much to promote health at a communitywide level by working to enact policies and programs that assist people who are taking care of others, whether children, elderly impaired, or others with reduced function, by providing the supports they need to do well. The clear message is that mutual support and cohesion at the local level are most helpful and should be facilitated with organizational policies that enhance local community mutual support systems.

Hafen and colleagues (1996), in a textbook dealing with the biopsychosocial model, noted:

> As defined by most researchers, social support is the degree to which a person's basic social needs are met through interaction with other people. It's the resources, both tangible and intangible, that other people provide. It's a person's perception that he or she can count on other people for help with a problem or for help in a time of crisis. (263)

The following are the five components of social support:

1. Feeling cared about, and a sense of shared intimacy
2. Feeling valued and respected by others and oneself
3. Having a sense of belonging, companionship, communication with others
4. Having access to informational support, advice, and guidance
5. Having access to material and physical assistance as needed (Amick and Ockene, 1994:260-261, cited in Hafen et al., 1996:263)

I think we sometimes forget that information itself can be supportive. One study (Telfair and Gardner, 1997) found only one variable was a statistically significant determinant of support group attendance (at better than .001 percent) among seventy-nine study subjects who participated in a total of twenty different support groups for teenagers with sickle-cell disease: learning how to solve personal problems. In short, this suggests that learning coping skills through watching and talking with other people can be experienced as a form of social support. Information and education are sources of empowerment, which contributes to a sense of mastery and competence, like having a map to find one's way in the world. Learning directly from the experience of other people who are on the same path can be especially supportive.

In addition, it may be that cultural variables, such as the extent to which a society values the well-being of the family, group, or community relative to the well-being of the individual, may be social support variables. For example, Japan (see Table 8.1 in Chapter 8), whose culture is family and community oriented more than individually oriented, has one of the lowest infant mortality and longest life expectancy rates in the world, even though the Japanese people have high rates of cigarette smoking, pollution, overcrowding, and stress. Thus, a strong sense of social cohesion and community may go a long way toward moderating the otherwise adverse effects of negative health behavior.

The extent to which a society provides for its people through social security programs may also be experienced as a form of social support. For example, the Scandinavian countries (Denmark, Sweden, and Finland) which have "cradle to grave" social welfare systems, such as comprehensive national health systems, family support allowances to all families with young children, and lengthy paid family leave (see Chapter 8), have relatively low infant mortality and longer life expectancy rates.

In short, whatever forces in the social environment cause us to feel cared about, respected, and competent; to have access to needed resources; and to be part of a larger whole may be viewed as forms of social support. Social

---

Main Components of Social Support

1. Feeling cared about, and a sense of shared intimacy
2. Feeling valued and respected by others and oneself
3. Having a sense of belonging, companionship, communication with others
4. Having access to informational support, advice, and guidance
5. Having access to material and physical assistance as needed (Amick and Ockene, 1994:260-261)

---

support is empowering. It is an adjunct to our own resources and makes us feel stronger. It may derive from satisfaction with our roles in society, family, work, religion, and other community organizations. Wherever it comes from, it makes us feel worthwhile, valued, respected, and secure.

Empowerment and social support seem closely related to a sense of control. It may be that stress is not something external to ourselves, but rather the perception of having inadequate resources to effectively protect us from some perceived threat. Thus, stress is a feeling of vulnerability, of lack of sufficient strength or power to cope with some challenge. On the other hand, having people and external resources to call upon, when needed, becomes an obvious source of empowerment and stress reduction. In fact, anything that contributes to feeling more competent, protected, strong, and allied with other sources of strength is experienced as empowering. Thus, religion, the support of the group, learning karate, or earning a PhD could all promote a sense of empowerment.

It may be that the fundamental struggle in human life which motivates much of human behavior—for good or evil—is a search for a comfortable sense of being empowered. Martin Seligman (1975), a psychologist famous for his theory of "learned helplessness," discovered that much of a relative sense of competence and empowerment is learned (conditioned) from past experience.

INTERDISCIPLINARY TEAMWORK

The need for collaboration across disciplines obviously derives from the theoretical perspective of primary health care. However, as often happens, practice does not always keep pace with theory. "Some models of primary care include a team of physicians only, some also include representatives of other disciplines, such as nursing, social work, physician extenders, nurse practitioners, and nutritionists" (Miller, 1987:321). However, Miller also noted that "to accomplish the goals of the primary care model, the interdisciplinary team is not only desirable but essential. . . . However committed to the biopsychosocial approach, the physician alone cannot be the sole provider" (1987:324).

The Institute of Medicine Committee acknowledges that knowledge of the family and community may also help the primary care clinician better understand the health problems and health risks faced by the patient. In addition, personnel in primary care teams and settings often may be able to act on behalf of their patients in settings and circumstances outside the traditional health environment (Donaldson et al., 1996:59).

Clearly, primary prevention and health promotion are rooted in the recognition that a broad range of forces influences the health of both individuals and communities and the subsystems within communities, including culture, age, gender, socioeconomic status, genetics, opportunities to develop and thrive, the quality of the physical ecosystem, the level of social integration, political perspectives, and the extent to which all sectors of the population are included and represented in the political process. This multiplicity of health determinants implies that a wide range of disciplines are appropriately involved in health prevention and health promotion efforts, including physicians and other health care providers, political scientists, economists, politicians, psychologists, sociologists, social workers, and health educators.

As Raczynski and DiClemente (1999) have noted,

> First, the science of health promotion and disease prevention is an emerging science of diverse disciplines. Much will be gained by bringing the breadth of perspectives to bear from these different disciplines; however, it is incumbent on both researchers and practitioners in the area not only to embrace the breadth of perspectives but to work toward convergence of theories and methodologies if the goal of achieving a defined science is to be realized. (661)

Perhaps the goal should be not so much a convergence but an integration of theories and methodologies to reveal a clearer picture of how each is an integral part of a whole, like puzzle pieces that fit together to reveal an illuminating picture.

ORGANIZATIONAL CONSIDERATIONS

The role and function of social work in primary health care, including public health and primary prevention, will greatly depend on (1) funding sources, (2) whether the host setting of primary care is public tax supported, voluntary nonprofit, or private for profit, and (3) if private, what, if any, sectarian influence there is. In addition, the geographical location of the organization in terms of whether rural or urban and the cultural influences in the surrounding community will impact on the social worker role and function.

Funding sources for social work in primary health care settings, depending on the host organization, include Medicare and Medicaid, private health insurance, private out-of-pocket fees, and administrative overhead approaches (Ell and Morrison, 1981:39s).

Another significant organizational variable is by which standard-setting organization it is accredited, if any. The requirements concerning social work services tend to vary and to impact greatly on whether the organization employs social workers, how many it employs, the extent to which social work services are viewed as essential and integrated with the whole program, and the degree requirements for social work services.

CLIENT PROBLEMS AND SOCIAL WORKER FUNCTIONS

Client Problems

Some Causes of Biopsychosocial Health Problems

Most of the health problems we face today are substantially caused by destructive human behavior, ignorance, unrelieved environmental stress, social injustice, and other social or emotional conditions, which are the arena of social workers more than physicians.

Although the tendency today is to equate population risk factors with individual risk factors, evidence suggests that this is not a valid step. Concepts of risk factors and causes in epidemiology are not good indicators of health outcomes at the individual level. "Furthermore, the equating of risk factors with the causes of individual cases fosters an indifference to the social determinants of risk factor distributions and thus contributes to ineffectual disease prevention policies at the population level" (Rockhill, 2001:367-368).

Examples of Biopsychosocial Health Problems

Examples of common biopsychosocial health problems requiring social worker participation in treatment include drug and alcohol abuse, child abuse and neglect, domestic violence, elder abuse, teenage pregnancy, sexually transmitted diseases, suicide, depression, homicide, motor vehicle accidents, tobacco addiction, eating disorders such as anorexia, bulimia, and obesity, obsessive-compulsive behaviors, panic disorders, agoraphobia, social isolation, emotional withdrawal, and self-mutilation behavior.

Some Links Between Psychosocial Factors and Physical Health Problems

Overweight. Persons who are obese, or even overweight, are at higher risk for heart disease, diabetes, gallstones, hypertension, and stroke, according to the Nurses Health Study for women and the Health Professionals Follow-Up Study for men (American Public Health Association, 2001a). An estimated 32 percent of the U.S. population is overweight, with an *additional* 25 percent considered to be obese (American Public Health Association, 2001a:32). That over one-half of the American population is at higher risk for some of the major chronic diseases because of health behavior is appalling.

Not controlling for ethnicity, among the twenty to seventy-four age group, females are more likely than males to be obese, while males are more likely than females to be somewhat overweight. (Obesity was a subset of the overweight groups.) However, comparing ethnic groups in terms of the percentage classified as of "healthy weight," white females ranked highest (48.0 percent), then black males (40.2 percent), white males (38.7 percent), Hispanic (Mexican) males (31.6 percent), Hispanic (Mexican) females (29.8 percent), and, last, black females (28.9 percent) (U.S. Government Printing Office, 2000a, Table 68).

Presumably, being overweight or obese are most often the result of overeating, especially high-fat, high-cholesterol, high-sugar, and high-salt comfort foods, compulsively consumed in an effort to relieve long-term underlying emotional distress, or perhaps as part of a pattern of one's family or group culture or socioeconomic class. The lack of a consistent pattern across sex and race reflects perhaps some statistical interaction between ethnicity and sex.

A study of knowledge and attitudes about health among American and Swiss adults found that in both countries women and persons with more education were more health conscious, but despite similar exposure to health-related information in the two countries, significant differences existed in areas of knowledge that were emphasized (Girois et al., 2001). In particular, the Swiss were more attentive to weight control, avoiding sugar and salt, and maintaining a high-fiber diet. Americans were more concerned about limiting fat and cholesterol intake.

Cigarette smoking. Cigarette smoking has been identified as the health behavior with the most damaging impact on the health status of its participants, and as the single largest contributor to the nation's health costs. Smoking cigarettes is believed to be a major cause of not only lung cancer but also COPD and other lung disorders, heart disease, and various types of cancer.

Official data (U.S. Government Printing Office, 2000b, Table 61) indicate that in 1995, 1997, and 1998, among the eighteen and over age group, age-adjusted, the highest rate of cigarette smoking was among the American Indian and Alaska Native population, with 28.9 percent of females and 40.5 percent of males smoking, and lowest among Asian and Pacific Islanders, with 11.0 percent among females and 18.1 percent among males. Among white non-Hispanic females, cigarette smoking declines with age but is generally the highest rate among the three female groups compared; among black non-Hispanic females, cigarette smoking increases with age, peaking in the thirty-five to forty-five age range, and then declines; among Hispanic females, cigarette smoking increases somewhat in the thirty-five to forty-four age group and then declines but is consistently the lowest consumption rate of the three compared female ethnic groups.

When educational level of persons is considered, cigarette smoking is found to be inversely correlated with years of education. The difference between adults age twenty-five and over who have no high school education or GED compared to people who have at least some college education is a multiple of 2.4 for white males, 1.9 for black males, 1.7 for Hispanic males, 2.4 for white females, 1.6 for black females, and 1.0 for Hispanic females. Curiously, smoking increases somewhat for Hispanic females with a high school education or GED compared with those without a high school diploma or a GED, but then declines among those with some college education to about what it was among those with no high school diploma.

However, cigarette smoking is not only a U.S. problem but a global one. Satcher (2001) noted:

> Globally, about 4 million deaths per year are attributable to smoking. . . . Over the past 20 years, there has been a gradual decrease in cigarette smoking in the developed countries and an increase in the developing countries. . . . As the large transnational tobacco companies such as Phillip Morris and British American Tobacco move into new markets around the world, they spend enormous amounts on advertising and promotion. (192)

Alcohol consumption. Alcohol consumption is generally highest in the late teen years and early twenties and has been found associated with violence, date rape, accidents, academic problems, and family conflict. However, the findings of a study of college students conducted in 1990 indicated that a single brief counseling intervention with a random sample of students who had earlier revealed that they had a heavy drinking pattern produced a significantly reduced difference in their drinking, compared to a control group from the same population of college students who did not receive the intervention (Beer et al., 2001:1310).

The study findings suggest that early intervention with excessive alcohol consumption patterns may be effective in reducing the likelihood of a lifelong pattern of heavy drinking, which is known to be associated with liver disease, poorly controlled diabetes, and a host of problems of functioning in daily living, such as auto accidents, violence, sexual impotence, a high rate of work-related tardiness and absences, and failure to keep commitments to family members. Clearly, more knowledge is needed about individual and population risk factors and their interaction before we can effectively address them. The clear call is for heightened research efforts.

Social Worker Functions

The functions of social work in a public health program include the following:*

1. Participation in the planning and implementation of programs for the protection of communities from health hazards, the promotion of improved personal health care, and the prevention of ill health, including the promotion of positive health behaviors
2. Use of the epidemiologic approach in determining the association between social factors and the incidence of health problems and planning intervention strategies to promote health, protect against specific diseases, provide early intervention, prevent avoidable disability, and maximize comfort and function of impaired persons
3. Alleviation of social stress associated with having health problems and utilization of social supports to promote well-being and health protection
4. Participation in outreach to at-risk persons to ensure access to health care and needed social services
5. Participation in promoting consumer involvement and leadership in the planning and delivery of health care and relevant social services. (NASW, 1987:12-14)

Thus, it would appear from the NASW standards that, depending on the population using primary care services, social workers may be engaged in program planning and policy formulation, community needs assessment, outreach to members of high-risk populations, health education to individuals and groups, formation and facilitation of self-help groups, and conducting epidemiological research to identify high-risk groups (Miller, 1987: 322).

---

*Copyright 1987, National Association of Social Workers, Inc., NASW Standard for Social Work in Health Care Settings.

Social Worker Functions in Primary Medical Care Settings

However, most social workers in primary health care are in direct service roles, providing clients with counseling and linkage to community resources (Green and Kulper, 1990; Oktay, 1984). For example, social workers in primary care may provide appropriate services to address the psychosocial needs of patients who would otherwise present somatic complaints and misuse primary medical care.

In the medical clinic of one urban hospital adjacent to an impoverished African-American community, a group of social workers reported on their project to empower patients through the social support of the group (Dobrof et al., 1990). According to the authors, the support groups were effective, both in reducing physical symptoms and in engaging clients in a more active role in their own health care. The social workers saw themselves as role models, facilitators, teachers, skill builders, and change promoters (Dobrof et al., 1990:36). Groups were developed to address specific psychosocial problems:

1. A men's stress management group for those with anxiety leading to psychosomatic symptoms
2. An empty nest syndrome group for middle-aged women who need to discover life outside the empty nest
3. Senior socialization for isolated elder women
4. Support groups for people with a common physical disease
5. Support groups for people with a common psychiatric disorder
6. A housing advocacy group to teach people how to self-advocate to get action on environmental issues (Dobrof et al., 1990)

Most social workers continue to seem to prefer clinical social work with individuals and lack interest in, and/or knowledge of, more macrolevel interventions. In one study of social workers in the primary care setting of family practice residency programs (Hess, 1985), the social workers reported that most of the patients had a cluster of psychosocial problems rather than just one, and the problems identified covered a wide range of types. However, the social workers were selective in their choices of which client problems to address: "Respondents' descriptions of their clinical work conveyed a general tendency to select emotional/interpersonal conflict client problems rather than social/environmental problems; interventions within the therapeutic type; and an individual rather than a family, agency, or community focus" (Hess, 1985:60).

In addition, in the Hess study (1985), many of the social workers were engaged in educating the physicians through their clinical practice. However, since the social workers tended to self-select a limited range of client problems rather than making a representative selection of the clients' actual problems, the implication is that their teaching of the physicians would also tend to present a biased picture, one preoccupied with emotional and individual problems, to the exclusion of social-environmental and family-centered ones (Hess, 1985:61-62).

Zayas and Dyche (1992) describe their social work practice in a primary care medical clinic and residency program, where they teach physicians about attending to four main, essentially clinical, concepts:

1. The concept of process (development of events), including beginning "where the patient is" in their concerns and interpretations
2. The helping relationship and "conscious use of self"
3. The person-in-situation perspective (what is going on in the patient's life situation when the health complaints ebb and flow)
4. The context of practice (from the clinical setting to the community, home, school, or workplace, as well as the patient's own demographic characteristics)

Lesser (2000) described an experience of collaboration between a community mental health center and a family medicine practice, citing the broad range of common psychosocial problems they invited the primary medicine service to refer to the social workers, including "school and learning difficulties, parenting concerns, intercultural and interfaith family issues, adolescent adjustment, work stress, mid-life transitions, marital and family problems, depression, alcohol and substance abuse, chronic illness, bereavement, and elder care" (121). A wide range of interventions were also employed, including linkage with other needed community services, group work with parents to address child development and parenting issues, a caregivers' support group, a women's group for midlife transition issues, and a chemical dependency recovery support group. Lesser (2000) notes that many managed care companies have expressed interest in this collaborative arrangement.

Those of us who remember when the United States had a network of publicly supported community mental health centers will recognize the Lesser report as quite typical of the extensive mental health promotion, prevention, and treatment services that those CMHCs once provided in America on a sliding scale basis.

Rock and Cooper (2000) describe a student practicum of Fordham University in a not-for-profit primary medicine clinic in an economically and socially oppressed neighborhood in New York City. The practicum purpose was to demonstrate to physicians and managed care payers the utility of having social workers within a primary care setting, using screening tools, rapid assessment instruments, and high-risk indicators, and to give the students the experience in what was predicted to become a frequent setting of social work in health care in the future.

The aim was early identification and social work intervention with patients having psychosocial problems that, if not addressed, were likely to complicate and impair the effectiveness of medical treatment. To measure their effectiveness, the social work students utilized single systems design, which involves graphing the frequency or intensity of a target behavior before, during, and following an intervention period, to determine the behavior pattern across these periods and infer the effect and duration of the intervention. The students selected for the project had the advantage of speaking a range of foreign languages common to patients using the clinic. The students used a variety of clinical interventions with the clients, such as ventilation, cognitive therapy, assistance in strengthening social supports, desensitization training, grief therapy, and referral back to the physician for increased antidepression drugs. This report includes recommendations for further development of this interesting social work model.

Netting and Williams (2000) report the findings of a qualitative evaluation of a demonstration project involving nine primary medical care sites around the United States that examined the use of social workers in collaborative practice with physicians. The study revealed that the social workers were particularly helpful to and accepted by the physicians in cases of elderly patients with psychosocial problems. The project was funded by the Hartford Foundation, which has made extensive financial contributions to the social work profession to promote gerontological social work. As the elderly population increases and people live longer, many more older Americans with largely chronic health conditions will need medical and social work services to enhance functioning and quality of life. Netting and Williams report:

> We learned that these physicians and their staffs were eager to have professionals to whom they could refer older clients with complex problems. . . . Social workers, as well as other professionals, are logical collaborators with primary care physicians. Social workers, therefore, should seize these opportunities by demonstrating their value in dealing with the seas of troubles, nebulous issues, and cans of worms that characterize geriatric practice for physicians. *To do this, social workers will need knowledge and skills in working with older people.* (2000:241) (emphasis added)

Constraints on Social Work in Primary Health Care

According to Miller (1987:323), barriers to social worker participation in primary health care include the following: (1) physicians lack understanding of the knowledge, functions, and skills of social workers and of the biopsychosocial model; (2) as primary care becomes competitive, a challenge may emerge for primary care practitioners in medicine to retain a large enough patient load, thus providing a disincentive to employ people such as social workers who could effectively contribute to health promotion and the prevention of health problems; (3) most primary care will probably be provided through HMOs, which are likely to serve a predominately economically comfortable sector of the population, which the medical staff may not perceive as needing social work services. Yet another barrier to social worker involvement in primary health care may be social workers' lack of educational preparation for this type of work (Oktay, 1995:1891).

Furthermore, there has been a general lack of funding for social work in primary care. Most health insurance plans provide minimal coverage for mental health services or for preventive services in general. With the current focus on cost control, case management service (assessment, referral, and coordination of services to be provided by others) is more likely to be funded than direct provision of needed services (Oktay, 1995:1892).

A still greater barrier to social work in primary care may be the lack of qualified social workers, especially in rural areas. In 1985, the Task Force on Social Services in Primary Care was organized to study a sample of both rural and urban community health centers funded through Section 330 of the U.S. Public Health Service Act and ascertain the use of, and need for, social work services in these centers (Young and Martin, 1989). They found that although the patients were reported to have many of the same types of social problems in both rural and urban centers, the social work support available to address them was different. The rural centers employed far fewer social workers for the size of the patient load and also hired far fewer MSW-level social workers, even to direct the social work program, and rural centers made fewer referrals to community resources other than hospitals. Many of the rural primary care centers were staffed by only one BSW-level social worker to handle all the psychosocial problems presented.

However, primary care practice of physicians varies between rural and urban areas in its use of social worker assistance. Rural primary care physicians are unlikely to employ social workers to assist with addressing patients' psychosocial problems, and social work practice in primary care is much more common in urban areas. A study of rural primary care physicians to explore their current and potential use of social workers indicates that they tend to perceive social workers as specializing in resource referral and linkage tasks (Badger et al., 1997). This was also the finding of an earlier study of physicians' and nurses' perceptions of the hospital social worker role (Cowles and Lefcowitz, 1995).

There is unquestioned need for qualified social workers in primary health care. A recent study of the extent to which primary care physicians encounter psychosocial problems of patients found that primary care physicians are, indeed, the gatekeepers for an array of psychosocial problems (Gross et al., 1996:89). Zayas and Dyche (1992) expect increased federal funding for primary care, including increased demand for social workers, whose functions would include a greater role in medical education.

KNOWLEDGE REQUIREMENTS

Given the complex theoretical perspective of primary care in the health field and the associated necessity of interdisciplinary teamwork, various areas of knowledge are required for optimal social work practice in primary care. Ell and Morrison wrote, "the social worker in a primary health care setting is truly a generalist and must be prepared to intervene at many levels—individual, family, group, or community." They continue:

> The knowledge base in primary care social work is unique in its breadth. The array of medical and emotional problems presented in different primary care settings requires social workers to have an unusually extensive knowledge of medicine, psychopathology, and organizational theory. Knowledge of epidemiology, the etiology of illness, psycho-social dysfunction, and the sociology of medicine provides the foundation for decisions about which patients to treat and with what technology. (1981:37s)

Given this array of needed knowledge, a model curriculum for social work in primary care has been proposed as follows.

A Model Curriculum for Social Work in Primary Care

A model primary care curriculum for schools of social work and other professional schools to adopt is recommended by the Michigan Prevention Training and Curriculum Development Project, explaining that

> [t]he Public Health Social Work Forward Plan documents the need for graduate schools of social work to incorporate increased public health content into their curricula to prepare practitioners to work in a broad

range of practice settings beyond those traditionally associated with public health. (Siefert, Jayaratne, and Martin, 1992:18)

The following principles provide the foundation for the recommended curriculum:

1. health and mental health conceptualized holistically as positive well-being, not merely the absence of disease;
2. a developmental perspective emphasizing competence and mastery as well as vulnerability over the life cycle;
3. knowledge of the impact of individual and environmental risk factors in the etiology and prevention of health and mental health disorders;
4. an understanding of the protective function of social support;
5. concepts and strategies from epidemiology;
6. comprehension of research design and methodology appropriate to prevention; and
7. appreciation of the need to intervene at multiple levels using a range of preventive strategies. (Siefert, Jayaratne, and Martin, 1992:19)

The proposed curriculum plan has been integrated with the CSWE required core curriculum of human behavior and the social environment, social welfare policy and services, social work practice, social work research methods, and field practicum (Siefert, Jayaratne, and Martin, 1992:19). One of the most interesting aspects of the proposed curriculum is that the participating graduate students are required to design a social work intervention project aimed at prevention and to test its effect (Siefert, Jayaratne, and Martin, 1992:22).

In an editorial on public health social work, Siefert (1995, cited in Poole, 1995:244) was quoted as saying:

Social workers will need to be prepared to engage in practice that is collaborative, culturally competent, community-based, and oriented to prevention and early intervention. Preventive intervention in public health social work requires that social workers engage in multiple methods of intervention simultaneously, ranging from the provision of direct service to community planning and advocacy. This poses a challenge for schools of social work, which tend to track students into micro or macro methods and discourage an integrative approach. . . . Collaborative practice also poses a challenge to social work education; specialization within the curriculum often perpetuates the lack of interchange across fields of service that characterizes practice in the real world. Long-standing barriers to interdisciplinary education will also require innovative approaches.

Need for Conceptual Integration of Physical and Mental Health

In addition, the proposal challenges schools of social work to recognize that the traditional separation of health and mental health is no longer workable (Siefert, Jayaratne, and Martin, 1992:25). Shannon also wrote, "A biopsychosocial model of health care—in which disease is seen as an interplay between environmental, physical, behavioral, psychological, and social factors—can integrate mental health services into the primary care sector" (1989:32). Tessie Cleveland added:

> The historical division between medical social work and psychiatric social work has been serious and divisive, perpetuating a caste system within the social work profession. . . . Social workers have not yet recognized forthrightly that the division, which may serve some ego needs, confuses colleagues outside social work and undermines the profession. . . . Social workers must move to present uniform definitions of health and mental health practice and must seek reform in social work education and agency administration to solidify this uniformity. Social workers should be proud that . . . they can maintain a single identity and view the client holistically. To this end, each disease . . . with its accompanying psychosocial involvement, has import for social work practice. (1981:125)

The Need to Move Beyond Clinical Social Work

Addressing the subject of prevention, Pray (1995) noted that the trend today in national and international places with progressive health care approaches is to focus on community organization and community empowerment and policy changes, which go beyond one-on-one efforts to modify health behavior. Pray cites Bracht (1990) as a rich source of information about such projects. Bracht's (1999) second edition of *Health Promotion at the Community Level* is necessary for any serious social work student in the health field area.

Schools of social work must make a greater effort to lure future social workers from a preoccupation with one-on-one clinical work to greater interest and competency in community organization and social action approaches.

Need for Collaboration Between Classroom and Practicum

Finally, to develop the necessary knowledge and skills for effective social work practice in health care, it is imperative that social work education in the classroom and field practicum employs coordinated and cooperative educational efforts. These efforts should include

1. the classroom and practicum exchanging information concerning their curriculum content and changes;
2. classroom faculty providing field faculty with written descriptions of areas of concentration, course descriptions, and research programs;
3. field instructors providing classroom faculty with information about their agency programs, field curricula, and seminar presentations;
4. more joint programs between the two to exchange information and share ideas; and
5. seminars by the schools for field instructors to promote information exchange between agencies and between agencies and schools. (Marshack, Davidson, and Mizrahi, 1988:231)

Summary

Ideally then, social work practice in primary care in the health field requires knowledge of the following: health behavior, illness behavior, social aspects of illness, generalist social work practice (including how to work at all social systems levels of person, family, group, organization, community, and society), medicine, psychopathology, organizational theory, epidemiology, the etiology of illness, psychosocial dysfunction, the sociology of medicine, the WHO concept of health, empowerment and the strengths perspective, individual and environmental risk factors, the protective function of social support, epidemiology, experimental research methodology to test the effect of interventions, and the biopsychosocial model of health care.

As described in Chapter 2, the health care social worker requires specific knowledge in the areas of client population and problem, organizational setting, the community and its resources, specific intervention modalities, and specific methods of research, evaluation, and documentation appropriate to the setting.

VALUES AND ETHICS CONSIDERATIONS

More than any other area of health care, primary care, in the sense of primary prevention and health promotion, must attend to adverse social environmental conditions. According to the current NASW Code of Ethics:

The *primary mission* of the social work profession is to enhance human well-being and help meet the basic human needs of all people with particular attention to the needs and empowerment of people who are vulnerable, oppressed, and living in poverty. . . . Fundamental to social work is *attention to environmental forces* that create, contribute to, and address problems in living. Social workers promote *social justice and social change* with and on behalf of clients. "Clients" is used inclusively to refer to individuals, families, groups, organizations, and communities.* (NASW, 1996:1) (emphasis added)

Social justice is listed as one of the six core values of the social work profession, whose associated ethical principle is stated as follows:

Social workers *challenge social injustice.* Social workers *pursue social change,* particularly with and on behalf of vulnerable and oppressed individuals and groups of people. Social workers' social change efforts are focused primarily on issues of poverty, unemployment, discrimination, and other forms of social injustice. These activities seek *to promote sensitivity to and knowledge about oppression and cultural ethnic diversity.* Social workers strive *to ensure access to needed information, services, and resources, equality of opportunity, and meaningful participation in decision making for all people.** (NASW, 1996:5) (emphasis added)

Given the organizational pressures that increasingly are felt by all professionals in health care settings today to compromise their values and ethics, it is important for social workers to remember that their responsibilities begin with *a primary responsibility to promote their clients' well-being.* "In general, *the clients' interests are primary"** (NASW, 1996:7) (emphasis added).

In addition, the social worker has an *"obligation to promote the client's right to self-determination and to understand and respect the client's culture and social diversity"* (NASW, 1996:9).

SKILL REQUIREMENTS

Ell and Morrison (1981) listed among the skills needed by social workers in primary health care: decision making, differential diagnosis, counseling the resistant patient, team building, consultation, and education. Other needed

---

*Copyright 1996, National Association of Social Workers, Inc., Code of Ethics.

social work skill areas include case finding, discriminating between various biopsychosocial sources of patient anxiety, the ability to help some patients recognize the source of their symptoms as social or emotional rather than organic, facilitating the learning and application of psychosocial assessment and treatment skills by other professions in addition to social work, and teaching skills, especially about how to interview and about how psychosocial issues affect health and illness. Primary care social workers also need to be skilled in the use of community resources for health promotion and prevention of health problems, such as referring primary care clients to particular programs, for example, weight control, cessation of smoking, Alcoholics Anonymous, support groups, and training in such skills as effective parenting, self-assertion, nutrition, and child development.

Research and evaluation skills are also needed by social workers, especially in primary care, to develop tools for assessing clients' need for social work services so that referrals to social work are not limited to the physician's judgment of need (Ell and Morrison, 1981:38s). Finally, research skills are needed to evaluate practice in order to refine primary care social work practice by developing knowledge concerning what are and are not effective social work interventions in primary health care. By so doing, social workers can develop credibility and gain funding to support the work.

Hess examined social work practice in a primary care setting and concluded that

> social work graduate education needs to strengthen its ability to promote excellence in areas of teaching, health care coordination, and health team participation, [as well as in] areas of physical illness, health behavior, and social aspects of illness, [in addition to] methodology for work with families. [Note that] *an effective practice model of social work in primary health care settings is needed.* (1985:64) (emphasis added)

Goel and McIsaac (2000:6), in writing about health promotion in the clinical practice setting, include among required skills (1) communication skills, (2) the ability to identify the social context in which patients live, (3) integrating cultural or behavioral factors that influence a patient's response to disease or to recommendations, and (4) recognizing the role of families.

HELPING INTERVENTIONS

Ell and Morrison noted the following about social work interventions in primary health care settings:

Interventions used with patients include evaluation, information and referral, outreach, case management, short-term psychotherapy, family and group therapy, crisis intervention, family planning, genetic counseling, behavior modification, patient education, and facilitating and advocating system or community development and change. Interventions with [interdisciplinary] teams include consultation, staff development, in-service education, administrative analysis, and professional research. (1981:37s)

Bloom (1995) suggests a variety of potential interventions for social workers to use in primary prevention work at the micro level, such as problem-solving, coping, and social skills education, self-efficacy development, assertiveness training, cognitive reframing, anticipatory coping, parent effectiveness training, and social support groups. Although such interventions would doubtlessly help, they do not address the adverse social institutional conditions that seem to be at the root of poor health, such as social inequality and unequal opportunity, illuminated by Evans, Barer, and Marmor (1994), Kozol (1991, 1995), and Kawachi, Kennedy, and Wilkinson (1999).

The Need for Macrolevel Change

Social workers will not be able to change the economic system, educational system, political system, or health care system unless they become more involved in community organization and other macrolevel approaches directed to empowering the public (Dunlop and Holosko, 1992).

The public must be engaged in demanding a dramatic reduction in both absolute and relative poverty, the development of national health insurance or some other national health care system that ensures access to primary medical care, and more early identification of, and intervention in, family and community situations that threaten the mental and physical well-being of their members. Only then will it be possible to prevent the damage to human development that results in behavior that is destructive to self and others:

The philosophy of primary health care emphasizes prevention, health education, community participation (not token, but listening to all local viewpoints with respect), the importance of environmental factors, and the need to reach out to even the most remote areas and to all parts of the population, including the poorest. (Smyre, 1993:59)

Social Mapping

All intervention in primary care must be rooted in sensitivity to human diversity. Community participation, community organization work, must employ what Cochrane (1979, cited in Green, 1995:100) termed *social mapping,* a kind of inventory at the macro social level, including the following:

1. Identification and location of an ethnic group in an area
2. Description of the community's social organization
3. Description of the residents' beliefs and ideological characteristics
4. Identification of patterns of wealth, its accumulation, and its distribution
5. Description of the patterns of mobility, both geographical and social
6. Information on access and utilization of available human services

Green wrote the following about the result of social mapping:

> The product of social mapping should be a short document containing one or more physical maps and descriptive information for each of the six items listed above, provided in sufficient detail that a stranger could read it and gain some general sense of: (a) who lives in the area; (b) how they live; (c) what they believe and do; (d) how they use social services. The document should also make clear the outstanding needs of the community, especially as they are perceived by the residents themselves. (1995:100-101)

Caring at the Primary Health Care Level

> Health is created and lived by people within the settings of their everyday life, where they learn, work, play, and love. *Health is created by caring for one-self and others,* by being able to make decisions and have control over one's life circumstances, and by ensuring that the society one lives in creates conditions that allow the attainment of health by all its members. (WHO, 1986:3) (emphasis added)

Caring at the primary health care level is directed at primary prevention and health promotion. It is comparable to the nurture of children or plants or anything else we value and wish to do well. It means that we must determine what is needed in order to do well, and then we must assume responsibility for their provision. Although caring is rooted in *caring about* something, that is a shallow sentiment unless followed up by assurance that needs are met. To do otherwise is "care-less."

Therefore, it seems careless for a society to ignore the social conditions that are adverse to the prevention of health problems and the promotion of health. It is my conviction that the entire field of social work in health care needs to awaken to the social-structural conditions in the etiology of health problems. For example:

- A society is not "healthy" if, as of 2000, 16.9 percent of its children are without economic means to live according to even minimal standards of decency and health (U.S. Census Bureau, 2000).
- A society is not "healthy" if it relies on the local property tax base as the primary source of public school funding, which results in vast differences in the quality of public education from one locality to another.
- A society is not "healthy" if the percentage of its citizens incarcerated in prisons and jails is the highest in the world.
- A society is not "healthy" if 15 percent of its members have no health insurance, despite the majority of them being employed full-time.
- A society is not "healthy" if over 50 percent of its citizens who are poor, according to its own poverty index, are not covered by its Medicaid health insurance program for the poor.
- A society is not "healthy" if its own low standard for distinguishing the poor from the nonpoor is itself considerably higher than the legally required minimum wage.
- A society is not "healthy" if its government will not allocate enough funds to employ a sufficient number of adequately trained staff to competently address the problems of physical, emotional, and sexual child maltreatment.
- A society is not "healthy" if it is so morally insensitive that it allows members of its federal legislature to have comprehensive health insurance, subsidized by the taxpayer, while these same persons fail to enact policy providing the same to the rest of the citizenry.
- A society is not "healthy" if it claims to be the "best in the world" and yet continues to be the only industrialized nation in the world without any system of national health care, and still claims that medical care ought to be purchased from providers who are in the business primarily to make a profit.
- A society is not "healthy" if it attempts to achieve cost control in health care through a system that allows the chief executive officers of managed health care organizations to receive multimillion-dollar annual incomes from the profits derived from withholding needed medical interventions to their patients.

- A society is not "healthy" if its legislature does not take action to ensure that Medicare reimbursement to medical supply companies is based on competitive bids, as is done in the Veterans Administration, but instead continues to allow the Health Care Financing Administration to pay claims, without challenge, which are sometimes hundreds of times higher than over-the-counter costs, because the legislature has succumbed to the lobbying and political contributions of this supply industry, and seeks, instead, to compensate for this total waste of taxpayer money by increasing out-of-pocket cost sharing of elderly and disabled Medicare recipients.

How Health is Created

"Health is created and lived by people within the settings of their everyday life, where they learn, work, play, and love. Health is created by caring for oneself and others, by being able to make decisions and have control over one's life circumstances, and by ensuring that the society one lives in creates conditions that allow the attainment of health by all its members." (WHO, 1986:3)

The major danger for the future of primary health care in the United States is that the goal of cost control will be achieved through using public funds and legislative policy to promote a profit-making industry that will be extremely lucrative to stockholders and CEOs. This will cause the general public in America to experience a reduction in the quality and quantity of health services and make members of the medical profession salaried employees of business and industry. As a result, the health of the nation will continue to decline.

Perhaps social work in health care in the twenty-first century needs to consider a return to settlement house social work as practiced at the turn of the twentieth century, as described at the beginning of this chapter—essentially helping communities to build social structures that promote a sense of well-being and healthy living.

COMMENTARY

Hopefully, U.S. health care system administrators will finally realize that the only effective route to cost control is through greater focus on primary prevention of health problems—thoroughly rooted in addressing the underlying social problems of poverty, racism, environmental pollution, lack of education, and general lack of taking care of ourselves and one another. This recognition will mark the end of what has often been referred to as "the medicalization of social problems." When this awakening happens, social workers will be employed as one of the important groups of agents needed to achieve the goals of primary care.

Chapter 4

Social Work in Hospitals

HISTORICAL BACKGROUND

The Development of Hospitals in the United States

Originally, hospitals in the United States were almshouses for the poor, and many of them later became well-known, public tax-supported hospitals. For example, Bellevue Hospital in New York City was founded in 1736 as the second almshouse in the country. The first almshouse was established in Philadelphia in 1713 (Nacman, 1977:407).

During the second half of the 1700s, private nonprofit hospitals began to emerge, on demand of the middle class, who saw the need for hospitals but were repelled by the squalor of the almshouses. One reason for their emergence at this time was the need for treatment facilities for those injured in the Revolutionary War (Nacman, 1977:408).

After the Revolutionary War, immigration and urbanization increased and were accompanied by epidemics and other public health problems (Rosen, 1958:182, 201). Consequently, more public hospitals were built, such as Massachusetts General in 1821 and the Lincoln Hospital in 1840, built in New York City for the care of elderly and disabled African Americans (Nacman, 1977:408).

However, even by the mid-1800s, almshouses continued as centers of care for most of the economically dependent population. Recognition was spreading, though, that the conditions in almshouses were extremely bad, and specialized care facilities began to emerge for subgroups seen as "deserving" of being saved from almshouses—such as children, the elderly, the mentally ill, and the developmentally disabled. Thus, society saw the growth of orphanages, homes for the aged (often for specific religious or ethnic groups), and state hospitals for the mentally ill and developmentally disabled (Nacman, 1977). In addition, "outdoor" relief assistance programs, in cash or in kind, also arose to save specific religious or ethnic group members from almshouses.

143

Although hospitals emerged in the second half of the 1700s, they did not become the center of medical practice until around the end of the 1800s, when the germ theory of disease began to be widely accepted (Cannon, 1923).

The Emergence of Social Work

The need developed for some system to oversee and set standards for these new institutional care facilities, as well as to coordinate the multiple outdoor relief charities that were emerging. The people who filled these positions on the state boards of charities and corrections and with the charity organization societies later came to perceive themselves as having a common function and philosophy, and they adopted the title "social worker." Settlement house staff were the third set of new workers responding to similar conditions.

Social Work in the Health Care Field

Social work in the health care field is usually traced to the entry of social work into the general hospital. However, from the time social work emerged in the mid-1800s, its practitioners were involved with the multiple health-related problems of poverty, overcrowding, and the lack of proper water and sewage systems that accompanied urbanization and immigration, unregulated and unplanned industrialization, and lack of acceptance of the emerging germ theory of disease (Rosen, 1958:348-349, 353, 360-364; Trattner, 1989:133-134).

Growth of Hospital Social Work

In 1984, there were 6,872 hospitals in the United States, of which 6,302 (92 percent) responded to an annual survey of the American Hospital Association (AHA). Of those that responded, 5,209, or 83 percent, reported having social work services. Of the reporting hospitals, 5,801 were general and nonpsychiatric specialty hospitals, and about 82 percent of these had social work services. The remaining 501 reporting hospitals in 1984 were psychiatric hospitals, and 95 percent of them had social work services (American Hospital Association, 1985).

In 1994, there were 6,374 hospitals in the United States, of which 5,387 (84.5 percent) responded to an annual survey of the American Hospital Association. Of those that responded, 4,533 (84 percent) reported having social work services. Of the total reporting hospitals in 1994, 4,926 (85 percent) were general and nonpsychiatric specialty hospitals, and 4,184 (85 percent) of these had social work services. The remaining 461 reporting hospitals in 1994 were psychiatric hospitals, and 349 (76 percent) of them had social work services (American Hospital Association, 2002).

In 2000, of the 4,856 reporting hospitals, 86 percent had social work services. Of the 4,525 general or nonpsychiatric specialty hospitals, 3,900 (86 percent) employed social workers. Social workers were employed by 76 percent of the 333 psychiatric specialty hospitals. Table 4.1 depicts the comparison for all three years.

The U.S. Department of Labor estimated that in 1992, a total of 26.2 percent of social workers were employed in the health care field, and 14.13 percent alone were employed in hospitals, both public and private, by far the largest employer of social workers in health care (Ginsberg, 1995:355).

THEORETICAL PERSPECTIVES

Curing

When the germ theory of disease began to be widely accepted, medical practice recognized the desirability of aseptic conditions for surgery and wound care and the possibility of preventing and curing infection, though antiseptic was not demonstrated until 1867 by Joseph Lister, a surgeon (Rosen, 1958:317). However, it was not until the last decade of the nineteenth century and the first decade of the twentieth century that the germ theory of disease was well developed and accepted (319).

The modern hospital became the seat of medical practice when this was occurring, and medical practice began a transition from *social medicine* to the *medical model,* and from *caring* to *curing.* Indeed, the hope of conquering human disease grew ever larger during the twentieth century, eventually resulting in a hospital-centered health care system whose costs of high technology and specialization were rising so much faster than those of other industries that the U.S. government began to take steps to reduce the use of hospitals and medical specialists.

Cost-Effectiveness

Cost control became the overriding concern of U.S. hospitals as the health care inflation rate rose from 5.1 percent of the GDP (gross domestic product) in 1960, to 7.1 percent in 1970, to 8.9 percent in 1980, to 12.2 percent in 1990, and to 13.4 percent in 1994—when it began to stabilize. In 1998 total national health expenditures were still "only" 13.5 percent of the GDP (U.S. Government Printing Office, 2000a:322, Table 115). Nonethe-

TABLE 4.1. Number and Percentage of Reporting Hospitals with Social Work Services, 1984, 1994, and 2000

Reporting Hospitals	1984		1994		2000	
	number	percent	number	percent	number	percent
Psychiatric specialty hospitals N = 501 (1984) N = 461 (1994) N = 333 (2000)	478	95	349	76	253	76
General/nonpsychiatric hospitals N = 5,801 (1984) N = 4,926 (1994) N = 4,525 (2000)	4,731	82	4,184	85	3,900	86
Total hospitals N = 6,302 (1984) N = 5,387 (1994) N = 4,856 (2000)	5,209	83	4,533	84	4,153	86

Source: 1984 data are from American Hospital Association (1985). *Hospital Statistics.* Chicago: Author, Table 12A, 194; 1994 data are from American Hospital Association (1995). *AHA Annual Survey.* Chicago: Author; 2000 data are from American Hospital Association (2002). *Hospital Statistics.* Chicago: Author, Table 7, 161, and unpublished data from the AHA annual survey.

less, the United States continues to expend both a higher per capita amount and a higher percentage of its GDP on health care than any other country in the world, including those with national health care systems (U.S. Government Printing Office, 2000a:321, Table 114).

National health expenditures totaled $1,149.1 billion in 1998 in the United States. The largest percentage of the total, 33.3 percent, or $382.8 billion, went for hospital care (U.S. Government Printing Office, 2000a: 325-326, Table 118).

Only since the DRG system went into effect in 1984 has the annual rate of increase begun to decline. From 1975 to 1980 it peaked at 13.6 percent, from 1980 to 1985 the annual rate of increase in national health expenditures dropped to 11.6, and between 1995 and 1996, it declined to an all-time low annual rate of 4.6 percent. However, by 1998 it had begun to rise again, to 5.6 percent (U.S. Government Printing Office, 2000a:325, Table 118).

Of the total expended for hospitalization in 1998, 80 percent went to general medical and surgical hospitals, 8 percent to psychiatric hospitals, and the remaining 12 percent to other specialty hospitals (U.S. Government Printing Office, 2000b:120, Table 181). The financing of hospital care in

1998, including hospital-based nursing home and home health agency care, is shown in Table 4.2.

The Biopsychosocial Model

Since at least the beginning of hospital social work, social workers have recognized that biological, psychological, and social-environmental variables impact one another. The *mission of social work in the acute-care medical hospital* is delineated by the National Association of Social Workers (1990) as follows:

> Social work services are provided to patients and their families to meet their medically related social and emotional needs as they impinge on their medical condition, treatment, and recovery, and safe transition from one care environment to another.* (NASW, 1990:4)

However, the focus of hospital social work has tended to shift back and forth between psychological, social, and psychosocial as the profession as a whole responded to changing professional and national political priorities. Thus, hospital social work started in 1905 with a social medicine view of the social roots of health problems when infectious and contagious diseases were predominant. In the 1920s, social work shifted to a Freudian view of individual-seated problems, in response to Abraham Flexnor's concept of "professional status," to which the medical profession had already adapted by shifting from a social medicine perspective to the medical model (Smith and Anderson, 1995:248).

During the 1930s, the focus of social work moved to an acknowledgment of the force of macrolevel political and economic conditions, as the suicide rate skyrocketed and the general population ate at soup kitchens during the Great Depression. In the euphoric era of post–World War II, social work again moved back to a more individual-centered approach. Then, during the social justice and antimaterialistic movements of the 1960s and 1970s, hospital social work switched back to a more social action orientation. Finally, · during the conservative backlash of the 1980s, social work again returned to a more individual focus, where it and society generally remain lodged. Although lip service is given to psychosocial intervention, the emphasis appears mostly to be on the "psycho" part—less as a result of conviction than from a sense of powerlessness, perhaps.

---

*Copyright 1990, National Association of Social Workers, Inc., NASW Clinical Indicators for Social Work and Psychosocial Services in Nursing Homes.

TABLE 4.2. Financing Hospital Care, 1998

Source of funds	Percent
Government programs	61.0
Private health insurance	30.8
Out-of-pocket payments	3.4
Other private funds	4.6
Total ($382.8 billion)	99.8

Source: U.S. Government Printing Office, 2000b. *Statistical Abstracts of the United States.* Washington, DC: Author, Table 156, 110.

Unfortunately, this early lack of consensus concerning the focus of hospital social work and the profession in general led to a division within the profession, creating a separation between "medical" and "psychiatric" social workers, so that throughout much of the twentieth century, many hospitals maintained separate social work departments, one a department of medical social work and the other a department of psychiatric social work, despite their role and function being more alike than different (Nacman, 1977). "The problem is that the patient's need for care is a composite of physical, functional, emotional, social, and medical levels. Unfortunately, the skilled services directed to demonstrable acute needs are frequently not sufficient *to care for* the aggregate needs of patients" (Greenlick and Brody, 1997:112) (emphasis added).

Caring

Caring at the acute level, that is, secondary level of health care, refers to providing needed assistance to support comfort and function while the person is temporarily impaired by illness or injury to enhance or facilitate the curative or recovery process. Such care interventions may be directed to either physical, psychological, or social comfort and function aspects by addressing

1. barriers to admission to the acute care service or facility;
2. problems of adjustment to the acute care service or facility;
3. problems of adjustment to the diagnosis, prognosis, or treatment plan;
4. lack of information to make informed decisions and to feel in control;
5. lack of resources to meet needs; and
6. barriers to discharge.

However, care interventions provided by social workers at the secondary level of health services are rooted in individualizing and personalizing the client, in part by attending to his or her human diversity characteristics.

HUMAN DIVERSITY RELEVANCE

As indicated elsewhere, human diversity variables, such as age, gender, ethnicity, sexual orientation, disability, rural or urban residence, religion, and social class, can influence health behavior, illness behavior, and sick-role behavior and can interact rather than being merely additive. That is, one cannot assume that within each group people are alike, and so the traits of a "typical female" can merely be combined with those of a "typical elderly person" and a "typical African-American person," for example. Instead, females differ across class, ethnicity, sexual orientation, age, health status, and so on. Likewise, African Americans differ across class, gender, age, health status, and sexual orientation, and so forth. Nonetheless, the hospital social worker needs to have some familiarity with broad health-related differences across class (income, education, and occupation), ethnicity, gender, age group, and so on, yet not assume that such differences are true of all members of a particular group. A recent and excellent text dealing with these complexities of ethnicity and health care is *Multicultural Awareness in the Health Care Professions* (Julia, 1996).

It is always important for the hospital social worker to understand the client's view of the nature of his or her health problem, its causes and effects, and the appropriate treatment. Otherwise, the client may simply appear to agree, when, in reality, he or she has another perspective and plan. Of course, this difference in perspective may be due to a discrepancy in any one or a combination of variables, such as values, beliefs, customs, attitudes, resources, experience, or simply understanding.

African-American Health Beliefs

Congress and Lyons have discussed some of the cultural differences in health beliefs and their implications for social work in health care settings. Although many contemporary African Americans may be unfamiliar with their cultural traditions, Congress and Lyons point out that part of the African-American cultural tradition includes the conceptualization of health problems as falling into three categories: natural, occult, and spiritual (1992:83), with associated intervention types. For example, natural illness was often treated with herbal remedies, occult health disorders with witchcraft or "rootwork," and spiritual problems with prayer and the laying on of hands (Congress and Lyons, 1992). Black Americans of Haitian origin may attribute their health problems to supernatural causes and employ voodoo interventions.

Hispanic-American Health Beliefs

On the other hand, Hispanic-American people have tended to think of health problems as either natural ones that God has willed or unnatural ones that other people have caused through evil intent (Congress and Lyons, 1992:84). In either case, the idea that individuals have the power to greatly influence their health through their own health behaviors may be outside the belief system of Hispanic-American persons. Hispanic Americans see mind and body as a unity and health as dependent upon harmony with one's social and physical environment; thus, their emotional problems tend to manifest as somatic complaints (85).

The description of symptoms and interpretation of the health problem that the Hispanic-American patient or family member gives the health care provider may be misleading, if the provider is unaware of these kinds of cultural differences. Hispanic-American people of Puerto Rican background may seek assistance from a folk healer or spiritualist *(curandero)* before a physician, and it may be more beneficial to the patient for both traditions to be included in treatment (Congress and Lyons, 1992:85).

Asian-American Health Care Beliefs

There is much diversity within the Asian-American population due to the many different countries and cultures of origin, although many utilize home remedies and believe in a yin-yang food group system (Congress and Lyons, 1992:86).

Similar to Hispanic people, the Chinese tend to express their mental health problems somatically and to describe them in physical terms (Congress and Lyons, 1992:86). However, as with all ethnic groups, their traditions are more often found among the older generation and among those who are less assimilated into U.S. mainstream culture. In addition, people of lower socioeconomic status are more likely to seek informal family and folk remedies, partly because they are more accessible financially. As the Clemens (1995) study of hospital social worker discharge planning with an elderly ethnic population found, "the poor, and especially the ethnic poor, are particularly vulnerable to paternalistic interventions" (Congress and Lyons, 1992:89).

Whenever any patient has preferences for care which are important to them but which deviate from the hospital's usual approach, effort should be made to accommodate them, as long as it does not pose a significant threat to the functioning of the hospital or the well-being of the patient. Examples include food, clothing, or bathing preferences, religious ceremonies, or having loved ones nearby. Presumably, such accommodations can affect the patient's mental attitude, will to live, and sense of social support and empowerment.

INTERDISCIPLINARY TEAMWORK

Ross (1993) has argued that "[o]ur claim to a place on the interdisciplinary team must be based on expertise. Communication with other providers about issues related to patient and family adjustment requires more than a shallow grasp of biopsychosocial aspects of an illness" (1993:245). A key to survival in hospital social work is learning to collaborate and cooperate with other professional groups in the setting in such a way that staff members complement rather than compete with one another (Ruster, 1995).

However, the problem of a lack of clear role identity within the hospital social worker community has become compounded in recent years by indications that hospital physicians and nurses also have increasingly moved away from the medical model and toward a biopsychosocial perspective (Cowles and Lefcowitz, 1992). This appears to have led to increased overlapping of roles among professional groups in interdisciplinary teamwork. For example, Cowles and Lefcowitz, in their study of interdisciplinary expectations of the hospital social worker role, found that at least 60 percent of the physicians and nurses expected to at least equally share with other professional groups, including social workers, responsibility for the assessment of both emotional and social-environmental problems of their patients and for helping patients examine solutions to their emotional problems (1992:63).

As Donnelly (1992) pointed out:

> Under the impact of the knowledge explosion, increasing members of the interdisciplinary team share a common knowledge base. . . . Nurses, psychologists, physicians as well as a growing variety of counselors and therapists have often read the same books, undergone similar training and share many of the same skills as social workers . . . [in short] the psychosocial [arena] is by no means the exclusive domain of social workers. (108-109)

Still, recent research has also found considerable interdisciplinary consensus concerning the expected roles and functions of physicians, nurses, and social workers in urban hospitals (Cowles and Lefcowitz, 1992, 1995) and between nurses and social workers in rural hospitals (Egan and Kadushin, 1995). The main difference is a tendency for social workers to expect more *exclusive* responsibility for assessing patients' emotional problems, while the other professional groups expect this to be a task that is shared.

The Need for Biopsychosocial Expertise

"[Social workers'] claim to a place on the interdisciplinary team must be based on expertise. Communication with other providers about issues related to patient and family adjustment requires more than a shallow grasp of biopsychosocial aspects of an illness." (Ross, 1993:245)

DeCoster and Egan (2001) studied the views of over 200 physicians in an effort to understand how they perceive and respond to the emotions of their patients. The findings from the respondents' interpretation of a series of vignettes suggest that physicians may in fact be less likely to react to patient emotion with psychotropic drugs and may instead be more likely to take time to talk with them and attempt to address their perceived concerns, apparently considering the attitudes and feelings of patients as a legitimate arena for physician concern and attention. This supports the earlier findings of Cowles and Lefcowitz (1992, 1995) that physicians tend to perceive the emotional problems of their patients as their own domain, and that both physicians and nurses tend increasingly to see the psychosocial arena as a shared one.

There is growing recognition today that responsibility for addressing psychosocial needs of patients and families is not confined to any one professional group. This is reflected in an excellent article by Lauria and colleagues, who published a protocol for "clinicians charged with providing psychosocial care" (1996:1345) to child cancer patients and their families. The article offers a conceptualization of a systematic process of examining and helping with common psychosocial needs of child cancer patients and their families at various stages of disease course, for use by a multidisciplinary team of specialists in cancer care, including a pediatric oncologist, oncology nurses, oncology social workers, and pediatric psychologists (1347). The article provides an outline for the psychosocial assessment of both patient and family as well as an extensive list (protocol) of client issues and needs and associated clinical interventions that are relevant at various stages in the course of the condition.

A recent study by Mizrahi and Abramson (2000) involved lengthy interviews with fifty pairs of hospital social workers and physicians who had worked together on inpatient cases requiring unusually lengthy hospital stays. The purpose of the study was to ascertain the extent to which they agreed or disagreed with each other's amount and type of participation in the cases in question. The study findings indicate that the majority of physicians valued the social workers' participation in the collaboration. However, physicians perceived fewer psychosocial problems in patients than did social workers, and both groups "generally agreed that almost no physicians referred a patient or family for social work counseling" services (11). This tends to support the finding of a previous study (Cowles and Lefcowitz, 1995) that the only form of counseling which physicians in hospitals perceive as primarily a social worker role is counseling with the family concerning social-environmental problems.

Curiously, the Mizrahi and Abramson study found that 68 percent of the social workers thought they were the case coordinators when only 12 percent of physicians perceived the social workers as case coordinators. These recent findings of Mizrahi and Abramson (2000) suggest that physicians continue to recognize the need for social workers to assist with certain problems that patients and their families face, but that physicians and social workers continue to have somewhat discrepant perceptions of the nature of patient and family problems, and of the abilities of social workers to address certain of those problems, such as one which would require patient counseling.

ORGANIZATIONAL CONSIDERATIONS

Politically Conservative Hospital Roots

Hospitals tend to be conservative organizations, especially today, when more are for profit, but the medical profession has always been dominant in hospitals and its members traditionally have an upper-middle-class conservative perspective. Medical practice addresses health problems in individuals, not adverse social conditions that may have produced the health problems.

The Challenge to Hospital Social Workers

Thus, the organizational environment of the hospital tends to produce a conservative culture, which is difficult to ignore and survive. Social workers in hospitals need to recognize this influence in order to try to resist it when appropriate. Otherwise, the social worker is likely to become a tool of the system—resulting in becoming an agent for facilitating hospital and medical professional survival goals and objectives, at the expense of both client (patient and family) health and well-being and social work professional values, ethics, and autonomy—without which, professional status is questionable. Social work students preparing for hospital social work need to be taught how to set limits in carrying out institutional policies in order to avoid compromising professional autonomy and responsibility (Kadushin and Kulys, 1995:184).

Intraorganizational Variation in Culture

However, hospitals vary not only from one another but across intra-organizational units. Each medical and surgical service tends to have a culture of its own, reflecting a mixture of variation in characteristics of the health conditions served, the types of interventions provided, the usual prognosis, and patient and staff characteristics. For example, pediatric and obstetric units are likely to differ considerably in culture from cardiac care and oncology units (James and Studs, 1987), and surgery and orthopedic units from medicine units. This is sometimes referred to as patient-oriented services as compared to procedure-oriented services. The assumption has been that, in general, health services that involve procedures, such as the use of machinery and surgery, tend to produce a somewhat different atmosphere from health services that revolve more around nurturing kinds of interpersonal interactions. In a sense, this is one distinction between curing and caring.

Vertical Integration of the Modern Hospital

Robinson (1994) noted:

> The delivery system of the 21st century might remain centered around the hospital, albeit a vertically integrated system where acute care beds play only a modest role. . . . Hospitals have integrated rapidly into outpatient facilities that diagnose patients prior to admission, into subacute care facilities that shelter patients after discharge, and into many forms of health care that are not directly linked to acute in-patient care at all. (259, 262)

Increasingly, community hospital social work departments are achieving recognition by expanding into areas where they are needed and can complement rather than compete with other professions and health care organizations. These areas include joint nursing and social work discharge services, consultation to home care agencies and nursing homes, and health education to the community (Ruster, 1995), spanning the hierarchy of primary, secondary, and tertiary care levels.

A nationwide study of hospital social work reported by Berger and colleagues (1996) revealed that hospitals in the United States today have diversified; while 89 percent of those reporting offer both acute and ambulatory services, 48 percent also offer subacute or extended care; 62 percent, home care; 36 percent, durable medical equipment; and 29 percent, home infusion services (1996:168). Such vertical integration of the continuum of health care services may raise issues concerning free-market competition to achieve cost control (Robinson, 1994:265).

Horizontal Integration Within Hospital Organizations

There also is a trend toward hospitals in the United States moving from bureaucratic structures, with a hierarchal chain of command across various levels of management, to a new model of a horizontally integrative organization with a flattening of administrative structure, involving a reduction in middle management and professional group boundaries across functions and organizational units. The objective is an increase in cost-effectiveness through collaboration, coordination, and shared resources (Globerman and Bogo, 1995). In such a horizontally integrative organization, an interdisciplinary work group is organized around a level of care, such as trauma, or a client category, such as aging, and its management is referred to as the program management (5).

Globerman and Bogo (1995) argue that such an integrative organization is more compatible with social work values than a bureaucratic one, but does raise the question of how a particular professional group will retain its identity and standards in this atmosphere. Globerman, Davies, and Walsh (1996) report that although hospital social workers surveyed in Ontario, Canada, expressed concerns about the effect of the new integrative organizational model on control over the nature of their work and role, and on changes in whom they report to, they also felt it was important for hospital social workers to develop understanding of the new types of organizational structures, in terms of their theory, rationale, and positive potential (182).

Elsewhere in the literature, a hospital social work director has described her participation in a leadership training program that taught her how to engage all of the staff in brainstorming solutions to department problems. This allows line staff to replace the traditional middle manager role so that participatory democracy becomes a reality, compatible with the integrative organizational concept (Mayer, 1995).

Impact of Organizational Changes on Hospital Social Work

The percentage of freestanding hospitals, which was 62.5 percent in 1992, dropped to 45.2 percent by 1994, with a commensurate increase in multihospital systems. Although most of the reporting hospitals continued to have a centralized social work department, there was some increase in decentralized social work services. In addition, there appeared to be some decrease in middle management, and 21 percent of social work departments had merged with a non-social work department. Nearly one-third had experienced formal reviews by management of, for example, staffing and productivity. Although most (77.5 percent) hospitals still had MSW social work managers or directors, many reported some increase in nursing staff in social work departments. Most hospitals also reported similar changes occurring in other areas of the organization. Some decrease in social work responsibility for discharge planning was also reported. Overall, most reports did not regard the changes as negative (Berger et al., 1996:172-173).

In 2001, Mizrahi and Berger reported additional data from the 1994 study reported by Berger in 1996. The data indicated one-third of the hospital social work directors reported "pressure on social work" (indicating a general experience of being required to do a lot more with a lot less resources), while nearly one-fourth reported "devaluation or nonrecognition of social work" (citing turf conflict with nursing staff over the psychosocial problem arena and continued demand that social workers see only patients referred by physicians). The general impression from the reported findings is that as hospital resources continue to diminish, conflict and struggle for survival and control over what resources remain tend to increase. In such an environment, pressure to accept responsibility for functions outside of one's professional arena are likely to seem increasingly attractive in order to survive. Other themes that social work directors reported included expanding ambulatory and community settings, outpatient services, and home visits; increased case management; less clinical work and more discharge planning; cross-training initiatives for more teamwork; increasing lack of appropriate, affordable, and quality community resources for patient and family aftercare; and the replacement of MSWs with BSWs.

On a more promising note, one of the most frequently used terms by hospital social work directors in the study (Mizrahi and Berger, 2001) was *primary care*—and usually in a positive context. This may reflect a shift in the health-related literature from a preoccupation with the acute or secondary level of care intervention with well-developed health problems toward greater interest in and attention to the primary level of disease prevention, health promotion, and early identification and intervention with budding health problems.

A follow-up study of hospital social work by Berger and Mizrahi (2001) examined the issue of what effect, if any, the organizational changes in hospitals and in hospital social work may have had on supervision of hospital social workers. Three models of social work supervision were examined: (1) traditional (another senior social work staff person functions in the formal role of a supervisor), (2) peer supervision (two or more line social workers consult with each other in an individual or group format), and (3) non-social work supervision (the person who serves in a formal supervisory position does not hold a social work degree). They found that the traditional model continues to predominate but has decreased, accompanied by some increase in use of the alternatives and their combinations.

Despite the overall loss of 944 hospitals in the United States between 1980 and 1998, beginning soon after the introduction of the prospective payment system in 1984 with 86 percent of these being community hospitals, there was an increase of forty-four for-profit hospitals during the same period. Still, nonprofit community hospitals continue to predominate, constituting all but 15.4 percent of the industry (U.S. Government Printing Office, 2000b:127, Table 194).

However, in this age of increased profit-making hospitals, the issue may be raised as to the comparative costs and quality of services of for-profit compared to nonprofit hospitals. Ortiz and Bassoff (1988) reported that for-profit hospitals employ a significantly lower percentage of social work directors who belong to the social work in health care major professional organization, the Society for Social Work Leadership in Health Care. Furthermore, none of the proprietary hospitals were university affiliated and were more likely to be in urban than rural areas. Far fewer hospital social work directors had degrees in social work, and they generally had lower levels of formal education. The authors concluded that the same array of social services was offered by both for-profit and nonprofit hospital social work staff, but were provided by persons with less education in the for-profit organizations.

These changes in hospital social work are part of a general shift from acute care to primary and tertiary level care, and from inpatient to community-based care.

CLIENT PROBLEMS AND SOCIAL WORKER FUNCTIONS

Client Problems

The NASW (1990) has categorized the major problems of hospital patients and their families addressed by hospital social workers as including the following:

- Problems related to care and activities of daily living
- Environmental problems
- Patient and family adverse reactions or dysfunctional adjustment to illness and changes in functional status
- Problems related to physical, sexual, and emotional maltreatment
- Relationship problems
- Problems of behavior and cognition and mental disorders, including substance abuse
- Vocational and educational problems
- Legal problems (NASW, 1990:4-5)

Social Worker Functions

The hospital social worker role has evolved over time, resulting in a wide range of expectations for the position (Caputi, 1978). This fact, coupled with the traditional division between medical and psychiatric social work in hospitals, combined with a long history of lack of agreement between social workers and physicians and nurses concerning role expectations for hospital social workers, tends to produce a poorly defined professional identity (Germain, 1980).

According to the AHA Profile of United States Hospitals (American Hospital Association, 1993/1994), "organized social work services" means:

Services that are properly directed and sufficiently staffed by qualified individuals who provide assistance and counseling to patients and their families in dealing with social, emotional, and environmental problems associated with illness or disability, often in the context of financial or discharge planning coordination. (xxviii)

The Health Care Financing Administration (HCFA), which administered Medicare and Medicaid prior to their recent transfer to the Center for Medicare and Medicaid, defined *qualified social worker* as a person with an MSW degree or its equivalent from a social work educational program accredited by the CSWE; the HCFA defines *social work assistant* as a person with a bachelor's degree in social work or a related field who is supervised by a person with an MSW (NASW, 1997).

The *principle* of social work in health care in general has been articulated by NASW as follows:

Social work services shall be an integral part of every health care organization. The services shall be provided to individuals, their families and significant others; to special population groups; to communities;

and to special health-related programs, and educational systems.

To provide comprehensiveness and continuity of care, social work services shall encompass the following:

1. The promotion and maintenance of physical and psychosocial well-being
2. The promotion of conditions essential to assure maximum benefits from short- and long-term care services
3. The prevention of physical or mental illness
4. The promotion and enhancement of physical and psychosocial functioning, with attention to the social and emotional impact of illness or disability
5. The promotion of ethical responses to address the often conflicting value positions held by various parties involved in health care settings* (1987:3)

Hospital Social Work Defined

Organized social work services means "[s]ervices that are properly directed and sufficiently staffed by qualified individuals who provide assistance and counseling to patients and their families in dealing with social, emotional, and environmental problems associated with illness or disability, often in the context of financial or discharge planning coordination." (American Hospital Association, 1993/1994:xxviii)

NASW has also developed *clinical indicators* for social work services in the acute care medical hospital, which include the following (note that a clinical indicator refers to a criterion or benchmark for knowing whether a standard has been achieved in practice):

1. *Case finding and access:* patients needing social work services receive them
2. *Discharge delays:* the amount of care received is not excessive
3. *Patient and family involvement in planning:* social workers involve patients and families in making their own decisions about posthospital care
4. *Timeliness:* patients receive social work services early in the hospitalization

---

*Copyright 1987, National Association of Social Workers, Inc., NASW Standards for Social Work in Health Care Settings.

5. *Teamwork:* patient discharge occurs with the knowledge of the social worker coordinating discharge planning* (1990:6)

The Principle of Social Work in Health Care

"Social work services shall be an integral part of every health care organization. The services shall be provided to individuals, their families and significant others; to special population groups; to communities; and to special health-related programs, and educational systems.

To provide comprehensiveness and continuity of care, social work services shall encompass the following:

1. The promotion and maintenance of physical and psychosocial well-being
2. The promotion of conditions essential to assure maximum benefits from short and long-term care services
3. The prevention of physical or mental illness
4. The promotion and enhancement of physical and psychosocial functioning, with attention to the social and emotional impact of illness or disability
5. The promotion of ethical responses to address the often conflicting value positions held by various parties involved in health care settings" (NASW, 1987:3)

Case Finding—High-Risk Screening

For many years, hospital social workers depended largely on referrals from physicians and nurses for identification of patients needing social work services. However, as early as 1977, the AHA published indicators of *high social risk* in acute-care hospitals as a tool for professional standards review for hospital social work (American Hospital Association, 1977). Although the indicators used vary somewhat among hospitals, in many hospitals today patients are identified and automatically referred to hospital social work if the patient characteristics include any of the following: age sixty-five or over and living alone; terminal or chronic illness, disability, disfigurement, or accidental injuries; suicidal tendencies; mental retardation or mental health problem; unusually passive or aggressive behavior; health problem-induced employment limitations; low-income, unwed, minor mother (Becker and Becker, 1986:27); and lack of social supports (Berkman et al., 1991). Screening may be done at admission or prior to admission (Coulton, 1988).

---

*Copyright 1990, National Association of Social Workers, Inc., NASW Clinical Indicators for Social Work and Psychosocial Services in the Acute Care Medical Hospital.

Coulton (1988) pointed out that the ideal screening mechanism rates high in both sensitivity and specificity. *Sensitivity* refers to the ability of the process to identify people needing help with discharge planning and is referred to in program evaluation as target effectiveness, whereas *specificity* is the ability of the screening mechanism to exclude persons who do not need help with discharge planning, what research methodology calls target efficiency. In other words, a good high-social-risk screening system in a hospital will identify a high percentage of persons of the type the system intended to identify and will not falsely identify many of those which the system did not intend to pick up. Wolock and colleagues (1987) found that screening tools current at that time needed to be refined to improve both sensitivity and specificity.

Evans and Connis (1996) developed a simple index for VA hospital social worker use as a tool in screening for high risk of placement, death, or readmission—and therefore of need for early social work intervention—and determined that, of the variables they included, the ones that best predicted outcome were *comorbidity* (more than one health problem), mental status, living arrangement, prior institutional admission, prior hospital admission, *iatrogenic* (secondary to treatment) trauma, and pending litigation. However, they admitted that their tool rated highly on sensitivity but low on specificity.

Other Sources of Case Finding

In spite of the increase in high-risk screening, nearly one-half of hospital social work cases still may be referred by non-social workers. One large study of elderly posthospital patients found that 26 percent were identified by the social workers through screening admission summaries, and another 20 percent were picked up through social workers making rounds with other professional staff, while nearly one-half (49 percent) had been referred to social work by another type of health care professional (Oktay et al., 1992:294).

Pray (1991:184) has noted that hospitals vary in the extent to which the social workers are dependent on physicians for referrals (a *closed referral system*) as compared to a system that allows anyone to refer patients to the hospital social workers (an *open referral system*). However, even in open referral systems, the physician (or nurse) can influence referrals by others to the social workers by interpreting the social worker role to patients and families, as the physician (or nurse) understands (or misunderstands) it (185).

Pray (1991) found variation in perceptions among physicians of what appropriate referrals to hospital social workers include. Still, Pray (1991), similar to Cowles and Lefcowitz (1995), found that physicians were far more likely to refer patients to hospital social workers for concrete-instru-mental or social-environmental problems, such as those involving financial needs, posthospital care, and transportation, than for primarily affective-expressive problems involving attitudes, feelings, or behaviors related to health.

Risk Factors for Prolonged Length of Stay

Reflecting current cost containment pressures, a large teaching hospital in New York City sought to identify the high-risk indicators associated with prolonged hospital stays, which the social workers hoped to address pro-actively to reduce those stays and, subsequently, save the hospital social work program from being downsized (Auerbach et al., 2000).

The key indicators of prolonged length of stay (past acute care need) were found to be these:

1. Admission through the emergency department
2. Problems with memory
3. Difficulty climbing stairs
4. Waiting for a nursing home placement
5. Family problems relating to discharge planning
6. Medicaid pending (Auerbach et al., 2000)

These findings actually led to the social workers' obtaining increased staffing in the ER, where patients were screened to identify these indicators. This led to a more efficient Medicaid eligibility office being established within the social work department instead of in financial aid and to an acute special care unit being established for geriatric patients and another for stroke patients, both of which resulted in more appropriate care delivery with less patient deterioration (and thus fewer aftercare problems). Finally, the social work department established a computerized social work infor-mation system that proved to save time and facilitate a tracking and out-comes measures system. The development of the management information system was financed through an outside grant, but ongoing funding was pro-vided by the hospital, which was so impressed with the computer consultant the social workers had used that the hospital employed the same person to develop a similar system for another department in the hospital. One of the amazing successes of the new social work program in the ER was that 85 percent of patients seen by the social workers were diverted from being un-necessarily admitted to the hospital; another 5 percent were admitted to nursing homes directly from the ER.

A similar social work information system implemented in Israel in 1992 (Epstein et al., 2001) routinely identifies up to two reasons for delayed discharge from a list of eight choices:

1. Lack of patient cooperation with discharge planning;
2. Lack of family cooperation with discharge planning;
3. Hospital staff or procedure-related factors;
4. Policies or procedures of community or external institutional service providers, or lack of access to key providers;
5. Delay in availability of community aftercare resources;
6. Absence of the type of community care resources required by patient;
7. Change in status of patient or expected caregiver, requiring change in plans;
8. Other, for example, a patient with more complex care needs than available from current community resources

This article (Epstein et al., 2001) reported on a recent study to identify reasons for delayed discharge of cases handled by social work staff. Curiously, the study results indicated that, in general, an intake diagnosis of "injury" (especially road accidents) rather than "illness" was the main variable associated with extended length of stay across inpatient units. All other demographic variables, such as age, gender, marital status, living arrangement, and health insurance seemed to vary across inpatient units in terms of their relationship to length of stay, indicating that the nature of both disorder and treatment interacted with demographics. For example, in medicine and orthopedic units, increased age was correlated with increased length of stay, but in surgery departments, lower age was correlated with increased length of stay. Overall, neurosurgery patients had the longest length of stay.

The implication, of course, is that identification of patients at high risk for prolonged length of stay means that the social workers responsible for discharge planning need to prioritize the order and frequency of visits with patients they serve, based on the indicators relevant to their particular inpatient units.

Discharge Planning: The Central Function
of Hospital Social Work

Assisting patients with timely arrangements for their posthospital care continues to be a, if not *the,* central function of social workers in many hospitals, especially since the 1984 onset of the *prospective payment system* (PPS), according to which hospitals are reimbursed by Medicare in a preset amount based on the estimated number of inpatient days required, given the particular diagnosis and planned procedure, that is, diagnosis-related group (DRG).

Social work satisfaction with discharge planning. Despite increased pressure for rapid discharge, Resnick and Dziegielewski (1996) report, from their 1993 survey of hospital social workers and others doing discharge planning, that most claim satisfaction with their work and with client termination and outcome.

Client satisfaction with discharge planning. Furthermore, Stuen and Monk (1990) conducted a survey of 141 patients discharged from three acute-care hospitals in New York City and found that most patients were satisfied with their inpatient care, the discharge plan, and the posthospital care they received. However, among those who were not satisfied, a significantly higher percentage had chronic health conditions. Stuen and Monk speculated that the reason for this finding may be that the hospitals and home health care programs tend to be geared to acute care more than the ongoing functional limitations of persons with chronic health conditions (1990:161).

On the other hand, Clemens (1995) conducted a study in one teaching hospital with a high percentage of elderly patients of a variety of ethnic backgrounds, most of whom spoke English as their second language. Clemens found that although the social workers believed that they had done a good job with the discharge planning of the forty randomly selected cases, the family caregivers presented quite a different interpretation, with many feeling that the wishes of neither themselves nor the patients had been sufficiently heeded. Apparently, in this teaching hospital, the physicians decided within twenty-four hours whether patients were candidates for home care or nursing home care and referred them to one of two discharge planning departments, one staffed by nurses, the other by social workers, depending on the physicians' judgment. As a result, once the referral was made, the final decision tended to be a foregone conclusion.

The Clemens (1995) study reveals how the organizational structure of the hospital itself can significantly influence the process followed by departmental staff, with implications for professional autonomy and ethics. Worse yet, the family caregivers felt that their ethnicity had been responded to with a lack of sensitivity by discharge planners, and the discharge planning staff admitted they tended to make less effort to engage family caregivers when they presupposed there might be a language barrier, even though the hospital had foreign language interpreters available (Clemens, 1995:259).

Discharge Planning: Special Needs Categories of Patients

Psychiatric patients. All social workers who work with psychiatric patients with chronic mental illness need to become aware of the difficulties often faced by the families of these patients and to take appropriate steps to try to correct the reported problems. For example, a qualitative study of thirty-four such families found that most felt they were not provided with enough information by the hospital prior to discharge of patients to their care, that there was a lack of follow up by the hospital or mental health center, a lack of immediate service available when needed, and a lack of help in getting the patient to follow through with referrals to outpatient community services (Hanson and Rapp, 1992). The families' overall complaints suggest that hospitals are perceived as "dumping on families" through their discharge-planning procedures; this resembles some other study findings reported in this chapter of family members' perceptions of elderly patients concerning the discharge-planning process.

Dementia patients. Another increasingly common and difficult discharge-planning situation is that of elderly patients with dementia. Cummings (1999) examined the cases of 131 hospitalized patients with a diagnosis of dementia who were discharged within a seven-month period. Data were collected on a wide range of variables and examined both descriptively and via correlation and multivariate analysis. The findings indicated that having been transferred to a care facility not specializing in dementia patient care was the one variable that explained the most variance in outcome and was most likely to predict rehospitalization. Other significant predictor variables were (1) family caregiver did not accept the patient's diagnosis and degree of functional impairment; (2) family caregiver lacked caregiver support; (3) caregiver lacked needed resources; and (4) patient had a longer length of stay in the hospital prior to discharge. Presumably the last variable is a marker for patients requiring more extensive care, and whose aftercare is likely to continue to be extensive. This study highlights the need for further similar studies whose findings could serve as predictors of discharge-planning outcome for various categories of patients, thus helping to develop a science of discharge planning.

Coronary artery bypass graft patients. Ben-Zur and colleagues (2000) reported a study, also conducted in Israel, to examine discharged patients who were within two to twenty months of having had coronary artery bypass graft (CABG) surgery. The purpose was threefold: (1) to assess compliance with their rehabilitation program; (2) to assess their level of emotional functioning in terms of anxiety, pessimism/optimism, and coping strategies; and (3) to compare their level of emotional function with a comparison group drawn from the community who had not had CABG surgery (to establish a baseline for emotional functioning without the surgery factor).

The goal was to determine whether persons who have undergone such surgery tend to have higher levels of emotional distress than persons who have not had the surgery, and to determine whether the post-CABG surgery patients' level of physical functioning, prescribed for their rehabilitation, is correlated with their emotional functioning. The results of the study indicated that, in general, the postsurgery patients had significantly higher levels of emotional distress, and their level of distress was inversely associated with their level of functioning required for their rehabilitation. The postsurgery patients who did better in terms of their recovery and rehabilitation tended to rely more on problem-focused coping strategies and to have lower levels of distress as compared to those who were less compliant and were not functioning as well who tended to rely on emotion-focused coping strategies.

The study investigators (Rappaport, a medical social worker; Ammar, a physician and surgeon; Uretzky, a physician and surgeon; and Ben-Zur, a psychologist and lecturer at a school of social work) recommend the development of intervention procedures for medical social workers to offer to persons who are in various stages of diagnosis, treatment, and recovery from CABG surgery to teach them effective coping strategies, using such cognitive and behavioral techniques as

1. providing needed *patient information* that is both positive and believable, directed toward patient empowerment, such as what patients can do to positively impact their chances for a successful recovery;
2. implementing short-term intervention programs using cognitive and behavioral interventions, such as relaxation and cognitive coping strategies (e.g., consciously reminding oneself of certain positive and empowering thoughts or images), which also serve to increase the patient's sense of control; and
3. encouraging patient participation in social support groups, which have been shown to make positive contributions to patient length and quality of life and capacity for changes in health behavior to enhance QOL.

Congestive heart failure patients. A recent study (Proctor et al., 2000) found that quality of home care after hospital discharge was associated with whether patients were readmitted to the hospital. More specifically, they found that to obtain appropriate and adequate home care, it was necessary to do a thorough functional assessment in the hospital to identify specifically what the patient could and could not do without assistance in terms of activities of daily living (ADLs), such as bathing, dressing, grooming, toileting, eating, and ambulating and in terms of skilled nursing tasks, and to identify specifically what the formal and/or informal caregivers could and would do. Areas of special need include proper diet for congestive heart failure (CHF), proper intake of prescribed medications, and prescribed activity level maintenance.

Incidentally, some health maintenance organizations have employed nursing staff to telephone CHF patients on a regular basis to monitor their compliance with prescribed care and to check certain physical indicators, such as blood pressure and edema (tissue swelling from fluid retention), in an effort to prevent avoidable rehospitalizations, which are costly.

The Challenge of Discharge Planning

Many patients are considered ready for discharge and accordingly referred to hospital social workers and other discharge planners even though one or more of the following conditions exist:

- The patient may be insufficiently recovered from the acute health condition to take care of himself or herself.
- The patient may be mentally confused, emotionally depressed, or otherwise mentally impaired, permanently or temporarily.
- The patient may need oxygen, an indwelling catheter that requires irrigating and changing, assistance with eating, dressing, walking, bathing, toileting, and so forth.
- The patient may have a new baby with special problems but has never cared for an infant before.
- The patient now has a seizure disorder and his or her family has never seen a grand mal seizure before.
- The patient has been advised not to climb stairs, but lives in a second-floor apartment with no elevator access.
- The patient has AIDS and the family has not yet been informed.
- The patient is a young man, now permanently paralyzed from the waist down, and his only family lives in a rural mountain area several hundred miles away.
- The patient is a young mother with several children to care for, but she will be unable to do any lifting for several weeks, and the father is undependable.
- The patient will need to return to the hospital twice a week for an indefinite period of time for kidney dialysis treatments, and he or she has no personal transportation.

These are some examples of the challenge of discharge planning for the social worker or whoever else is assigned the responsibility. It should be evident from these examples that discharge planning requires much more than simply referring the client to a nursing home or home health care agency. The kinds of services often involved in hospital discharge planning include assessment, referrals, planning and coordination, family education, patient education, patient counseling, postdischarge follow up, and family counseling (Oktay et al., 1992:294).

Abramson and colleagues (1993) have concluded from their study of the level of disagreement among the various interested parties in discharge-planning situations that a high level of disagreement is not unusual, but rather the norm. This indicates the need for clinical social work skills in discharge planning to effectively elicit and explore the participants' perspectives and to achieve equitable conflict resolution (62).

Another study (Proctor et al., 1995) of pediatric discharge planning reported that their results also indicate the complexity of the discharge-planing process, which is influenced by family, resources, and teamwork. Nearly all (90 percent) of the 105 cases involved one or more complications, the most common (67 percent) being financial or lack of economic resources to obtain the needed services, largely reflecting the fact that at least thirty million American children have no health insurance, and one-fourth of all children in America live in families with incomes below the official government poverty line (Proctor et al., 1995:9, 15). (Note that the percentage of children living below the poverty line in the United States had declined to 16.9 percent by 1999, the lowest since 1979, according to the U.S. Census Bureau [1999].)

The significance of quality discharge planning to cost savings is indicated by study findings that the earlier the hospital social worker intervention with a patient, the shorter the patient's length of stay (Evans et al., 1989:277; Fillit et al., 1992).

A study (Soskolne and Auslander, 1993) conducted in Israel examined the comparative effect on patient posthospital care services of implementing *discharge-planning protocol training* of hospital social workers. The study found that a significantly higher percentage of patients in the group whose social workers participated in the departmental training program in discharge planning not only received formal home health care services but received them for a longer period of time than the patients served by the social workers before their discharge-planning training.

The importance of interdisciplinary collaboration is underscored by the findings of a study by Feather (1993) of discharge planners from a random sample of all U.S. hospitals to determine their perceptions of the variables determining effective discharge planning. Feather (1993) found that the single most important factor is "cooperation and support from the physician staff of the hospital" (1). Later Feather commented, "if discharge planners have power and clarity, almost any model of discharge planning can be effective, whether the hospital is large or small, rural or urban" (11). Feather suggests that hospital discharge planners focus more on strategies to enhance the understanding and cooperation of physicians and other hospital personnel concerning the discharge-planning function (12).

The Need for Improved Patient and Family Involvement in Decision Making

Coulton (1990) has reviewed the research relating to patient and family involvement in decision making. Her concerns are as follows:

- Patients and families do not always understand what their options are and the implications of each.
- Patients and families may have difficulty focusing on the issues at hand because of anxiety about the health condition.
- Patients and families often have so little time to make important decisions concerning life-sustaining measures or posthospital care that they are unable to think them through adequately.
- Hospital records sometimes indicate a patient's choice about serious matters such as whether or not to resuscitate, with little or no documentation of patient or family involvement in the decision making.
- Several studies have found lack of agreement between the physician, social worker, patient, and family concerning perceptions of the patient's position on such issues.
- There is some evidence that a patient's decisions may be led so that it is questionable whether what is recorded is actually what the patient wants.
- A major problem suggested by study findings on patient and family involvement in decision making is whether their assumptions were accurate, that is, whether they fully understood both the pros and cons of each alternative.
- There also is some evidence that patients prefer a family member they trust to make decisions rather than their physician.
- The outcome for most patients improves the more they perceive that they were adequately involved in decision making concerning themselves.

Elsewhere, Coulton and colleagues (1989) reported that among patients with an *internal locus of control,* posthospital anxiety decreases with an increase in perceived control over the discharge plan.

Abramson (1990), too, has expressed concern about the danger of compromising the social work value of client self-determination and of the primacy of client interests; she reviews the evidence of the importance of feeling in control to well-being, health status, and even survival (54-55). Abramson recommends the social worker offer choices to clients and explore rather than ignore signs of conflict between the key participants, continually advocating for the patients' right to control over decision making concerning their own lives (56).

Advocacy in Hospital Social Work

One Canadian study (Herbert and Levin, 1996) of hospital social workers' perceptions of their own role, including advocacy, found that they reportedly spend the least time on advocacy, compared with assessment, counseling, resource linkage, and consultation/collaboration (71). The same finding was obtained by Oktay and colleagues in a study of Baltimore hospital social work (1992:294). Canadian hospitals are undergoing a similar reorganization process as U.S. hospitals, with similar effects on their social workers. The general consensus among social workers seems to be "don't make waves," which reflects a general sense of disempowerment (Herbert and Levin, 1996:82).

However, Dobrof (1991) commented on the findings of past research on the impact of the DRG system, stating that "[i]t is imperative that the social work profession use its expert advocacy skills to promote both an increase in post-hospital health care resources and to develop mechanisms for financing this care" (50).

Still, Holliman, Dziegielewski, and Datta (2001) reported from their study of tasks performed by social work discharge planners that advocacy (in the sense of efforts to influence decision makers to change policies or laws on behalf of patients or caregivers) was seldom or never done, as reported by about 63 percent of the respondents.

Critical Incident Stress Debriefing (CISD)

In efforts to survive hospital reorganization, downsizing, and demands for evidence of value, some hospital social work departments have found inventive ways to demonstrate their importance to the hospital system. One example of this is described by Spitzer and Neely (1992) and Spitzer and Burke (1993), who played a leadership role in developing a statewide system in Oregon for providing *debriefing* services to providers of emergency services in crisis situations.

The premise is that service providers such as police, firefighters, emergency medical technicians, and emergency room personnel, often suffer personal trauma from their battlefield-like experiences, and need help to release their subsequent feelings, which otherwise can accumulate and cause harm to themselves and others in the form of reactions such as depression, violence, and physical illness.

Spitzer and Neely (1992) describe the six stages in the debriefing process, which lasts about three hours. This is an excellent article that should be read by anyone interested in learning more about how to develop such a stress-debriefing service, which its authors report brought state and national recognition to their hospital social work department and "united local fire, ambulance, clergy, mental health and medical professionals into one of the largest critical stress debriefing teams in the U.S." (56).

Crisis Intervention in the Emergency Room

In 1996, the Task Force on Adolescent Assault Victim Needs of the American Academy of Pediatrics published a model protocol for providers of hospital-based pediatric emergency and trauma care, out of concern for the increase in adolescent victims of violent assault being seen in hospital emergency departments, often attended by personnel with a lack of understanding of how to deal with the psychosocial aspects of such situations. The protocol includes specific steps for social workers, pediatric psychologists, and psychiatrists to follow, such as critical incident stress debriefing (CISD) for the victim and family, if needed; evaluating the circumstances of the assault; evaluating the victim's psychological functioning before the injury and his or her response to the incident; arranging for follow-up mental health services, if needed; assisting the family with discharge planning (which may include a change of residence and/or schools); ongoing supportive assistance to the victim and family if they are required to identify the assailant or testify in court; and periodic postdischarge assessment of victim and family follow through with needed services and of the status of possible post-traumatic stress disorder (Task Force on Adolescent Assault Victim Needs, 1996:998).

Bloch (1996) has written about her experience as chief of clinical social work services in the emergency department of a large urban medical center in terms of how the social worker can help family members when the patient is critically ill or injured, likely to die, and does die in the emergency room. Bloch (1996) stresses the importance of providing these families with a special room in which to wait, of keeping them informed of medical efforts and the patient status and interpreting the condition to them, and of the social worker remaining when the physician enters and provides a brief review of what has happened, concluding with a simple but gentle statement informing the family of the death. Bloch (1996) also shares what she has learned from experience about such issues as the family viewing the body, initiating discussion of organ and tissue donation, a coroner exam or autopsy by the hospital, the funeral arrangements, and care of the closest or most distressed family survivor.

Other common social work services in hospital emergency departments include brief counseling and referral and resource finding for patients and families with such presenting problems as attempted or threatened suicide, child abuse, domestic violence, chemical dependency, acute psychiatric problem behavior, rape, assault and battery, and homelessness. Such social work services can be cost effective for the hospital (Ponto and Berg, 1992) and more effective for the patients, who otherwise tend to keep coming back because, without social work intervention in such cases, the underlying psychosocial problems often are not addressed by medical personnel (Keehn, Roglitz, and Bowden, 1994).

Another group of people who tend to use hospital emergency department medical services inappropriately, who can be more effectively and efficiently helped by social workers instead, consists of certain elderly people who tend to seek help for physical complaints when the problem is a mental health one and those with chronic health problems in acute episodes because of noncompliance associated with psychosocial problems (McCoy, Kipp, and Ahern, 1992). Social work intervention can reduce repeat utilization of this sort.

Hospital emergency departments are excellent places for social work students to obtain training in the assessment, treatment, and disposition of patients with psychiatric problems (Walsh, 1985).

Other Hospital Social Worker Functions

Elder abuse. Of course, many patients with psychosocial problems who are first seen in the emergency room are subsequently admitted to inpatient care and seen by social workers assigned to special medical or surgical units, as a result of high-risk screening systems or referrals to social work. Elder abuse is another problem that may be increasing, as a result, perhaps, of both the growth of the elderly population and the shortened hospital stays and increased burden on family members to provide personal care services to sometimes severely impaired family members. Such situations are an example of the need for collaboration between the medical and social work staff of hospitals (Hazard, 1995).

Child sexual abuse. Child sexual abuse is another psychosocial problem that is sometimes identified among pediatric patients in hospitals. Dubowitz,

Black, and Harrington (1992) reported the findings of a study to determine which types of evidence collected by an interdisciplinary team, including a pediatrician, child psychologist, and pediatric social worker, best helped to diagnose child sexual abuse. The results indicated that the child's disclosure of having been sexually abused and positive physical examination findings most influenced team members' conclusion, whereas sexualized behavior of the child, somatic problems, and the child's response to the physical exam did not contribute (688), as these may be indicative of life experiences other than sexual abuse. In this study,

> The [hospital] social worker assessment included a history of the alleged abuse, the family's response to the allegation, the involvement of public agencies, and sources of support to the family. In addition, the social worker assessed the functioning of the family, parental concerns regarding the child, and access to services. (1992:689)

KNOWLEDGE REQUIREMENTS

Specific Client Populations and Problems

Hospital social workers need knowledge concerning the medical and social implications of specific health conditions, in terms of their prognosis and treatment and probable psychosocial problems, appropriate resources to address the needs, and information about how to access them (Rauch and Schreiber, 1985:215; Ross, 1993:244-245).

Fahs and Wade (1996) found that AIDS patients significantly benefit from being hospitalized in specialized units with an interdisciplinary team having expertise regarding this health condition. This team should include a social worker with specialized knowledge and skills who can facilitate discharge planning through knowledge of specialized resources (29). Furthermore, Beckerman and Rock (1996), through a survey of hospital social workers who specialize in working with AIDS patients, found that some common themes emerge from their experience, pointing both to the challenges and rewards of their work. One of the reported rewards is that the interdisciplinary team tends to become more mutually supportive and cooperative than usual in hospitals, apparently as a result of the emotional intensity of the shared experience (86).

The hospital social worker also needs to have knowledge of "response patterns of particular ethnic and cultural groups and be able to intervene with them appropriately" (Ross, 1995:1373).

The Organizational Setting

In addition, hospital social workers need to understand the cultures, roles, and functions of other professionals in the setting and how to work collaboratively with them; they must have mastery of the vocabulary of the health care world and know the community resources for various types of health problems and how to access them (Rauch and Schreiber, 1985:215).

Community Resources

Having knowledge of community resources is more than knowing which resources exist for which particular need; it is also important to develop and continually strive to update more intimate knowledge of the *quality* of such resources, such as nursing homes, home care agencies, and medical aids and appliances providers. Hospital social workers who link clients with such resources need to visit these places (Dobrof, 1991:51), get to know the people who work in them, and do follow-up studies of referred clients. Such studies should include asking patients and family members their opinions on the quality of the services they received, in terms of timeliness, interpersonal treatment, the condition of physical equipment, and the competence of the personnel.

Nursing homes and home health care agencies presumably receive a sizable portion of their intake of new patients from referrals by hospital social workers. Thus, to improve the quality and timeliness of the care services of these community resources, hospital social workers could not only telephone patients and/or family members to follow up but also make home visits for this purpose. This could have a positive public relations effect for the hospital and serve as a stimulus to the aftercare service providers to do better. Continuity of care, a common term in health care social work, implies that the patient and family may benefit from a sense that they are not simply shifted from one level of care to another but progress along links between them. (People need to feel respected and cared about to maximize their potential comfort and function.)

Intervention Modalities

Since discharge planning is often central to the hospital social worker role, it is essential that hospital social workers understand what is involved in effective and efficient discharge planning and recognize that it is not simply a concrete service, but one requiring considerable clinical skill (Donnelly, 1992:108). Rauch and Schreiber (1985) present a framework for training in discharge planning that is directed toward demonstrating its clinical aspects.

Needed Research, Evaluation, and Documentation

Ross (1995) argues that hospital social workers need to have a sufficient grasp of existing knowledge in a particular area to plan and conduct research for knowledge development (1373-1374).

As has been noted elsewhere in this book, the current focal interests in the field of health services research are *outcomes and effectiveness* (Marcus, 1990). That is, cost effectiveness continues to be the name of the game, and social work research in health care needs to continue to improve its management information systems, which are essential sources of research data, and also continue to improve its research quality, attending especially to issues of external validity (generalizability of findings) and instrument reliability (consistency of results obtained with the instrument) (84).

Hospital social workers must learn what is required of them in terms of documentation of their work for use by other health professionals in the setting, for Medicare and Medicaid reimbursement purposes, and for quality assurance and peer review purposes. Clearly, if social work is to survive and achieve its potential in the hospital setting, it must demonstrate that it is cost effective—that the cost of the services it provides is considerably less than what the hospital saves as a result of what the social workers do. This is often measured in terms of timely discharge planning, but it could also be measured in terms of avoiding relapses and rehospitalizations. Thus, some hospital social work programs are now offering *crisis lines and case management services* to patients in home care, often with family caregivers, who encounter dilemmas and crises with which they need timely intervention as well as *outpatient support groups,* to provide needed information and self-care training, to enhance emotional well-being, and to encourage positive health behavior modification.

Social work has tended to take the position that it cannot ethically apply experimental design research to the practice issues it seeks to answer in terms of comparative outcomes. Why we should think that our issues are more critical than those confronted by physicians, nurses, psychologists, and other professions is puzzling. If we are currently using a particular approach and do not know whether an alternative approach might be more or less effective, all we need to do is randomly assign our clients to the "usual" and the "alternate" and then compare the results. This is, in fact, the only way we will be able to develop a scientific body of practice knowledge that will enhance our credibility and influence with other professional groups.

Furthermore, the use of experimental design is the only way that hospital social work can demonstrate its cost effectiveness. If what we do, or might do, matters, we must demonstrate that by testing it against an alternate approach, which need not be "no intervention," but rather the "usual intervention."

The Need for Outcomes Research

The Bartlett and Baum (1995) follow-up study of hospital patients discharged by hospital social workers to nursing homes implies the importance of social workers evaluating their practice and provides a brief interview guide to use in follow-up phone interviews to assess discharge outcomes. The wide variation in outcome raises questions about their determinants. Did they get the services they needed? Were they satisfied with their placements? They found that of 136 patients followed up, 28 percent were still in the nursing home, 23 percent had died, 21 percent were readmitted to the hospital, 12 percent were excluded for reasons of missing data or unusable data, 10 percent had been discharged from the nursing home, and 6 percent were transferred elsewhere (75).

Still another study (Travis, Moore, and McAuley, 1991) examined the social work records of 480 discharged patients and found that 84 percent of the total returned home after discharge, 11.5 percent went to institutional placements, and the remainder died before they could be discharged. What these studies do not tell us is which variables may be predictors of the outcome of patient discharge arrangements.

Practice Experience in Knowledge Development

Ideally, future hospital social workers should have a field placement in a hospital in order to enhance their experience and desire to remain in hospital social work. Showers (1992) found five aspects of field practicum in which students' satisfaction with their field placement was most predictive:

1. satisfaction with the supervisory relationship was most predictive of satisfaction with the field instructor;
2. supervisory teaching was most predictive of satisfaction with the learning experience;
3. variety of opportunities was most predictive of satisfaction with the program;
4. stress level was most predictive of satisfaction with the hospital; and
5. the level of field program organization and coordination between field instructors was found most predictive of the overall fieldwork experience. (31)

In relation to the third area identified, another study (Cuzzi et al., 1996) also found that social work students who experienced three rotations during their hospital field placement reported greater satisfaction with their experience than a control group of social work students who remained on the same medical or surgical service throughout their placement. Cuzzi and colleagues (1996) attribute this finding to the fact that hospital social workers today have more diverse caseloads and the profession needs "expert generic social work practitioners" (76).

The University of Iowa School of Social Work has developed an innovative approach to teaching practice research skills to MSW students in an advanced research methods course. It involves giving students the option of doing a research practicum at a local medical center where they would work closely with a social work practitioner in health care. The union of student and practitioner proved productive for both, as the practitioner could identify issues for practice research while the student had the research skills to design an appropriate study (Hall et al., 1996).

Holliman, Dziegielewski, and Datta (2001), based on their 1997-1998 study of hospital social work discharge planners, recommend that since hospital social work, now more than ever, revolves around discharge planning, which is largely carried out with little supervision, and consists predominately of generalist social work functions that require considerable skill in interaction and working cooperatively with other health care professionals, that "courses and field preparation for these workers should maximize independence and autonomy" (15), and that "these findings support advanced generalist preparation and the interdisciplinary/multidisciplinary nature of current discharge planning activities (14). The four main skills and types of training the social work respondents identified as key to their work were: (1) communication skills (writing, public speaking, listening, reading nonverbal behaviors, assertiveness, and motivational techniques); (2) knowledge of community resources; (3) social assessment skills (including financial assessments); and (4) field experience and continuing education.

VALUES AND ETHICS CONSIDERATIONS

Foster and colleagues (1993) surveyed 255 hospital social workers concerning how they deal with certain ethical dilemmas in practice and what they perceive as their needs for training in bioethics. They found that most social workers felt well prepared to deal with ethical issues in practice situations, but still expressed a desire for more training, particularly concerning the rationing of health care.

Foster and colleagues (1993) note that although rationing of health care is associated with such issues as who will and will not receive organ transplants and other high-cost procedures, such rationing is, in fact, also involved in social work high-risk screening and discharge planning in the sense that the process of selecting certain patients for service implies an exclusion of others. In addition, discharge-planning decisions clearly involve rationing, as determined by reimbursement policies of public and private health insurance as well as out-of-pocket financial resources of clients. For example, Morrow-Howell and Proctor (1994), in their study of the determinants of hospital discharge-planning destination, reported that patients with Medicaid coverage were eleven times more likely to be discharged to a nursing home (493).

Abramson (1996) explores four alternative approaches to ethical understanding in social work, which she labels (1) the principles approach, (2) virtue ethics, (3) feminist ethics, and (4) Afrocentricity. Abramson (1996) presents the principles approach as rooted in the false notion that there is consensus about the relative importance of underlying values or principles that can be discerned dispassionately. In comparison, virtue ethics revolves around efforts to discern and weigh the underlying motivations of the players. Feminist ethics, the third approach, takes a variety of forms revolving around combating oppression at both the micro and macro levels. Finally, Afrocentricity is depicted as reflecting concern for the well-being of the family and community and for past and future generations, as well as respect for human feelings and dignity.

Abramson (1996) reminds us that an emerging trend today is to have a more flexible and receptive attitude toward alternative *paradigms* (worldviews). This can serve to enrich and sensitize health care social workers' capacity for relatedness to diverse human dilemmas in today's health care environment, which can be fraught with glib rationalizations for unethical actions.

Although the Clemens (1995) study discussed earlier under Discharge Planning is only one small study, which may in no way be considered representative, the fact that the reported findings occur at all supports the concern that professional social work ethics are at risk in hospital practice. Judith Ross (1993) asked, "it is imperative that a social work presence in health be sustained, but if it means relinquishing our commitment to the profession and to social work values, principles, and goals, is the expense too great?" (244). Dobrof (1991) also has expressed concern about the possible negative impact of the DRG system on the role and satisfaction of the hospital social worker and on the well-being of the discharged patient and his or her family, whose right to self-determination may be seriously compromised by the pressures of cost containment (46).

Landau (2000a) recently reported her interesting study of ethical issues in hospital social work conducted in Israel. She examined the professional experience of fourteen directors of hospital social work and eighteen line hospital social workers by having them identify the most frequent types of ethical dilemmas they encounter, rank them in the order of their importance, and indicate how they go about resolving them. Most surprising was that the two groups identified the same basic dilemmas but ranked their importance in reverse order. The online social workers tended to be most troubled about conflicts between their own personal or professional values and ethics and those of the client, family, physician, or hospital policy, which they related to concrete case situations, while the directors seemed to have a more abstract approach and concern for ultimate issues of life and death. All agreed that ethical dilemmas in hospitals are appropriately resolved through a multidisciplinary team approach, but they lacked protocols for addressing ethical dilemmas. Landau (2000a) suggested that it could be helpful for hospital social workers to document the ethical dilemma resolution procedures they follow, including a detailed accounting of how they resolved them (a sort of "process recording"), which could eventually lead to the development of protocols for future staff and for teaching and training purposes.

Commenting on other findings of her study (Landau, 2000b), the author reports that "they imply that in order to gain more power and be accepted as equal partners on multidisciplinary ethics teams, hospital social workers should improve their communication skills when interacting with representatives of other health care professions" (75). This report notes that the ward social workers who participate in interdisciplinary (ID) team decision making, sometimes involving ethical decisions, sense that they lack status on these teams. It also suggests that other professional groups do not always perceive the social workers' qualifications as the social workers themselves perceive them. This seems to be partly a by-product of an increased rivalry in recent years between social workers and nurses for control of the psychosocial turf arena, and partly a lack of social worker skill in clarifying to nurses and others their own perceived role. At the same time, the report acknowledges that the nurses and other team members appear to hold the social work directors in higher regard than the line social workers and attributes this to the social work directors communicating greater respect for the nurses and other team members. In other words, the sense of insecurity of the online social workers may cause them to interact more competitively, thereby antagonizing the nurses. Perhaps this is the case, but it may be recalled that short-term, acute-care hospitals tend to be patriarchal and competitive, both within and between professions and disciplines, reflecting perhaps status-conscious personnel in a place where social status is highly valued. This necessarily leads to considerable political interaction. The earlier discussion in this chapter on interdisciplinary teamwork speaks, I think, to the experience of the online social workers who reported frustration in their efforts to gain an appropriate foothold on their multidisciplinary teams that dealt with ethical issues. In short, growing evidence suggests that various health professions have overlapping concepts of their areas of expertise, especially when it comes to the psychosocial arena.

End-of-life decision making plays a prominent role in ethical decision making. Csikai and Bass (2000) conducted a study of NASW members to determine the extent to which they were aware of the NASW policy statement issued in 1996 titled "Client Self-Determination and End of Life Decisions," which highlights the right of clients to self-determination concerning their end-of-life care, as well as their own and their families' rights to be made aware of all options. The study was conducted to assist NASW in assessing the extent to which social workers know of the policy and accept its major assertions. It is anticipated that the study findings will contribute to NASW development of practice guidelines to assist social workers in end-of-life case situations. Such situations frequently revolve around health conditions and issues of when life begins and ends, especially in relation to its quality, in addition to such issues as truth telling, confidentiality, health care rationing, client competency, and requests for euthanasia and assisted suicide. Additional competing issues may include questions of money, suffering, and fear of the clients' wishes being disregarded.

The Csikai and Bass (2000) study findings indicate that the respondents, who all were social workers with at least some experience with client end-of-life decision making, *shared very similar views on the situations that most contributed to ethical dilemmas in end-of-life decisions.* These included, in the following order:

1. lack of advance directive,
2. not sure if client is competent to decide,
3. patient and family had never discussed the patient's wishes,
4. the patient and doctor had never discussed the patient's wishes,
5. patient and family disagree about it,
6. not clear about what constitutes an "advance directive,"
7. promotion of self-determination,
8. the patient does not clearly grasp the implications of treatment versus nontreatment,
9. lack of resources in the home for end-of-life care,
10. patient/family disagree with the health care providers,
11. lack of adequate coverage under managed care,
12. confidentiality issues,
13. patient wants information about assisted suicide. (11)

Surprisingly, however, even among the social workers who said they worked more than half their time with end-of-life issues, none was familiar with the NASW policy (Csikai and Bass, 2000:12). Twenty-seven percent of all fifty-nine participating social workers had no knowledge of the policy.

Respondents also agreed on ten activities that they viewed as "very important" for social workers to attend to in end-of-life care situations:

1. Promote the client's right to self-determination in the matter.
2. Serve as a liaison between patient, family, and health care providers.
3. Provide ongoing support.
4. Help the client identify his or her end-of-life options.
5. Serve as a liaison between patient and family.
6. Encourage the family's and friends' involvement in decisions.
7. Connect patient and/or family to other health care providers if they express discomfort in discussing end-of-life issues with the social worker.
8. Be open to discussing with the patient whatever he or she wishes to discuss, including assisted suicide.
9. Examine one's personal values concerning end-of-life issues.
10. Be open to discussing all available options, regardless of one's personal views. (Csikai and Bass, 2000:13)

Also, unfortunately, about one-half of the respondents indicated that in their formal social work education they had not experienced exposure to ethics and ethical decision making throughout the curriculum, as the CSWE requires.

Another recent study (Baker, 2000) found that a large majority (82 percent) of over 300 health care social workers in Ohio indicated they were fairly familiar with advance directives, such as the Durable Power of Attorney for Health Care Form and The Living Will (Directive to Withhold or Provide Treatment) Form. In addition, nearly all of them (98 percent) expressed positive attitudes about advance directives. Two multiple regressions were done: knowledge scores were regressed on four variables—age, years worked with elderly clients, years worked in social work, and primary work setting—and attitude was regressed on the same four variables. Number of years worked with the elderly was found to be a significant determinant of level of knowledge of advance directives, while primary work setting was found to be a significant determinant of attitude toward advance directives. Baker (2000) recommends:

Health care social workers can continue to encourage competent adults of all ages to consider the options contained in advance directives and to exercise their right to self-determination by: 1) educating individuals and families about advance directives whenever the opportunity arises; 2) facilitating open discussion between individuals, families, friends, and other allied health professionals around proxy appointments and related concerns; 3) incorporating discussion of advance directives into the routine psychosocial assessment process, in health care settings, as a means of opening conversation around important end-of-life matters. (72)

In the end, professional ethics may already be compromised when external factors such as reimbursement policies limit decision making based on client needs and preferences.

Causes of Ethical Dilemmas in End-of-Life Decision Making

1. Patient lacks advance directive.
2. Social worker unsure if client is competent to decide.
3. Patient and family have never discussed the patient's wishes.
4. Patient and doctor have never discussed the patient's wishes.
5. Patient and family disagree about it.
6. Social worker is not clear about what constitutes an "advance directive."
7. Social worker is conflicted regarding promotion of self-determination.
8. Patient does not clearly grasp the implications of treatment versus nontreatment.
9. Patient lacks resources in the home for end-of-life care.
10. Patient and/or family members disagree with the health care providers.
11. Patient lacks adequate coverage under managed care.
12. Confidentiality issues exist.
13. Patient wants information about assisted suicide. (Csikai and Bass, 2000:11)

SKILL REQUIREMENTS

Bennett, Legon, and Zilberfein (1989) have suggested that hospital social workers try to counteract the potentially negative effects of aggressive discharge planning by exercising greater empathy with clients. They regard this as a skill that can be developed with supervisor assistance in heightening worker self-awareness and understanding of the client's position concerning discharge-planning preferences.

However, consideration should perhaps be given to the possibility that a profession may be better off not to continue in certain settings when conditions there prevent them from practicing in accordance with their professional knowledge and/or their professional values and ethics. Even if social work does not survive in hospital settings, it may be that it could be more appropriately utilized elsewhere in health care. For example, Ross (1993) proposed that as hospitals reduce length of stay and inpatient acute care, they will increasingly compete for survival with providers of other levels of care, such as primary care and prevention, where social work may fit very well:

> Relationship building and counseling and communication skills that are integral to our work should be appreciated in primary care and health prevention and could contribute to developing consumer-oriented strategies beyond the current conception and practice as competition for patients intensifies. Understanding of and ability to negotiate systems will help position social workers to assume new roles and new assignments. (Ross, 1993:246)

HELPING INTERVENTIONS

Among the many available interventions for social workers to use in their work in hospitals are screening and case finding, crisis intervention, psychosocial assessment and intervention planning, brief counseling, bereavement services, discharge planning, postdischarge follow-up and outreach, group work, emergency services through on-call programs, documentation and record keeping, and collaboration (Ross, 1995).

Case Management

According to Naleppa and Reid (2000), "[m]ore and more hospitals integrate case management into the practice functions of hospital social work and nursing." This three-part model includes (1) a case management model, (2) a task-centered model, and (3) a modular treatment model. The case management part is described as contributing the "structure of case management core functions," while the task-centered part is described as adding "clearly described and structured intervention strategies that aided case manager and client," and the modular treatment part is described as adding "task plans (modules) for typical problems encountered by elderly clients in case management" (2000:3). This third part appears to consist of suggested, but flexible, protocols for dealing with specific types of problem situations.

As with most of what hospital social workers do, the cost-control rationale for this particular service is prevention of unnecessary rehospitalization. At the same time, the program apparently provides helpful services that assist clients and families to sustain function and comfort in the community. This is achieved through intervening early when needs arise and troubleshooting problems that otherwise could become compounded. This particular case management program focuses on elderly patients living in the community and is provided by three MSW social workers, who meet weekly with an interdisciplinary team of nurses, discharge planners, home health care workers, and physicians on an as-needed basis. The program is also assisted by a professional ethics committee. Referrals come from hospitals, community agencies, physicians in the community, and other clients.

Group Work

In addition to those interventions discussed earlier in the section Social Worker Functions, Glassman (1991) reminds us of the varied uses of social group work in health care settings and of its special healing potential, such as self-help, mutual support, education, coping with crises, self-esteem and empowerment building, and family and significant other support development, as well as being a medium for interdisciplinary teamwork through co-leadership or rotating leadership of group sessions.

Hanson and colleagues (1994) found that hospital inpatients being treated for alcoholism were significantly more likely to follow through with outpatient support group participation and to have lower rates of recidivism if they began their participation in such a support group with other recovering alcoholics prior to hospital discharge, thereby facilitating the transition from inpatient to outpatient status.

Perhaps the most common use of social group work in the hospital setting is to help victims of certain health problems learn more about their condition and how to cope with it, to ease unnecessary anxiety that stems from misinformation, to increase their sense of control, and to reduce social isolation and increase social support from others with whom they can identify. Thus, such social group work in hospitals is often addressed to a small group of patients and/or family members who share a common health problem. One such group work experience was reported by Posen et al. (2000). They described a twelve-session psychoeducational support group held for sixteen women with early onset Parkinson's disease. The program design aimed both to address feelings and attitudes about their condition and to provide needed information to enhance coping with their disease. This report is a classic description of the pervasive impact of a disease on a person's self-image, relationships with significant others, and sense of control, as well as the beneficial nature of social group work with victims of health problems, evidenced by these women meeting even after the formal group sessions had ended, and then requesting a continuation of the formal sessions.

Innovative Interventions

Gentry (1993) has reported on an innovative service provided by a hospital in Philadelphia. The service came about as a result of a growing problem of boarder babies, or newborns in fragile health as a result of prematurity and/or alcohol and drug absorption in utero. The babies' parents are generally unable or unwilling to assume responsibility for their care, so these babies remain in the hospital for a prolonged period of time. When the local child placement agencies were unable to rapidly find foster homes for the infants, hospital employees began to inquire about whether they might serve as foster parents. The social work department discovered that it was able to expedite the placement process by providing an information and referral service to the employees concerning the procedure for applying to become a certified foster parent (Gentry, 1993).

COMMENTARY

One cannot read the hospital social work literature today without sensing a sort of desperation and determination to do whatever it takes to hold on. As suggested by Ross (1993), the profession needs to examine the alternative to continued practice in some of the current settings of social work in health care and consider refusing to practice in settings which force us to compromise our values and ethics in order to retain our positions.

Chapter 5

Social Work
in Home Health Care/Home Care

HISTORICAL BACKGROUND

The Concept of Home Care

The term *home care* is used here as an umbrella concept to include both home health services that provide skilled services, such as nursing, physical therapy, and speech therapy, and the so-called unskilled services, such as homemaker, chore, and personal care services, that provide assistance with *activities of daily living* (ADLs). As the NASW Standards for Social Work in Health Care Settings state:

> [H]ome care cannot be viewed as only medical service. Home health care includes an array of services—nursing, rehabilitative therapies, social work, personal care, homemaking—to aid the individual in achieving and sustaining the highest level of health, activity, and independence.* (NASW, 1987:27)

In the literature, the terms home health care (HHC) and home care are sometimes used interchangeably, sometimes to refer to distinct types of services, and sometimes to refer to home health care as a subdivision of home care, the use employed here.

The Growth and Development of Home Care

The home was the original location of most health care, which was provided by family, friends, and neighbors with the support and supervision of a physician who visited occasionally.

---

*Copyright 1995, National Association of Social Workers, Inc., NASW Standards for Social Work in Health Care Settings.

Beginning in the latter half of the 1800s, voluntary, nonprofit agencies, such as visiting nurse organizations, began to provide *formal home care services* (i.e., other than family or friend provided) in the form of maternal and child care (Balinsky, 1994:1). The concept of home-visiting nurses was the forerunner of public health nursing, now called community health nursing, and preceded what we now call home health care (Clemen-Stone, Eigsti, and McGuire, 1987:8). The first Visiting Nurse Association was organized in Buffalo, New York, in 1885, and many others soon emerged around the United States and continue today to be significant providers of home health care (158). The VNA provides about 14 percent of all home health care services in urban areas and 5 percent in rural areas (Kenney, 1993).

Public health nursing has its roots in the early work of a leader in the history of nursing and social work, Lillian D. Wald, who founded the Henry Street Settlement House in New York City in 1893 (Clemen-Stone, Eigsti, and McGuire, 1987:9-10). However, the concept of public health nursing originally was not associated with government funding or service; only later was it gradually adopted by cities, states, and finally the federal government as, appropriately, a public tax-supported service (14-15).

Public health nursing, as well as social work, emerged in response to the multiple social and health problems of the latter half of the 1800s that accompanied industrialization, urbanization, and immigration in America. Infant and maternal mortality and contagious and infectious disease were rampant as a result of the social change of the period (Clemen-Stone, Eigsti, and McGuire, 1987:14).

Historically, although private, nonprofit nursing agencies could provide hands-on care, such as changing dressings and catheters and bathing patients, the public health nurses were legally required to confine their interventions to supervision, instruction, and monitoring communicable disease functions. Today, both types of agencies provide hands-on care through their home health care services.

Around the beginning of the twentieth century, the seat of health care shifted from the home to the hospital (Cannon, 1923). Now, as we enter the twenty-first century, the trend is toward moving health care back to the home and community (Balinsky, 1994:1; Simmons, 1994). In 1955, the U.S. Public Health Service endorsed the physician-oriented home care program, designed to provide medical and social services to patients at home through a professional group minimally composed of a physician, nurse, and social worker (NASW, 1987:27).

The Growth of the Proprietary Sector in Home Care

Although the first hospital-based home care service was established in New York City in 1947 at Montefiore Hospital (Balinsky, 1994:1; Blazer,

1988), as of 1967 there were only 133 hospital-based home care agencies and no proprietary freestanding home care agencies (Balinsky, 1994:2). After Title XVIII (Medicare) and Title XIX (Medicaid) were enacted by Congress in 1965, proprietary (for-profit) home care programs began to increase gradually, to a total of forty-seven in 1975 and 186 in 1980 (National Association for Home Care [NAHC], 2000:2).

Still, until about 1985, formal home health care services were largely provided by nonprofit organizations, such as the Visiting Nurse Association (VNA), and public agencies, such as public health departments. In fact, as of 1980, public health departments were the major providers of home health care services, the VNA was next, and other nonprofit HHC agencies were third (NAHC, 2000:2).

Remarkably, by 1985, proprietary home care agencies had become the most frequent type of home care agency and continue to retain that status today. Presumably, this sudden increase by more than tenfold between 1980 and 1985 reflected the introduction of the hospital prospective payment system in 1984, which resulted in significant reductions in length of hospital stays and associated discharges of patients with continuing care needs.

However, the Balanced Budget Act of 1997 (PL105-33) that introduced a prospective payment system into nursing homes also applied to home care organizations. That is, the system of reimbursement changed from a fee for service to a flat rate, based on classification of patient condition and associated needs, including exceptions for cases of unusually high need levels. As a result, reimbursements to Medicare-certified home care agencies decreased significantly and freestanding proprietary agencies declined markedly, from 5,024 to 3,192, or by nearly 37 percent, between 1997 and 1999, and even VNA home care agencies declined from 553 to 452, or 18.3 percent, during that period. In fact, all types of HHC agencies declined in numbers following the reduction in Medicare payments (NAHC, 2000:2). In addition to the reduction in HHC agencies, the NAHC reports that about 500,000 fewer persons received HHC services via Medicare between 1997 and 1998, apparently due to "beneficiary access problems" (NAHC, 2000:7).

By 1999, freestanding proprietary agencies numbered 3,192, or 41.2 percent of all 7,747 Medicare certified home health agencies, while hospital-based home health care agencies numbered 2,300, or nearly 30.0 percent (29.7 percent) of all certified HHC agencies. VNA home health agencies declined to only 452, or 5.8 percent of the total, and public health department home care agencies accounted for only 918, or 11.8 percent of total Medicare-certified home health care agencies in 1999 (NAHC, 2000:2)

Statistical Abstracts of the United States (U.S. Government Printing Office, 2000b:132, Table 205) reports that in 1998, 53.9 percent of all 13,300 home health agencies were proprietary, 36.2 percent were voluntary nonprofit, and the remaining 9.9 percent were government owned. In addition, 84.5 percent of all home health agencies were Medicare certified, and 85.1 percent were Medicaid certified.

Home health care has proved to be one of the lucrative human service alternatives to the reduction of manufacturing in the United States (Karger and Stoesz, 1994:227). (Profit-making enterprises sometimes turned to running health service businesses after the manufacturing sector began to diminish.) Part A of Medicare includes coverage for home health care services under medical supervision, provided that (1) the patient requires *skilled* care (professional nursing services, physical therapy, or speech therapy), (2) the patient is essentially homebound, and (3) the physician certifies that conditions (1) and (2) do exist (Balinsky, 1994:3).

In 1998, $29.3 billion of all national health expenditures in the United States went for revenues to home health care organizations. However, this represents a 4.0 percent reduction since 1997, reflecting the effect of the 1997 Balanced Budget Act. However, until 1996, revenues paid to home care agencies had been increasing at a rate of between 17 percent and 20 percent per year, indicating the urgency of some kind of cost containment action (U.S. Government Printing Office, 2000a:325, Table 118).

Social Work in Home Care

Social work service through Medicare-funded home health care is only provided if the physician orders it on the basis of a need directly related to the medical condition (Balinsky, 1994:3). In 1993, the U.S. Department of Labor (DOL) reported that about 26 percent of social workers employed in all industries were employed in health services, distributed as shown in Table 5.1, which indicates that slightly less than 1 percent of social workers are employed in home health care services.

Whereas Medicare mandates social worker participation in Medicare-certified hospice programs, in home health care, Medicare mandates only that social work services be available if the physician deems them necessary and medically related, which is largely dependent upon the attending nurse informing the physician of such a need, if perceived.

Other Constraints in Home Care Coverage

Home health care through Medicare is not provided twenty-four hours a day. Instead, a family member, friend, or other caregiver must be available. As a result of these restrictions, Medicare only pays for a small part of the home care that exists (Balinsky, 1994:3). Only the very affluent in America who can afford to pay out of pocket for these services receive round-the-

TABLE 5.1. Percentage Distribution of Social Workers Employed in Home Health Care Relative to Other Settings of Health Service

Practice Setting	Percent
Hospitals, public and private	14.13
Health and allied services	5.28
Nursing and personal care services	2.99
Offices of physicians	1.48
Offices of other health practitioners	1.22
Home health care services	.90
Medical and dental laboratories	.01
All health care settings	26.01

Source: Ginsberg, Leon (1995). *The Social Work Almanac* (Second Edition). Washington, DC: NASW Press, 355. Data obtained from U.S. Department of Labor, Bureau of Labor Statistics, November 1993.

clock home health care. Thus, a dual-level system is created, in which the services rendered are determined by individual economic ability rather than need for service (Olson, 1994:30).

The findings of two surveys of home health care agencies conducted in 1986 and 1987 (Binney, Estes, and Ingman, 1990) indicate that medical services had increased most, while social/supportive services were the most commonly requested services that home health care agencies could not provide (761).

Costs and Payers of Home Health Care

In 1998, personal health care expenditures in the United States totaled $1,019.347 billion. Of the total, approximately $29.255 billion was expended in 1998 for HHC, of which $15.515 billion, or 53 percent, was paid by government programs; $6.037 billion, or 20.6 percent, was out of pocket; $4.008 billion, or 13 percent, was private health insurance; and the remaining $3.695 billion, or 12.6 percent, was "other," which includes nonpatient revenues and industrial plants (see Table 5.2) (U.S. Government Printing Office, 2000b:110). Personal health care expenditures combined with costs for administration, construction of medical facilities, and medical research totaled $1,149.100 billion in 1998. This larger figure is referred to as "national health expenditures" (U.S. Government Printing Office, 2000b:108, Table 152).

TABLE 5.2. Home Health Care Expenditures, 1998

Expenditure	Percent
$15.515 billion government funded	53.0
$6.037 billion out of pocket	20.6
$4.008 billion private health insurance	13.0
$3.695 billion "other"	12.6
$29.255 billion total home health expenditures	100.0

Source: U.S. Government Printing Office (2000b), *Statistical Abstracts of the United States,* Washington, DC: Author, 110, Table 156.

In 1998, Medicare expended $12.888 billion for home health care services for persons age sixty-five and over and for persons with disability secondary to end-stage renal disease, while Medicaid expended a total of $2.702 billion for home health care services during that year. Thus, together, Medicare and Medicaid expended about $15.590 billion for home health care in 1998. (Data extracted from various tables do not equal 100 percent when added.)

Medicaid payments for home health services amounted to about 2.0 percent of total payments for all Medicaid paid health care services in 1998, while Medicare payments for home health services amounted to about 7.6 percent of total payments for all Medicare paid health services that year.

When all sources of payment for home health care services are considered—Medicare, Medicaid, other government programs, private health insurance, and out-of-pocket payments—home health care costs constitute about 3 percent (2.869 percent) of all personal health care expenditures in the United States (U.S. Government Printing Office, 2000b:110, Table 156).

Reasons for the Growth of Home Care

Although home health care represents only a small fraction of spending for all personal health care services, it has, until the recent Balanced Budget Act of 1997, been the fastest growing segment of the health services industry in the United States. The reasons for this growth include the following:

1. The aging of the population, especially the *old-old* (people age eighty-five and older) with a high rate of functional disability
2. The shift from acute infectious diseases to *chronic diseases* (incurable but not terminal) as the major health problems

3. Efforts such as the *prospective payment system (PPS)* introduction of *diagnosis-related groups (DRGs)*, initiated in 1983 by Medicare to reduce the use of high-cost hospital services and to reduce the spiraling cost of nursing home care paid for by Medicaid
4. The increase in technology that allows people to be cared for at home in spite of the need for medical equipment such as IVs, catheters, suction machines, portable oxygen, ventilators, and infusion pumps (Balinsky, 1994:9-15; Braus, 1994)
5. The AIDS epidemic (Balinsky, 1994:45-70)
6. The alarming growth in numbers of medically fragile children (Balinsky, 1994:23)
7. The lack of economic access to alternative forms of care, such as nursing home care, for many elderly people
8. The poor quality of nursing homes in the United States, which prompts people to choose home care instead (Garner, 1995:1627; Olson, 1994)
9. By 1993, the transition from using home health care primarily for subacute care of posthospitalization cases to using it to care for chronically ill persons (Welch, Wennberg, and Welch, 1996), making the distinction between normal Medicare-covered acute care and long-term care benefits less clear (Kane et al., 1997)

In 1994, Allen I. Goldberg, president-elect of the American Academy of Home Care Physicians, wrote:

> Home health care is the next frontier of medical practice and is rapidly being explored for its limitless potential opportunities. . . . Explosive growth has occurred in advance of the definition of public policy, determination of social consensus, and the establishment of a scientific foundation for the state of the art practice. (Goldberg, 1994:911)

THEORETICAL PERSPECTIVES

Although not a clear and developed rationale for home health care, the values and objectives reflected in the U.S. home health care system include (1) cost control through the encouragement of family caregiving; (2) elevation of political concessions to the medical profession and the profit-making business sector over concern for the needs and wishes of patients and families or for issues of social justice and humane caring; and (3) perpetuation of a two-level system of health care, dependent on economic status, that determines the appropriateness of service interventions.

Caring

"Ideally however, the objective of home care is to maximize the independent functioning of the client and the caregiver and to maintain the person in the community. All of the assistance provided is focused on ameliorating problems that impede this functioning" (Cox, 1992:180).

Presumably, home care is for patients of any age, when they want to be at home, and when resources are available to adequately provide for their needs there. Most people feel more secure and comfortable at home (Garner, 1995), which, at least theoretically, optimizes their potential sense of well-being and, hence, health status.

Cost Control

In addition, home health care may be less expensive than nursing home care, if family, friends, or neighbors volunteer the basic supportive care services, which are only supplemented by part-time formal home care. As a result, both public and private health insurance programs limit home care to part-time services.

In estimated Medicare charges, the average home care visit cost $93 in 1998, compared to $523 for an average day in a skilled nursing home care facility, or $2,401 for an average day in the hospital (NAHC, 2000:22).

In 1998, total expenditures for HHC from all sources was $29.255 billion, or 33 percent of total expenditures of $87.835 billion from all sources for nursing home care, and 55 percent of the government's share ($53.023 billion) of nursing home care (U.S. Government Printing Office, 2000b: 110, Table 156).

The Medical Model

Home health care in the United States is a prime example of what has been termed "the medicalization of social problems" (Binney, Estes, and Ingman, 1990).

"Home health care is the next frontier of medical practice and is rapidly being explored for its limitless potential opportunities. . . . Explosive growth has occurred in advance of the definition of public policy, determination of social consensus, and the establishment of a scientific foundation for the state of the art practice." (Goldberg, 1994:911)

Although many elderly people do have health problems requiring so-called skilled care, more simply need supportive assistance for functional impairments, such as difficulty ambulating, dressing, bathing, eating, and taking medications as directed. However, this type of care is not reimbursable by Medicare, either in a nursing home or at home, and is only reimbursable by some state Medicaid waiver programs if the person is financially indigent (Cox, 1992).

As a result, elderly or disabled people who require such supportive assistance frequently exhaust their personal economic resources in order to become eligible for Medicaid for the very poor. The United States is the only nation in the world for which the leading cause of personal bankruptcy is health care costs (Garner, 1995:1629).

This medicalization of formal home health care services resulted from an effort, when Medicare was introduced to Congress in the mid-1960s, to make the proposed legislation politically palatable to the American Medical Association, which had long resisted any type of government intervention in health care that appeared to threaten the interests of the medical profession. As a result, home health was proposed as only reimbursable through Medicare if it were recommended as medically necessary and under physician authorization and supervision. "In sum, Medicare and other health policies for the elderly, e.g., Medicaid, from their origin to the present day, reflect medicine's monopoly in the control and management of the care of the aging" (Binney, Estes, and Ingman, 1990:763-764).

HUMAN DIVERSITY RELEVANCE

Significant differences are found among age groups, gender groups, socioeconomic status groups, ethnic groups, rural/urban groups, and so on, in regard to health behavior, illness behavior, and sick-role behavior, and these diversity variables interact with one another, so that group characteristics are not additive (Corin, 1994). In addition, considerable evidence suggests that a sense of empowerment or of being in control plays a significant role in health outcomes (Evans, Barer, and Marmor, 1994), and this seems to be influenced by such things as social supports and being in a culturally integrated, congruent, familiar, and cognitively comfortable environment, one that is rooted in tradition and has status consistency (Corin, 1994). Therefore, to maximize the potential for positive health outcomes, it behooves social workers in the health field to attend to the clients' attitudes, beliefs, customs, and preferences concerning their health care options, which are often influenced by human diversity.

Ethnicity needs to be a major consideration in social work in home health care, since the nonwhite elderly population is expected to increase markedly. In 1990, 86.7 percent of America's population age sixty-five and over was white, but by 2050, this percentage is expected to decrease to 66.9 (U.S. Department of Health and Human Services, National Institute of Health, National Institute on Aging, 1993). Thus, the nonwhite elderly population is expected to increase from about 13 percent in 1990 to about 33 percent by the year 2050. Table 5.3 depicts these expected changes in the ethnic composition of the U.S. population from 1990 to 2050.

Erik Erikson considered cultural identity essential to achieving "ego integrity":

> For he [the older person] knows that an individual life is the accidental coincidence of but one life cycle with but one segment of history; and that for him all human integrity stands or falls with one style of integrity of which he partakes. (Erikson, 1959:98)

> The style of integrity developed by his culture or civilization thus becomes the patrimony of his soul, the seal of his moral paternity of himself. (Erikson, 1956, cited in Giordano, 1992:24)

Ethnic sensitivity is a manifestation of the social work value of individualizing the client. Since the first step in sensitivity to human diversity is becoming aware of the person's differences, ideally, an *ethnic assessment* ought to be part of the psychosocial assessment in health care situations, including home health care. Fandetti and Goldmeier (1988) provide a framework for such an assessment at the micro, mezzo, and macro levels (see Box 5.1).

Three levels of population and program characteristics interact to determine whether geriatric services are equitably used: *appropriateness* to the

TABLE 5.3. Ethnic Distribution of the U.S. Elderly Population, 1990 and 2050

Ethnic Group	1990 (%)	2050 (%)
White	86.7	66.9
Black	7.9	9.6
American Indian	0.3	0.6
Asian	1.4	7.4
Hispanic	3.7	15.5
Total	100.0	100.0

Source: U.S. Department of Health and Human Services, National Institute of Health, National Institute on Aging (1993). *Profiles of America's Elderly: Racial and Ethnic Diversity of America's Elderly Population,* Number 3, November, POP/93-1-8.

health and functional status of the elder; *accessibility* given the social and economic characteristics of the group; and *acceptability* to group-specific norms and expectations (Damon-Rodriguez, Wallace, and Kington, 1994: 55). For example, about one-half of American Indian, Eskimo, and Aleut elderly live in rural areas (Damon-Rodriguez, Wallace, and Kington, 1994: 57), yet formal home health care services often are lacking in rural areas

---

BOX 5.1.
A Multilevel Ethnic Assessment Framework

Micro: The Person

1. Assess the person's cultural orientation: languages spoken, religion professed, and the generation of immigration of the primary client.
2. Evaluate the importance of within-ethnic-group variation affecting the person's orientation.
3. Consider the person's social class membership as a mediating factor.
4. Select ethnically compatible solutions to personal problems.

Mezzo: The Family, Client Group, and Care Provider Team

1. Assess the ethnically based dynamics of the family, client group, and care provider team.
2. Assess the responsiveness of the group or team whose members may themselves reflect different ethnic orientations.
3. Evaluate the importance of such within-ethnic-group variation.
4. Consider class membership as a mediating factor.
5. Select ethnically compatible solutions at the level of family, group, or care provider team.

Macro: The Community, Local and Nonlocal

1. Assess family boundaries with the larger community in intervention and planning.
2. Facilitate community responsiveness to ethnic cultural needs.
3. Be aware of local/state/national policies affecting the integration of the ethnic group.

Source: Fandetti, Donald V. and Goldmeier, John (1988). Social Workers As Culture Mediators in Health Care Settings. *Health and Social Work,* 13 (3):171-179.

(Kenney, 1993), meaning appropriate care may be unobtainable to these ethnic elderly.

One consideration to take into account regarding ethnicity is that poverty rates are higher among all ethnic minority groups of elderly Americans than among white Americans, and many elderly members of ethnic minority groups have no "medigap" insurance to cover the coinsurance and deductibles of Medicare. Thus, formal home health services may be rejected in favor of informal family-provided caregiving, partly because formal services are not economically accessible.

A second consideration in deciding between home care and nursing home care is that most geographical areas of the United States lack ethnic nursing homes. Thus, people who have never been socially intimate with white society are not likely to be comfortable in a nursing home where most everyone else is white, and where the food, language, and decor is *culturally dissonant* to the ethnic patient, that is, not culturally acceptable.

Apart from cultural congruity, some evidence suggests that African-American elderly, for example, have poorer health status than white elderly and that both classism and racism in the health care system play a role in this (Wallace, 1990).

A third consideration in deciding whether to choose home care or a nursing home is ethnic difference in perspective of the optimal way to spend one's later years: European-American elderly people tend to see this as being able to function normally; Chinese-American and African-American elders usually see it as internal contentment and satisfaction; while Spanish Americans usually see optimal old age as being able to enjoy life, to be active, and to be with family (Wallace, 1996).

Aranda (1996) enumerates the main ethnocultural factors that need social work assessment in the process of acquiring the needed information to develop an appropriate care plan (see Box 5.2).

All cultures have traditions concerning family responsibility for the care of dependent family members, especially elderly parents (Mindel and Wright, 1982). It is important for the social worker, during the home care assessment, to explore client and family attitudes and feelings concerning such family responsibility.

The literature indicates consistently that African-American families may underuse services that could enhance the quality of their care (Morrow-Howell et al., 1996). African-American clients and their families are significantly more likely to prefer home care over nursing home care than are white clients and their families. The reasons for this are not yet entirely clear (138). In addition, African-American clients use significantly less formal home health care services and significantly more informal home health care services than white clients after hospital discharge, yet they rate the quality

---

BOX 5.2.
Ethnocultural Factors in Health Care Assessments

- Language
- Norms regarding hierarchical relationships
- Cultural presentation of symptoms
- Cultural views on mental illness
- Appraisals of cognitive decline and "loss of faculties"
- Reactivity to or tolerance of cognitive decline and personality changes
- Coping styles and behaviors
- Informal social networks
- Caregiving norms
- Biomedical history
- Death and dying

Source: Aranda, Maria P. (1996). *Implications of Diversity for Practice.* Presented at the California Geriatric Education Center, Cultural Diversity in Aging, Faculty Development Program, UCLA, June 18.

---

and quantity of their care lower than whites (Chadiha et al., 1995). The practice implication of this finding is that discharge-planning social workers need to explore the realistic ability of the informal care network to adequately provide the needed services, not just whether such a network exists (238).

Another study examined caregiver practices of German, Irish, English, and African-American ethnic groups. One of the main differences found was that among African Americans, the amount of time the family caregiver devotes to caregiving is not related to the closeness of the relationship, while among the Irish, especially, hours of caregiving was inversely related to the distance in the relationship between caregiver and patient. This difference was attributed to the African-American tendency to include more distant relatives and even nonrelatives with whom they are emotionally bonded as "family," while the Irish have a tradition of duty to care for close relatives (White-Means and Thornton, 1990a). Furthermore, African-American family caregivers provided significantly more daily hours of caregiving than either German, Irish, or English family caregivers (White-Means and Thornton, 1990b).

Variation in reluctance to use nursing home care also was found among Japanese Americans, whose future intention to enter a nursing home rather than home care was significantly greater among women than men, among those with little or no social support system, and among those who were born in the United States and more acculturated to American lifestyles

(McCormick et al., 1996). Whereas only 12 percent would plan to enter a nursing home following a hip fracture, 53 percent would enter a nursing home if the disability involved dementia (McCormick et al., 1996:769). The authors noted that this high percentage of respondents intending to use nursing home care under certain circumstances may reflect the fact that King County, Washington, where the study was conducted, happens to have "an ethnically appropriate nursing home which is strongly supported by, and familiar to, this close-knit community" (McCormick et al., 1996:769).

In working with Asian and Pacific Islander elderly, it is essential for social workers to be sensitive to the fact that this category encompasses at least twenty-six ethnic subgroups, which vary widely from one another in culture and socioeconomic status (Tanjasiri, Wallace, and Shibata, 1995).

Applewhite (1995:248) points out that Mexican Americans are more likely to accept needed health services if the formal caregivers are aware and respectful of the culture of the patient and family, with regard to folk healing beliefs and practices and to the values of *confianza* (confidence), *respecto* (respect), and *personalice* (to personalize) on an interpersonal level: Mexican Americans "may avoid needed health care (such as formal home health care or nursing home care) because existing health care systems, with their emphasis on efficiency and impersonality, conflict with their cultural values, particularly *personalism*" (252).

INTERDISCIPLINARY TEAMWORK

In most formal home health care situations, the team consists of a supervising physician, professional nurse, nursing assistant, and family caregiver(s). Frequently, interaction among them is limited to intermittent contact between the nurse and physician, between the nurse and nurse aide, between the nurse and patient and family caregiver, and between the nurse aide and patient and family caregiver. However, rarely is there any interaction between the physician and nurse aide, and because the medical model dominates formal home health care, the relationships among staff tend to be hierarchical—with physician in charge, nurse reporting to physician, nurse aide reporting to the nurse, and patient and family caregiver interacting separately with each of them.

What was just described is not an interdisciplinary team, but a multidisciplinary team, at best, of the matrix model type (Mailick and Jordon, 1977). Interdisciplinary teamwork is not a hallmark of home health service in the United States. However, it is common practice in home health programs in many other nations that have more progressive health care systems and is highly recommended by geriatric specialists (Kane et al., 1997).

An experimental study (Zimmer, Groth-Juncker, and McCusker, 1985) of a home health care team, consisting of a physician, nurse practitioner, and social worker, to determine whether home health care patients served by the team would have a significantly different outcome than patients in a control group reported the following: (1) the experimental group patients spent significantly fewer days in either hospitals or nursing homes, (2) both they and their caregivers expressed significantly greater satisfaction with the care received than did the control group, and (3) the patients were significantly more likely to die at home, when that was their wish. However, there was not a significant difference in costs or in health status outcomes.

There is wide variation across HHC agencies in their utilization of social workers. Medicare requires that a physician authorize social worker services to an HHC patient on the basis that the need be related to the patient's acute medical condition. However, because Medicare will only reimburse for psychiatric nurse services when a psychiatrist is involved, it could be easier to gain authorization for a qualified clinical social worker than a psychiatric nurse when psychotherapeutic service is indicated. Unfortunately, however, turf conflict between the attending nurse and social workers can lead to underuse of social workers in home health care because both registered nurses and master's-level social workers have been professionally socialized to see psychosocial assessment and treatment as their own domain (Fessler and Adams, 1985).

Despite the underutilization of social workers in HHC and the barriers to effective teamwork, the NASW upholds the principle of the interdisciplinary team and describes its positive potential in Standard 4 of social work in home health settings:

> **STANDARD 4:** The home health social worker shall integrate social work intervention with that of other members of the interdisciplinary team.

Interpretation

The complex problems experienced at home by special populations should be assessed and addressed from a variety of perspectives. A collaborative team approach has the potential for being more comprehensive, more efficient and more responsive to clients' needs. The home health social worker must integrate the psychosocial plan and interventions with the other services being offered and educate the en-

tire team to the psychosocial needs of the client and client's family.*
(NASW, 1987:30)

ORGANIZATIONAL CONSIDERATIONS

There is an apparent association between organizational type and the extent to which professional social work services are used. Public HHC agencies, such as through public health departments and voluntary nonprofit HHC organizations, are more likely to employ full-time or part-time social worker staff, while the for-profit HHC agencies more often employ social workers only as needed, determined by the physician, sometimes with the recommendation of the attending nurse.

In general, social workers are underutilized by home care organizations. In 1999, the median hourly rate of compensation to social workers by home health agencies was $17.73, and the median rate per visit was $40 (National Association for Home Care, 2000:21), while the mean number of home visits per eight-hour day was three. However, when utilized, HHC social workers spend considerable time interacting with other members of the interdisciplinary care team and with community resource personnel.

Home health agencies must be certified by Medicare to be reimbursed by Medicare for skilled health care services. In 1998, about 15.7 percent of the 13,300 home care agencies in the United States were not Medicare certified and presumably were limited to providing homemaker-type services or obtaining out-of-pocket reimbursement for skilled care (U.S. Government Printing Office, 2000b:132, Table 205).

CLIENT PROBLEMS AND SOCIAL WORKER FUNCTIONS

Client Problems

The NASW lists the social work and psychosocial services in home health care as focusing on the following main categories of client problems:

- Patient and family adverse reactions or dysfunctional adjustment to illness and changes in functional status
- Vocational and educational problems
- Financial problems

---

*Copyright 1995, National Association of Social Workers, Inc., NASW Standards for Social Work in Health Care Settings.

- Caregiving problems, including caregiver stress
- Inadequate housing and living arrangements
- Barriers in access to medical care, including transportation
- Relationship problems, including social isolation
- Physical, sexual, and emotional abuse and neglect
- Substance abuse
- Other psychiatric illness, including depression and suicide
- Potential for institutionalization* (NASW, 1995:6)

These may be conceptualized as falling under the headings of

1. barriers to admission to the service or facility;
2. problems of adjustment to the service or facility;
3. problems of adjustment to the diagnosis, prognosis, or treatment/care plan;
4. lack of information to make informed decisions;
5. lack of needed resources; and
6. barriers to discharge from the service or facility.

Client Health Problems

Table 5.4 indicates a wide variety of health problems found among home health agency patients. Box 5.3 lists the ten leading causes of death in the United States.

It may be noted that the major primary health problems of home health agency patients do not correspond very closely with the major age-adjusted causes of death per 100,000 population in the United States in 1993. This presumably reflects the discrepancy between what often is functionally disabling, such as arthritis and diabetes, and therefore requires supportive assistance to function, and what is most likely to be terminal, such as cancer, but does not have a prolonged period of disability. One recent nationwide study found that the "patient's functional status seems to play a stronger predictive role in determining post-[hospital] discharge than do [disease] severity measures" (Kane et al., 1996:247).

The relevance of the client's health problem to the social worker in HHC is the issue of how the health problem impacts mental, physical, and social functioning, particularly ADLs, and conversely, how the client's mental, physical, and social functioning impacts the health problem. This is the reciprocal biopsychosocial interaction:

---

*Copyright 1995, National Association of Social Workers, Inc., NASW Clinical Indicators for Social Work and Psychosocial Services in Home Health Care.

For the chronically ill, frail elderly, homebound person, every aspect of life becomes affected and possibly changed as a result of the illness. Family relationships which may already have been strained become more so. The patient not infrequently is pauperized by the cost of medical care, raising issues of self-worth, pride, and dependency. Preexisting personality problems can become exacerbated and feelings of anger, self-pity and hopelessness are common. Further compounding the problem is the frequent inability of the patient to perform simple activities of daily living such as eating, bathing, and toileting. (Jacobs and Lurie, 1984:89-90)

TABLE 5.4. Primary Admission Diagnoses of Home Health Agency Patients, 1998

Primary Diagnosis	Percent
Diseases of the circulatory system (heart disease and cerebrovascular disease)	23.5
Injuries and poisoning	8.9
Musculoskeletal and connective tissue disease	8.2
Endocrine, nutritional, and metabolic and immunity disorders	8.2
Respiratory system diseases	7.9
Disease of the nervous system and sense organs	7.6
Malignant neoplasms	3.9

Source: U.S. Government Printing Office (2000a). *Health, United States.* Washington, DC: Author, 132, Table 206.

BOX 5.3.
Ten Major Causes of Death in the United States, 1998

1. Heart disease
2. Cancer (malignant neoplasms)
3. Cerebrovascular diseases
4. Chronic obstructive pulmonary disease
5. Unintentional injuries
6. Pneumonia and influenza
7. Diabetes mellitus
8. Suicide
9. Nephritis, nephrotic syndrome, and nephrosis
10. Chronic liver disease and cirrhosis

Source: U.S. Government Printing Office 2000a. *Health, United States.* Washington, DC: Author, 172, Table 32.

Client Funding Problems

One of the many nonhealth problems of clients needing home health care services is the current lack of financial resources to pay for services. Currently, a patchwork pattern of sources of funding for home care includes Medicare (Title XVIII), Medicaid (Title XIX), Title XX of the Social Security Act (Social Services Block Grant), Title III of the Older Americans Act, the Veterans Administration, and Civilian Health and Medical Programs of the Uniformed Services (CHAMPUS) (National Association for Home Care, 1996:5-6.) Private health insurance pays only a small fraction of the costs of home health care. As a result, about 21.0 percent of HHC costs are financed out of pocket by consumers (NAHC, 2000:4; U.S. Government Printing Office, 2000b:110, Table 156).

As with other areas of health services in the United States, home health care has considerable gaps in covered services:

- If one is elderly or disabled and eligible for Medicare, HHC may be available if a physician documents the need for *skilled care* (i.e., needing professional services, such as those of a registered nurse, physical therapist, or speech therapist).
- If the patient is poor and eligible for Medicaid insurance, he or she may be eligible for home care for either skilled care or homemaker/chore-type services, especially if the patient is otherwise likely to need nursing home care.
- However, for those who do not qualify for skilled care and are not poor enough to qualify for Medicaid assistance, but are age sixty-five or older, their AAA (Area Agency on Aging) may have funds to help with personal care services or homemaking services.
- Depending on state plans for use of Social Services Block Grant Funds (formerly Title XX), patients may qualify for some assistance to help pay for home care.

Family Caregiver Burden

Although several million Americans receive formal home care services, the Pepper Commission estimated that three-fourths of home care assistance to the elderly is provided free of charge by informal caregivers (family or other unpaid help) (U.S. Government Printing Office, 1990). Karen Pace, Director of Research for the Washington, DC–based National Association for Home Care, estimated that nine to eleven million elderly Americans need assistance to remain at home (Braus, 1994:41). Most functionally impaired elderly people rely exclusively on family and other informal sources (Wilcox and Taber, 1991). Eighteen percent of family caregivers of brain-impaired persons (due to, e.g., Alzheimer's disease, strokes [CVAs], Parkinson's disease, Huntington's disease, traumatic brain injury) had to quit their jobs in order to provide care, and another 42 percent reduced the number of hours they work because of caregiving. Informal caregivers provide an average of seventy-three hours of care each week, or more than ten hours per day; one-third report that they receive no help from family or friends; 58 percent have symptoms of clinical depression and are at increased risk for physical health problems of their own (California's Caregiver Resource Center, 2001).

Who are the informal caregivers? Spouses, mostly wives, are the largest group of caregivers of elderly people, and adult daughters are the next largest group (Brody, 1981; Horowitz, 1984; California's Caregiver Resource Center, 2001). However, single women devote more time assisting elderly parents than do other family members. Because society tends to see them as the nurturers, women continue to carry the majority of elder caregiving, whether or not they work outside the home. "Over one-half (53 percent) of the caregivers under the age of 65 also work outside the home" (California's Caregiver Resource Center, 2001). Most family caregivers themselves are middle-aged or elderly; about one-third are middle-aged; another 25 percent are age sixty-five or older (Braus, 1994:41). According to the California's Caregiver Resource Center, the average age of family caregivers is sixty years, and about 33 percent of family caregivers are wives, 29 percent are adult daughters, 14 percent husbands, 7 percent sons, 5 percent parents, 2 percent siblings, and 5 percent "other" (California's Caregiver Resource Center, 2001).

Although home care tends to be presented as a way to reduce government expenditures for hospital and nursing home care, this public cost savings is often obtained on the backs of family members, especially women. The cost to these volunteer caregivers can include time, loss of income and retirement funds, neglect of their own health, lack of recreation and social life, and postponed careers (California's Caregiver Resource Center, 2001).

A survey reported in 1988 (Linsk, Keigher, and Osterbusch, 1988) found that thirty-five states, in addition to the District of Columbia and Puerto Rico, provide some form of financial payment to family caregivers for providing home care to clients when the client is a high risk for institutionalization, in spite of the fact that both Medicare and Medicaid regulations prohibit the payment of family members for personal care services (206). This funding mechanism most often is state Supplemental Security Income payments, and the amount varies widely across jurisdictions. However, only thirteen of the thirty-five jurisdictions indicated that they sometimes allow payments to family caregivers of elderly clients. More often, the client is a mentally or physically disabled nonaged person. Besides state SSI funds, other funding sources sometimes used for caregivers of elderly clients include Title XX Social Services Block Grants, Title III Older Americans Act, Medicaid provisions other than personal care, or state general funds. The Medicaid Home and Community-Based Care waivers appear to be an increasingly important source of coverage (209).

Barnes, Given, and Given (1992) compared four groups of family caregivers—spouses with children, spouses without children, adult children with siblings, adult children without siblings—and found that spouses were most apt to suffer damage to their own health, while adult child caregivers were most apt to experience feelings of abandonment, especially if they had siblings. The findings have implications for social work in terms of the importance of an early needs assessment in home care situations to assist the family with caregiving plans (286-287).

The issue of whether home care is less expensive than nursing home care apparently is complicated, with the answer depending on a number of variables. However, one study found that when formal home care services were provided, there was a tendency for informal caregivers to reduce their own free services and to substitute formal ones. Although this raises the immediate cost of home care, it may enable family caregivers to keep the patient at home longer, thus reducing long-term costs (Ettner, 1994).

The new Family Caregiver Support Program. Apparently in response to the mounting evidence of informal caregiver burden in the United States, the National Family Caregiver Support Program (NFCSP) was established and approved by Congress in December 2000, including $125 million of new funding as part of the newly reauthorized Older Americans Act. The NFCSP is intended to provide critical support to families to assist them in maintaining their caregiver roles for their older family members who are ill or have disabilities and also to older adults who have primary care responsibilities for young children. The federal funds have been awarded to state Units on Aging who will work in partnerships with Area Agencies on Aging to implement the new program. The NFCSP is being implemented in a manner that provides significant flexibility to states. An initial step that will be required in most states will be to conduct a statewide needs assessment to determine caregiver demographic characteristics, caregiver needs, available resources, resource deficiencies, and associated infrastructure/program development requirements to create effective statewide policy (Center for the Advanced Study of Aging Services, School of Social Welfare, University of California, Berkeley, 2001).

Other family victims. It must be remembered that whether impaired people are cared for at home by family members, formal caregivers, or both, having a family member who has unusual care needs in the home is a strain on the rest of the family, including children. These family members are likely to become the unrecognized victims of home care. A recent study conducted in Israel of children with a sibling with cancer reminds us of this tendency (Hamama, Ronen, and Feigin, 2000). Disproportionate amounts of attention and time are often devoted to the family member with an illness or a disability, and other family members' needs are often neglected. Compounding the problem often is that neglected family members may often feel guilty for feeling left out and for sometimes resenting the ill or disabled family member. This phenomenon is one of the many reasons why social workers are needed in home care situations.

Social Worker Functions and Interventions

According to Jacobs and Lurie (1984):

> The social workers become an indispensable part of the home care team. They are able to provide *counseling, assist* the patient *with concrete* financial, housing, and medical equipment *problems, advocate* for the patient with welfare, the health care system, Medicaid, *support* the patient in *compliance* with the treatment regimes, help the patient understand and *deal with* strained *family relationships and* help the patient be reconciled to *chronic illness.* Indeed, in the absence of good social work care, home care services can be an exercise in the application of medical technology, while the patient remains miserable, kept alive physically but in turmoil and suffering emotionally.
>
> Social work in home care, by providing services in the home, returns to the origins of the profession, to that subtle, artful blending of support, counseling and advocacy which social workers do best. (90) (emphasis added)

Garner adds that other commonly needed social worker roles and functions include

1. helping the clients and/or families cope with their losses, including anticipated ones;
2. promoting medical compliance;
3. psychosocial counseling as needed;
4. advocating on behalf of the clients or families; and

5. discharge planning when clients no longer need the home health agency (HHA) services or when they need another level of service, such as a nursing home, hospital, or rehabilitation center. (1995:1632)

Silverstone and Burack-Weiss (1983) argue, as a rationale for social work in home care, that all human beings need someone in their life with whom they are emotionally bonded and on whom they can count to provide, or arrange for, their needs as they arise, termed "the auxiliary function" (11). This is a fundamental function that the social worker can provide when needed, alone or with other HHC team members and family of the client. This is an affectively and instrumentally *supportive* function, including both a supportive relationship and supportive roles, such as interpreting, mediating, advocating, and monitoring person-in-environment transactions (11) in collaboration with the client and family (22). The mobilization of helping networks, when needed, is a major function of the HHC social worker (23).

The NASW has noted the following about the social work function and role in home care:

> The social worker assists patients and their families to adapt and plan in the home environment. Relief of stress, crisis intervention, assistance with financial problems, advocacy with community agencies, information and referral, assistance with planning, emotional support, appropriate counseling, and interpretation of and education about family and patient's needs to other health care staff and services providers, are the components of the social work role in helping patients adjust to their situations and in helping families sustain the patient at home rather than resort to premature or unnecessary institutionalization.* (NASW, 1987:28)

In addition, the NASW Standard 6 for social work in home health settings (1987:30) states that the functions of the social worker in home health settings shall include specific services listed in Standard 4 of the core standards for social work in health care settings (see Chapter 1 of this text).

Elsewhere, NASW lists the functions and services provided by social workers in home health care as follows:

---

*Copyright 1995, National Association of Social Workers, Inc., NASW Standards for Social Work in Health Care Settings.

- Assess social, economic, environmental, and emotional factors that interfere with patient and family adjustment to illness and treatment.
- Explain social work services and contract goals with patient and family and develop a treatment plan.
- Provide counseling for long-range planning and decision making.
- Provide counseling, education, and support to the patient and his or her family related to the identified medical condition.
- Identify and obtain needed community resources on behalf of the patient.
- Advocate for services for patients at risk due to mental or physical limitations.
- Provide short-term therapy.
- Provide consultation, liaison, and interdisciplinary collaboration.
- Provide discharge planning.* (NASW, 1995:5)

"Social work in home care, by providing services in the home, returns to the origins of the profession, to that subtle, artful blending of support, counseling and advocacy which social workers do best." (Jacobs and Lurie, 1984:90)

Case Management in Home Care

Ideally, social workers ought to play a major role as case managers in home health care. Who knows better than social workers how to gather important information from relevant sources to assess the needs and resources of a client and then to engage the variety of appropriate community resources to help meet those needs? Who can better work cooperatively with clients, professionals, and paraprofessionals from various disciplines to coordinate the timely provision of those resources and to provide ongoing monitoring to ensure their continued appropriateness, making adjustments as needed?

The broker role. A primary role of the HHC social worker ought to be that of a broker, a part of being a case manager, to link the client and/or family with needed community resources, such as a support group, home-delivered meals, chore services, telephone reassurance, volunteer home visiting, adult day care, medical aids and appliances, home modification/environmental adaptation services, or respite care (Garner, 1995:1632).

Ensuring the timely delivery of home care services. The social worker who does discharge planning in a hospital or nursing home also impacts

---

*Copyright 1995, National Association of Social Workers, Inc., NASW Clinical Indicators for Social Work and Psychosocial Services in Home Health Care.

HHC services, insofar as he or she often makes the referral to the HHC agency and has arranged for particular services to be delivered by a particular time. However, one follow-up study to monitor the delivery of timely and appropriate HHC services found that in 40 percent of cases, one or more services was not delivered as planned; yet most hospitals do not follow up with patients following discharge (Proctor, Morrow-Howell, and Kaplan, 1996).

Common Social Worker Roles and Functions

1. Helping the clients and/or families cope with their losses, including anticipated ones
2. Promoting medical compliance
3. Psychosocial counseling as needed
4. Advocating on behalf of the clients or families
5. Discharge planning when clients no longer need the HHA services or when they need another level of service, such as a nursing home, hospital, or rehabilitation center (Garner, 1995:1632)

Furthermore, Egan and Kadushin (1999) found from their study of home health social work that only 20 percent of the home care social workers met with hospital social workers about the referrals they received from them, suggesting a lack of coordination between the hospital referral source and the home care agency that is supposed to be ensuring continuity of needed care. However, they also found that two-thirds or more of the social workers studied reported that at least twice a week they engaged in the following activities:

- service coordination
- direct assessment
- counseling patients and families
- collaborating between agencies
- making home visits after assessment
- advocating for patient services

An apparent downfall of home care is the lack of collaboration and coordination—between the hospital, home care agency, financing programs such as Medicare, NASW, and patient and family—regarding the role and functions of social work in home care. Incongruence exists between what is medically needed, what is desired by the patient and family for maximization of comfort and function, what is deemed affordable, and what the social work profession perceives as appropriate activity for social workers.

Still, NASW's Standard 5 for social work in home health settings states the following:

STANDARD 5: The home health social worker shall work to achieve an appropriate continuum of care, assuring the clients of ongoing services to meet their needs.

Interpretation

The home health social worker must consider all social work services as part of a continuum of care including the family, referring agencies and institutions and other community social workers. When possible, he/she must work closely with initial referral sources to insure the patient an appropriate discharge plan and safe transition into the home. Likewise, prior to the discharge of the patient from home care, when indicated, the social worker must establish the necessary linkages to community resources, or other facilities to assure that needs are met.* (NASW, 1987:30)

Needs assessment in home care. Of course, the first step in case management is needs assessment, and the first issue in needs assessment is determining the appropriateness and feasibility of home care. Some of the considerations to explore with the patient and family that are relevant to deciding whether to opt for home care include the following:

1. Could the patient's condition be properly managed in the home?
2. Are there family members willing and able to provide the needed informal care (physically, emotionally, time-wise, in terms of other work and family obligations)?
3. If the patient and/or family prefers home care over nursing home care, what are the reasons?
4. Is the patient eligible for any third-party payment of any needed skilled care?
5. If not, is the patient or family willing and able to pay, out of pocket, for the needed skilled care?
6. Would the patient and/or potential family caregiver prefer the patient enter a nursing home facility, if one were available that was culturally appropriate and/or provided high-quality care in the community?

---

*Copyright 1995, National Association of Social Workers, Inc., NASW Standards for Social Work in Health Care Settings.

7. Does the potential family caregiver really *want* to assume responsibility for the informal care of the patient, or does he or she simply feel that it is expected of him or her?
8. Does the patient and/or family have any strong preferences or prohibitions concerning the gender or ethnicity of the formal caregivers provided by the HHC agency?
9. Are there any cultural values, beliefs, customs, prohibitions, and so forth, of the patient or family that the HHC agency ought to know about, ones that might affect the acceptability of the formal services to the patient?
10. What is the patient's and family's interpretation of the meaning of the patient's health problem(s)? That is, what do they think contributed to it, and what do they think needs to be done to best deal with it?
11. Are the types of care services that the family caregiver will have to provide compatible with the family's cultural traditions concerning intrafamily relationships (for example, a daughter bathing her father's genital area)?

The home care assessment serves a dual function with elderly clients. It provides essential information for understanding their problems, needs, resources, coping mechanisms, and strengths. It also acts as a tool that enables clients to experience a life review, which can help to achieve ego integrity (Erikson, 1950), or a sense of wholeness and fulfillment, after telling their life stories to an interested and empathetic listener (Kerson and Michelson, 1995).

Social work in home health care should begin with a thorough psychosocial assessment, except in crisis-intervention situations such as elder abuse (Garner, 1995:1632; Silverstone and Burack-Weiss, 1983). The social worker assessment of the home care situation should, as always in contemporary social work, identify and understand both needs and strengths of the client system (Cox, 1992:180).

Depending on which other team members participate, the social worker's assessment may include not only the customary psychosocial areas of the client's history and current status, relationships, and significant life events, but also ADL functioning, assessment of need for modification of the home environment, for support services, for income supports, for tools and equipment, and for interpersonal supports.

The status of the patient's activities of daily living (ADLs) (eating, dressing, bathing, walking, transferring, toileting, going outside) and instrumental activities of daily living (IADLs) (housework, cooking, shopping, driving, paying bills, banking) are the primary determinants of the need for environmental modifications, support services, income supports, tools and equipment, and interpersonal supports. In fact, ADL status is one of the main determinants of the need for home care service (Fredman, Droge, and Rabin, 1992).

Assessment of mental status is also often desirable, since it is not always obvious how well oriented, depressed, or forgetful a person is, and these are common problems in older adults, especially among those who have been hospitalized and traumatized by medical procedures and a strange and often frightening environment such as a hospital or nursing home. Depression alone is common among home care clients, who often experience a devastating sense of loss and dependency. The outcome of an assessment of mental health status should be an important determinant of the service plan (see Box 5.4).

A variety of assessment instruments are available to examine ADL functioning, such as the Older Americans Resources Survey (OARS), or the Older Americans Research and Service Center Instrument (Duke University Center for the Study of Aging and Human Development, 1978). More recently, the second edition of an extensive volume of health-related research instruments, including several for measuring ADLs, was published by Oxford University Press (McDowell and Newell, 1996).

Assessment skills include empathetic communication, verbal following, synthesization of information, and ongoing feedback and evaluation (Aranda, 1996).

Client Outreach and Advocacy in Home Care

Many people, especially elderly people, who develop functional impairments are not familiar with the available community resources or are reluctant to ask for help (Blazer, 1988). Thus, the HHC social worker should ensure that the community has outreach services through, for example, the mass media, physicians, housing managers, postal carriers, hospital emergency rooms, and elders themselves, to provide information and referral for needed services (Silverstone and Burack-Weiss, 1983:27).

Advocacy is often related to outreach and is an important role for social workers in home care. Given the fact that most home care is provided by family and friends without benefit of formal HHC services, it is likely that many of these informal HHC situations involve either caregivers or care receivers who need someone to both reach out to them and advocate for them. Family caregivers often are overworked and overtired and can even damage their own health unless someone reaches out to them and offers to advocate for them, whether with the care recipient, other family members, HHC agencies, the family physician, or politicians. At the same time, care recipients sometimes accept services of family caregivers or formal home care

---

BOX 5.4.
Psychosocial Assessment of the Home Health Client

Traditional Psychosocial History Areas

Childhood family history and significant experiences
Marital family history
Educational history
Occupational and retirement history, income, and insurance
Current household and housing situation
Transportation resources
Health history and development of current health status
Current support system, formal and informal
Religious status and preference
Political status and preference
Recreation, talents, special interests, pastimes
Reflections

HHC Supplementary Assessment Areas

ADL functioning
Mental status exam
Customary coping style
Specification of what family caregivers can/will do
Tools and equipment needs assessment
Support services needs assessment
Home environment modification needs assessment
Income support needs assessment
Interpersonal support needs assessment

---

agencies when they would prefer a different arrangement, but hesitate to complain when they are so dependent.

Advocacy is especially needed with vulnerable groups of patients, such as those with AIDS (Marder and Linsk, 1995). It has been a long, slow process in the United States to ensure that nursing homes, home health care, and hospice programs accept and treat AIDS patients properly, and the battle is not over yet. Advocacy may require providing education and information to correct misunderstandings, teaching new skills to deal competently with a new situation, emphasizing the advantages of a previously rejected alternative, and using the force of law.

The National Association of Social Workers includes as a specific service to be provided by social workers in any health care setting, "Client advocacy within and outside the organization, including attention to fiscal constraints" (NASW, 1987:6).*

Counseling in Home Care

Kerson and Michelson (1995) describe the counseling work of a hospital-based elder care center providing case management services to individuals and agencies throughout the entire county where it is located and whose services are reimbursed by Medicare. Their premise is that elderly people, regardless of their physical limitations, are still capable of introspection, of learning from past experience, and of psychological and social growth (160).

A primary goal of the elder care center (Kerson and Michelson, 1995) is to help frail elderly people to remain in their own homes as long as it is safe for them to do so and to empower them to maintain the highest level of independence that their mental and physical status allows (160).

Some of the counseling activities provided by the elder care center include the following:

1. Efforts to help family members understand the importance of the client's maintaining control over decisions about accepting needed services
2. Building a relationship of trust and mutual respect with "guarded" (reluctant to form relationships) elders
3. Using pet therapy to engage certain clients
4. Helping the client to understand the family caregiver's need for relief through accepting supplementary services
5. Using life review and reminiscence therapy to facilitate ego integrity and reduce the dread of death
6. Engaging a resistant client in accepting a needed environmental modification to enhance quality of life, such as a ramp for a wheelchair-bound client
7. Using positive imagery and the relaxation response to reduce depression and anxiety, as well as the provision of books on tape and a tape player to help pass time enjoyably
8. Helping the client to reinstate ties with some previous sources of support, such as a former clergyperson
9. Working with family caregivers to reduce stress, through prioritizing and partializing problem sources and selecting alternative solutions, through expressing and examining emotions causing distress, and through linking caregivers with caregiver support groups

---

*Copyright 1995, National Association of Social Workers, Inc., NASW Standards for Social Work in Health Care Settings.

The challenge of counseling in home care is to be able to work with both client and caregivers and to enable both to feel cared about, while supporting the primary client (Kerson and Michelson, 1995:183).

It is important to remember that people who are in need of home health care often are experiencing increased dependency and may not readily accept offers of various kinds of help. The acceptance of dependency and assistance to compensate for one's dependency can be emotionally threatening (Cox, 1992). Thus, it is essential for the social worker to be sensitive to this resistance to dependency and to provide counseling to support the patient and family with the decision-making process and coming to terms with the need for supportive services (Simmons, 1994). A cognitive therapy approach might be useful here to help the client and family become aware of what dependency and acceptance of help mean to them, as well as to assist them in reexamining and reshaping those interpretations to become more realistic and generous to themselves.

Policy Activism

It is not enough that social workers advocate at the micro level; it is vital that social workers also voice their views about the current status of home care and the need to develop a model of home care that recognizes the significance of social needs as contributing factors to dependency. The first task of social workers must be to lobby for, make recommendations regarding, and participate in the design of a more humane policy, with appropriate program reforms, that promotes a client's right to live as autonomously as possible in the community (Cox, 1992:182).

NASW's Standard 2 asserts the following regarding home health care:

STANDARD 2: Social workers in home health settings should support and advocate for appropriate home health care for people with chronic, acute, and/or terminal illnesses.

Interpretation

. . . Home health care social workers must be advocates for the maintenance of these individuals, families, agencies and the community resources and programs to support them. Advocacy must also be pursued on a state and federal level in support of legislation promoting home care.* (NASW, 1987:29)

---

*Copyright 1995, National Association of Social Workers, Inc., NASW Standards for Social Work in Health Care Settings.

KNOWLEDGE REQUIREMENTS

In addition to knowledge of social worker roles, functions, and service interventions, NASW has stated the following:

STANDARD 1: Social workers in home health settings shall have knowledge of chronic, acute and terminal illnesses, physical disabilities and the resultant age-specific impact on individual and family systems.

Interpretation

Social workers in home health agencies must have knowledge of acute, chronic, and terminal illnesses as well as permanent and temporary disabling conditions. They must be familiar with the usual course of the illness or condition, therapeutic interventions, and adaptations which will be necessary by clients and their families. Social workers must also be familiar with the general concerns of special populations. They must be aware that these illnesses are often long-term and permanent, resulting in functional losses, social isolation and economic pressures which can impact on the individual's and family's ability to cope.* (NASW, 1987:28-29)

Again, these areas may be classified under the need for specific knowledge of (1) the client population and client problem(s); (2) the organizational setting; (3) the community and its resources; (4) the needed research, evaluation, and documentation; and (5) appropriate intervention modalities.

Client Population

Home health care has a gender-specific, gerontological focus, consisting primarily of elderly unmarried women (Kaye and Davitt, 1995).

In 1999, nearly 1.9 million persons (1.8818) in the United States were under the care of a home health agency on any given day. Of these patients, 68.7 percent were sixty-five years of age and over and about 66.4 percent were women (U.S. Government Printing Office, 2000b:132, Table 206).

Age and Sex

As age increases, especially among women, home health care agency utilization increases. The greater tendency of elderly women rather than elderly men to use home health agency services is largely attributed to both
women tending to live considerably longer than men and older men often
having informal caregivers, that is, being married, often to younger spouses.
In addition, because women tend to outlive men, they are more likely to develop functional disabilities, which tend to increase with advancing age, and
often require assistance with ADL functioning.

In 1998 nearly one-third (31.3 percent) of home health agency patients
were under age sixty-five and the remaining 68.8 percent were age sixty-
five or older (see Table 5.5). Although the data are not depicted here, *Statistical Abstracts of the United States* (U.S. Government Printing Office,
2000b:132, Table 206) indicates that within the sixty-five and over age
group, as age increases, the percentage of persons receiving formal home
health agency services also increases. For example, the HHC utilization *rate*
within the 85 and over age cohort is about 2.3 times that of the sixty-five to
sixty-nine age cohort.

Race and Marital Status

In 1998, in addition to the population of home health agency patients being primarily elderly and female, 69.5 percent of HHC agency patients were
white, 13.5 percent were black, and the other 17.0 percent were of undeter-
mined race (U.S. Government Printing Office, 2000b:132, Table 206). In
addition, 29.7 percent were married, 32.5 percent widowed, 17.4 percent
never married, 4.8 percent divorced or separated, and the balance, 15.6 percent, were of unknown marital status (U.S. Government Printing Office,
2000b:132, Table 206) (see Table 5.6).

Since about 75 percent of the U.S. population was classified as white in
2000 and an even higher percentage of the sixty-five and over population are
white, these data suggest that whites are underrepresented among home
health agency patients. This may reflect a higher rate of functional impairment among elderly blacks and Hispanics and/or may suggest that nonwhites are more likely to use home care than nursing home care services
(Morrow-Howell et al., 1996).

That the majority of home care clients are not married reflects the greater
likelihood of needing formal services when one is unmarried. As Kane and
colleagues (1996) recently reported in a nationwide study of predictors of
posthospital care destination, "the availability of informal care, at least as

TABLE 5.5. Age and Sex Distribution of Home Health Agency Patients, 1998

Patient Age Distribution		Patient Sex Distribution	
		Male	Female
Under age 45	15.5		
45-54	7.1		
55-64	8.7		
	(31.3 cum.)		
65-69	8.3		
70-74	11.5		
75-79	14.4		
80-84	15.5		
85 and over	19.1		
Total (%)	100.1	33.6	66.4

Source: U.S. Government Printing Office (2000b). *Statistical Abstracts of the United States.* Washington, DC: Author, 132, Table 206.

reflected in a person's not living alone, appears to play a substantial role in [hospital] discharge decisions" (247).

One study comparing the characteristics of elderly home care clients who received formal home care services with those who relied solely on informal helpers found that formal home care recipients had far more fragile informal helping networks, which may help explain why they turned to formal HHC initially (Wilcox and Taber, 1991:258). In addition, the closer the biological relationship, and especially the closer caregivers live to the elderly client, the more help provided by these informal caregivers (259). Still, 32 percent of elderly persons in solely informal home care situations were receiving their assistance from persons who were not family members (261). There was little or no evidence that formal HHC tended to reduce informal helping (264).

The Organizational Setting

As I have indicated elsewhere, social workers considering employment with a home health care service need to know its organizational characteristics before accepting the position, such as whether it is a public or private, voluntary (nonprofit) or proprietary (for-profit) agency, what its history and current practice is in terms of use of social workers, degree requirements for social worker staff, and role expectations relative to other professional staff.

In addition, the prospective HHC social worker ought to explore what, if any, unusual limitations may be imposed on social work practice as a result

TABLE 5.6. Distribution of Home Health Agency Patients by Race and Marital Status, 1998

Race	Percent	Marital Status	Percent
White	69.5	Widowed	32.5
Black	13.5	Married	29.7
Unknown	17.0	Never married	17.4
		Divorced or separated	4.8
		Unknown	15.6
Total	100.0%	Total	100.0%

Source: U.S. Government Printing Office (2000b). *Statistical Abstracts of the United States.* Washington, DC: Author, 132, Table 206.

of agency policy, secondary to its sources of support or affiliation, for example, religious dogma, or secondary to its organizational priorities, for example, profit making.

The Community and Its Resources

As in all social work practice settings, it is essential that the social worker be very familiar with the nature of the community and its resources, which is in constant flux and requires ongoing updating of information.

Every community has a set of both formal and informal resources—official resources and resources learned about through word of mouth. The informal sources may exist to serve the members of a particular religious, ethnic, or occupational group, they may be available in a crisis to supplement the formal resource system when it fails, or they may be ones that special individuals in the community sometimes give, under special circumstances, and are not widely known.

There is a rural-urban variation in the pattern of use of Medicare home health care services, including medical social work services (Kenney, 1993). Urban use rates are 9.1 percent higher than rural use rates. Population density is directly correlated with HHC use, and the number of nursing homes per Medicare enrollee is inversely correlated with HHC use rate. Rural areas have lower Medicare reimbursement ceilings, proportionately fewer Visiting Nurse Associations, and lower availability of auxiliary services, such as medical social work, and physical, occupational, or speech therapy. Whereas 21.8 percent of urban Medicare-certified home health care agencies reported that medical social services were not available, 62.7 percent of these agencies in rural areas reported the unavailability of medical social work services through their agency (Kenney, 1993:413). Kenney commented:

> the consequences for rural residents of the more limited availability of auxiliary services such as physical therapy and medical social services need to be assessed. What happens when the rural elderly need these services? Do they enter nursing homes? Or is there an unmet need for these services? (1993:413)

Needed Research, Evaluation, and Documentation in Home Care

Knowledge of research methods is needed by social workers in home health care, as in all settings of social work practice. In particular, experimental design and clinical trials research skills are needed to test the efficacy of social work interventions. Efficiency-oriented health care policymakers are not impressed with claims of effectiveness that are not supported by research (Ell, 1996).

In addition, monitoring the quality of home care is especially important because much of the care is being provided by nursing assistants with limited training, who often are without anyone to assist or oversee their actions or judgments. One process-oriented quality of home health care study found that 14.4 percent of reviewed cases of services provided by forty-seven different HHC agencies had quality-of-care deficiencies (Jette, Smith, and McDermott, 1996).

Kramer and colleagues (1990) propose a conceptual framework for assessing the quality of home health care that focuses mainly on two quality control measures, *process* and *outcome,* and to some extent the third, *structure;* they also think that HHC patients should be classified into homogeneous quality indicator groups (QUIGs).

The selection of outcome measures should reflect outcomes that HHC can reasonably be expected to impact, and this varies with diagnostic category. For example, for patients recovering from a hip fracture, functional status (bathing, dressing, walking) is an appropriate outcome measure, whereas for a patient with heart failure or diabetes, level of knowledge, compliance, and ability to take medications are more appropriate outcome measures (Kramer et al., 1990:416).

On the other hand, for patients whose outcome is difficult to measure, such as the mentally impaired or terminally ill, it is more appropriate to examine the *process* of HHC service delivery, that is, the extent to which the services were actually provided, such as comparing the frequency of provided services to the standard for that service frequency, which many individual HHC agencies and associations of HHC agencies have developed (Kramer et al., 1990:417).

Structural standards for measuring outcome include such issues as guidelines for organizational structure, qualifications of various types of staff, admission and discharge procedures, record keeping, and the provision of medications or equipment. These standards are useful indicators of organizational infrastructure but are generally weak indicators of quality of delivered services (Kramer et al., 1990:418). Structural standards have been developed by a variety of organizations, including the Joint Commission on the Accreditation of Healthcare Organizations (JCAHO), the National League of Nursing (NLN), the Texas Association for Home Health Agencies, and the Colorado Association of Home Health Care Agencies (442-443).

Kramer and colleagues offer sixteen categories of HHC patient conditions most commonly reimbursed by Medicare (1990:421) and a table for each category that lists the suitable outcome and process indicators. Among the outcome indicators that could be relevant to social work interventions are client knowledge, compliance, family/caregiver strain, and client satisfaction. Tebb (1995) presented a caregiver well-being scale and established its validity and reliability in another recent article (Berg-Weger, Rubio, and Tebb, 2000). An unusual feature of this scale is its measurement of caregiver strengths and sense of well-being, rather than a measure of deficits, reflecting a strengths perspective.

However, according to Lawlor and Raube (1995), currently there is a second stage of health care outcomes research in progress, with a variety of disciplines involved, whose focus is on studying the cost effectiveness of intervention outcomes to deal with health problems having a complex etiological mix of biopsychosocial factors as well as a complex mix of medical and psychosocial interventions. This approach appears directed toward producing specific protocols for specific health problems and has emerged in response to the discovery that medical interventions vary widely across geographic areas and providers. Furthermore, the psychosocial variables to be measured are not always observable in the individual, but are measured in terms of family supports, culture, community, and environment (391).

A thirty-six-item, short-form instrument (SF-36) (Ware and Sherbourne, 1992) is available that serves to standardize and assess *eight dimensions of health status and functioning:*

1. Physical functioning
2. Role limitations due to physical problems
3. Social functioning
4. Bodily pain
5. Mental health

6. Role limitations due to emotional problems
7. Vitality
8. Perceptions of general health (Lawlor and Raube, 1995)

Because the causes of health problems are often a mix of biopsychosocial factors, the interventions and research often need to employ a biopsychosocial approach too (Lawlor and Raube, 1995). The first step in such interdisciplinary research is to *describe* what the various professionals and paraprofessionals actually do in community health care settings, and later to *compare* their efficacy in addressing particular situations. The trend is toward measuring patient outcomes such as quality of life, patient satisfaction, and social functioning, especially in home care and hospice care (395).

Eight Dimensions of Health Status and Functioning

1. Physical functioning
2. Role limitations due to physical problems
3. Social functioning
4. Bodily pain
5. Mental health
6. Role limitations due to emotional problems
7. Vitality
8. Perceptions of general health (Lawlor and Raube, 1995)

Lawlor and Raube (1995) note the intimidating complexity of the variables that need to be concomitantly examined to determine the outcome of home health care interventions. They present a framework for the design of such research with five sets of variables:

1. Client characteristics (health status, economic status, social support, sociocultural and home environment)
2. Organizational characteristics (structure, sponsorship, incentives for employees working in the home, organizational culture, and community environment)
3. Provider characteristics (specialty, education, age, gender, race/ethnicity, and practice tenure)
4. Intervention characteristics (cost, quality, complexity, instrumentation, and compliance)
5. Outcomes characteristics (functional status, satisfaction, quality of life, medical outcomes, caregiver burden, and utilization) (398)

The medical effectiveness movement poses a reasonable and traditional evaluation question: Which health care interventions work (Lawlor and Raube, 1995)? In spite of the complexity of such multivariate research, Lawlor and Raube advise the following:

> The individuals, disciplines, and professions who ask and answer this question will predominately set the standards by which care is delivered in the next 25 years. By integrating the expertise of social science, public health, and medicine, the effectiveness of health services that involve medical and nonmedical interventions and outcomes can be evaluated. (1995:401)

A "quick and dirty" approach to evaluation of HHC services for purposes of agency self-monitoring is proposed by Fashimpar (1991), who published such an instrument (Fashimpar, 1983), which both surveys consumer satisfaction and assesses progress on achievement of case and agency objectives.

The new HHC social worker needs to be sure to clarify the documentation requirements of the agency for purposes of reimbursement and Medicare-licensing review and to keep other team members informed. Three recent volumes that may be useful to social workers in health care settings are *Outcomes Measurement in the Human Services: Cross-Cutting Issues and Methods* (Mullen and Magnabosco, 1997); *Measures for Clinical Practice: A Sourcebook,* Third Edition (Concoran and Fischer, 2000); and *Measuring Health: A Guide to Rating Scales and Questionnaires,* Second Edition (McDowell and Newell, 1996).

VALUES AND ETHICS CONSIDERATIONS

> An ethical dilemma occurs when social workers must choose between two contradictory ethical principles or directives, or when every alternative would result in an undesirable outcome for one or more individuals. (Loewenberg and Dolgoff, 1996, cited in Kadushin and Egan, 2001)

A study by Egan and Kadushin (1999) of social work in home health care in Wisconsin found that the most common ethical dilemmas the social workers faced concerned issues of client autonomy/self-determination, mental competence of the client, advance directives, and access to services. In addition, significant differences were found between nonprofit and proprietary agency social workers in that the latter more often reported concerns about barriers to access and the need to advocate for necessary services that were not always reimbursable.

"An ethical dilemma occurs when social workers must choose between two contradictory ethical principles or directives, or when every alternative would result in an undesirable outcome for one or more individuals." (Loewenberg and Dolgoff, 1996)

A subsequent study of social work in home health care (Kadushin and Egan, 2001) sought to determine the frequency with which home care social workers experienced ethical conflicts and their difficulty in resolving them, associated with characteristics of the social workers, their agencies and caseloads, the stakeholders involved, and the resources available to the social workers for consultation. This study was conducted after the Balanced Budget Act of 1997 introduced the early stages of the prospective payment system, which effectively reduced reimbursements to home health care agency services for Medicare-eligible clients.

In general, the study found that the greater the number of stakeholders, the greater the difficulty in resolving ethical conflicts. Most social workers reported that they usually consulted either nurses or other social workers but found other social workers most helpful. The most commonly cited reasons given for feeling that they had compromised their professional ethics were "reimbursement limits" and "government regulations," but most social workers reported that they "rarely if ever" compromised their professional ethics.

Interestingly, about two-thirds of the reporting social workers were with home health care agencies that had ethics committees, but only 46 percent of the social workers were members of their agencies' ethics committee. Of the home health care social workers responding, 80 percent had MSW degrees, more than two-thirds were in nonprofit agencies, and they averaged seven years of practice experience in home health services. Also interesting is that only a minority of social workers (12 percent) had caseloads limited to elderly clients. The remaining 88 percent had caseloads that also included children and/or HIV/AIDs clients. Nearly all had caseloads including clients receiving more complex medical care that required use of respirators, intravenous drips, and medication pumps.

Some unique issues are associated with home health care (Robbins, 1996:11-12), for example, the danger of theft of patient property by HCA employees:

> The home care environment offers greater autonomy for both patients and caregivers. This autonomy can be a double-edged sword. It is helpful sometimes not to have someone always looking over one's

shoulder, but occasionally it is essential to gain access to guidance and support, something not easy to do in a patient's home. (Robbins, 1996:2)

Community-Based Ethics Committees

Robbins (1996) notes that home health care providers are often faced with the dilemma of patients needing services that are not reimbursable, yet the providers hesitate to complain to funding sources—such as Medicare, Medicaid, HMOs, or private insurance companies—for fear they will be seen as simply seeking to line their own pockets. He recommends the establishment of a community-based ethics committee consisting of representatives of local health care organizations, community leaders, and local clergy. Such a committee can help resolve particular case situations, propose agency and state policy for dealing with similar situations, and compile data from cases referred to them for use in lobbying (158). The presence of a community-based ethics committee relieves the health care agency of having to deal with these kinds of issues and provides assurance to patients, their families, and the public that an impartial group of respected citizens is active in decision making.

Advance Directives

The Patient Self-Determination Act (PSDA) of 1991 requires that all health care service organizations, such as hospitals, nursing homes, and home care agencies, at or near intake, obtain their patients' *advance directives* regarding their wishes for resuscitation, treatment, and life support measures under particular circumstances (Davitt and Kaye, 1996). Advance directives are written documents such as living wills and power of attorney for health care. Whereas the living will specifies the patient's own wishes, the power of attorney for health care allocates responsibility to a particular other person to make such decisions, should the need arise and the patient is incapacitated.

Depending on the legal requirements of the state and the policy of the organization, the social worker may be involved in interpreting the meaning of advance directives to clients, answering their questions, and assessing patient competence to complete such directives (Davitt and Kaye, 1996). Discussing these matters with clients and helping them to make decisions and plans is an exercise in client self-determination and self-empowerment.

It is important that directives be very specific as to the type of health condition for which the patient would expect to be treated and which conditions he or she would want to progress without intervention. When patients are mentally incapacitated, such as with Alzheimer's disease, the designated family member who is the surrogate decision maker must make clear to the care facility and staff whether, for example, they do not want any curative treatment should the patient develop pneumonia, but would want treatment efforts should the patient fracture a limb or sustain a wound. Otherwise, nursing homes, for example, may simply assume that no intervention is desired under any circumstances, and later, the family members may experience distress that their loved one was allowed to suffer unnecessarily.

Advance directives need to be clear to all staff who will be caring for the patient and prominently located in the patient's room or on the cover of the care chart record. If a patient is transferred from one setting to another, it is important to be sure that the advance directives are transferred too (Robbins, 1996:7).

Analysis of Ethical Issues

Harry Moody (1982) has written about ethical dilemmas in home care and nursing homes; he uses an analysis framework from Reamer and Abramson (1982) that involves addressing the following issues in the process of resolving the dilemma:

1. Is the *source* of the dilemma the setting, the client health condition, or something else? (What makes it a "dilemma"?)
2. Is the issue truly an *ethical dilemma* or simply a *practical problem?* (Is it that we don't know what we should do or that we know what to do but are not able to do it?)
3. How do the perspectives of the involved professions influence understanding of the issue? (*Are differences in professional values and ethics contributing* to the dilemma?)
4. What *level of action* is *needed?* (Does the situation demand individual change, policy change, or professional practice change?)
5. How *do ethical theories clarify the dilemma?* (Does it shed light on the issue, regardless of whether you see it as one of rights, utility, personal virtue, or social justice?) (Moody, 1982:100) (emphases added)

SKILL REQUIREMENTS

The health field social worker needs a wide variety of skills. As stated earlier, any activity that the social worker performs in the course of his or her work may be considered skilled if it reflects social work knowledge, values, and ethics and is conscious, purposeful, disciplined, and responsible.

Questions to Ask in Resolving an Ethical Dilemma

1. Is the source of the dilemma the setting, the client health condition, or something else? (What makes it a "dilemma"?)
2. Is the issue truly an ethical dilemma or simply a practical problem? (Is it that we don't know what we should do or that we know what to do but are not able to do it?)
3. How do the perspectives of the involved professions influence understanding of the issue? (Are differences in professional values and ethics contributing to the dilemma?)
4. What level of action is needed? (Does the situation demand individual change, policy change, or professional practice change?)
5. How do ethical theories clarify the dilemma? (Does it shed light on the issue, regardless of whether you see it as one of rights, utility, personal virtue, or social justice? (Moody, 1982:100)

Simmons (1994) examined the future of social work in home care and described *the following skill requirements for social workers:*

1. Patient problems are multifaceted and require services from a host of providers. Social work skill in complex care planning and service coordination is crucial.
2. The multiplicity of care providers addressing health and personal care are paid from a blend of public, private, and out-of-pocket resources. Social work knowledge of payment regulation is very useful in coordinating care. Experience with a full array of income levels is relevant as well.
3. Families provide vast amounts of supportive care. Friends and neighbors provide other informal care. Social work skill in facilitating shared family decision making and properly partialized caregiving is very useful. Family counseling skills are well used in this work.
4. Self-care is a critical element in managing chronic conditions to assure maintenance of maximum feasible health status. Social work health education and counseling skills are essential.
5. Mental competence, emotional and mental status are crucial factors in self-care. Social work skill in assessment, treatment, and other related skills are valuable with this population.
6. Health social work experience in facilitating interdisciplinary care planning for ethically complex situations, and facilitating patient and family involvement in decision making, is an important arena of professional expertise. (39-40)

COMMENTARY

Currently, we are in the midst of a period of rapid transition in health care, in which hospital social work, which has been the center of social work in health care, is undergoing downsizing as part of the efficiency-oriented health care cost-control process in the United States. At the same time, the center of health care is shifting to the home and community, where professional social work has not been officially recognized as essential to the health care system—*if* it is to achieve efficiency.

According to Simmons (1994), social workers may need to move into community settings, such as primary care physicians' offices, home health agencies, skilled nursing home facilities, residential settings, and adult day care facilities, in order to identify and reach out to people who need ongoing case management and assistance (41). However, to achieve the objective that health care social workers need to be of maximum help to clients and to the overall objectives of the health care system, social workers may need to find some way to be independent of any particular sector of the continuum of health care organizations (Berkman, 1996).

When the social worker is employed by a hospital, nursing home, home care agency, or other organizational setting where social work is a secondary function, some limits are imposed on what the social worker can do. For example, nursing homes have a vested interest in keeping their beds full, and so timely rehabilitation and discharge to home or to another less restrictive setting is not likely to be a high priority to management. Hospitals are eager to discharge patients quickly so as not to exceed the DRG days and, if possible, to realize a profit by releasing the patient before the DRG time limit. Consequently, rapid discharge planning becomes more attractive than quality discharge planning, which requires that the patient and family feel in control of the plan and assured that arrangements are in place for continuity of care. If for-profit home health care agencies are functioning in a highly competitive community, they may be tempted to retain patients in their own homes when patient or family caregiver needs have emerged that indicate a transfer to a different care setting is required.

In any case, as Garner (1995) noted, "To date, social workers have played only a secondary role in home care" (1632). The main cause of this is that while Medicare mandates the availability of social work services to home health care agency patients, as needed, it does not mandate the participation of social workers in making client needs assessments. As a result, non-social workers determine whether social work services are needed. Medicaid programs vary across states, and there is no uniform requirement that social work services even be available in home care cases financed through Medicaid (Garner, 1995:1632).

Chapter 6

Social Work in Nursing Homes

HISTORICAL BACKGROUND

The Development of the American Nursing Home

Nursing homes in the United States today are a mix of proprietary (private for-profit), voluntary (private nonprofit), and public (tax supported and nonprofit). The history of nursing homes in America varies with each of these three organizational types.

Public Long-Term Care Facilities

The earliest institutional form of care for the elderly, mentally or physically ill or handicapped, and other dependent persons in America was the variously termed *county home, poorhouse, poor farm, or almshouse.* These were sometimes found in larger communities during the colonial era but became the principle form of care of sick and otherwise dependent persons by the early 1800s—after industrialization, urbanization, and immigration undermined the earlier informal mechanisms of family and community care of the sick and needy. These were public, local tax-supported institutions (Boondas, 1991). In many cities and counties in the United States, these almshouses continued to exist until at least the 1960s (Dieckmann, 1993).

However, by the mid-1800s, there was widespread recognition of the unfit conditions in many poorhouses, where theory and practice concerning the ability of the residents to take care of one another and to operate self-supporting farms proved to be discrepant. In response, during the latter half of the 1800s, many large specialized institutions sprang up, mostly public, state tax-supported facilities—such as for the mentally ill, epileptic, or mentally retarded. According to one psychiatrist who had worked as an orderly in a mental institution during the 1950s, these places served as much, if not more, to replace the poorhouses of the early 1800s in providing supportive care of the homeless, alcoholic, addicted, brain damaged, demented elderly, and other impaired people as to provide any specialized treatment for the population identified in the title of the institution (Vogel, 1991).

231

Voluntary Long-Term Care Facilities

In addition, by the mid-1800s, many benevolent care facilities emerged for specific populations, sponsored by voluntary organizations—often with religious, civic, or occupational affiliations. Thus, "homes for the aged" sprang up for specific groups, such as for Germans, Jews, Methodists, Lutherans, Baptists, Catholics, or Masons, Elks, or retired teachers. In general, the quality of care in nonprofit facilities for the members of a particular subgroup was very good and set a standard for the care of the elderly as traditional nursing homes developed (Boondas, 1991).

Proprietary Long-Term Care Facilities

As early as the colonial period, there also were some private for-profit boarding homes, which were the forerunners of today's proprietary nursing homes (Boondas, 1991). These boarding facilities continue today, generally providing supportive, nonskilled care for mild to moderately impaired persons, while today's proprietary nursing homes are mostly classified as skilled care facilities.

As the United States entered the twentieth century, a variety of forces pressed for federal government assumption of responsibility to aid the elderly: (1) the devaluation of the elderly with the transition from agriculture to industry and its emphasis on speed and efficiency, (2) the reduction in extended families due to migration from rural to urban areas, and (3) the transition to a wage economy with loss of social supports associated with close-knit rural community living. The Social Security Act was passed by Congress in 1935, providing for a variety of federal social insurance and public assistance programs, including a social insurance program of retirement pensions for the elderly, and the onset of "old age" was arbitrarily set at sixty-five years.

However, the Social Security Act stipulated that Social Security pensions to the elderly could not be paid to persons residing in institutional care. The effect of this provision was an exodus of elderly people from institutional care to privately owned boarding homes, some of which were operated by persons with at least some nursing training; and such places came to be called nursing homes (Boondas, 1991).

In 1946, the Hill-Burton Act was passed by Congress. This act provided direct grants to public and other nonprofit organizations to construct nursing homes and other health care facilities.

In 1960, the Kerr Mills Act was enacted by Congress, offering federal matching funds to states to help pay for health care for the elderly and poor (Karger and Stoesz, 1994:282). These funds were often used to pay for nursing home care, which at that time was commonly provided in the nursing home operator's own home.

In 1958, the Small Business Administration was established and offered loans to nursing homes. These developments helped to meet the need for long-term care of the elderly, but, unfortunately, also helped to promote the medicalization of the care of the aged (Boondas, 1991).

That is, after Medicare and Medicaid were enacted in the mid-1960s, states transferred many of the residents of large state-supported institutions to nursing homes, in an effort to shift state costs to the federal government. However, another effect of the passage of federal legislation to provide public financial reimbursement for nursing home care was that many nursing homes were transformed from mostly small homelike settings into large, institutional, motel-like facilities where rows of identical rooms, resembling the isolated cells of a beehive, housed patients to be processed in efficient assembly line style. Thus, long-term care in the United States traditionally has been determined by reimbursement policy (Olson, 1994:31). Olson commented:

> The number of for-profit institutions in most other nations is negligible. As a result, no other country has developed the American equivalent of the nursing home; it is truly a unique institution. (33)

Funding Sources and Nursing Home Care

Medicare expenditures for nursing home care are entirely for skilled care, which in 1998 was provided to 1,443,000 persons, age sixty-five or over, and to 75,000 persons under age sixty-five with end-stage renal disease (U.S. Government Printing Office, 2000b:114, Table 167). Because Medicare pays for only skilled care, it reimburses more generously than Medicaid. Consequently, many nursing homes prefer Medicare patients and avoid accepting those on Medicaid (Olson, 1994:29), producing a dual-track system of care (Boondas, 1991), one for the welfare dependent and one for the rest.

Curiously, not all nursing home residents are in what we think of as traditional nursing homes. The most recent National Nursing Home Survey (1997) data are reported in *Statistical Abstracts of the United States* (U.S. Government Printing Office, 2000b:134, Table 209) and indicate that the living quarters of all nursing home residents are distributed as follows:

Hospital: 44.5 percent
Private residence: 32.2 percent
Nursing home: 12.2 percent

Retirement home: 2.3 percent
Mental health facility: 1.3 percent
Board and room and/or residential facility: 4.6 percent

Note: Table 209 footnoted that persons in strictly board and room facilities were not counted as nursing home residents, so the 4.6 percent must refer to persons in facilities that provide some care services in addition to board and care.

Even today, the best quality nursing home care tends to be provided in retirement communities or homes for the aged that provide a range of care levels, including supportive living in houses and apartments as well as skilled nursing care units. These continue to be either the voluntary organizations that were started for members of religious, professional, or civic organizations or proprietary organizations for the affluent, both of which often require a substantial lump-sum payment upon entrance, in addition to monthly rates, with assurance of lifelong care. Presumably, these are included under retirement home residents, constituting only 2.3 percent of all our country's population receiving nursing home care.

In 1998, the United States spent $1,019.347 billion for personal health care, of which 8.6 percent, or $87.8 billion, was for nursing home care (U.S. Government Printing Office, 2000a:327-328, Table 119). About 60.4 percent, or $53.03 billion, of the total $87.8 billion expended for nursing home care was paid for by the government; $40.7 billion, or 46.3 percent, was paid through Medicaid for the indigent; $10.5 billion, or 11.9 percent, was paid through Medicare for the relatively few who qualify for skilled care; and the other $1.93 billion, or 2.2 percent, was paid through the Veterans Administration and state subsidies to hospitals (see Table 6.1). (U.S. Government Printing Office, 2000a:327-328, Table 119).

In 1998, Medicaid paid for both skilled and intermediate nursing home care for 1,646,000 recipients, excluding the mentally retarded (U.S. Government Printing Office, 2000b:116, Table 172). Together, Medicare and Medicaid helped pay for nursing home care for a total of 3,164,000 persons during 1998.

Thus we can see that the largest share (46.34 percent) of nursing home care is paid for through Medicaid—which requires that income and resources place an individual below the poverty line—and the next largest share (32.5 percent) is paid out of pocket. In fact, unless the individual is transferred directly from a hospital or within thirty days of being hospitalized and requires skilled care, that person is not eligible for Medicare coverage for nursing home care, and so must reduce his or her resources to at least the poverty level before becoming eligible for Medicaid.

TABLE 6.1. Nursing Home Care Expenditures, 1998

Payer	Dollars (in Billions)	Percent
Government	53.1	60.4
Medicaid	40.7	46.3
Medicare	10.5	11.9
VA and other government programs	1.9	2.2
Out of pocket	28.5	32.5
Private health insurance	4.7	5.3
Other private funds	1.6	1.8
Total	87.8	100.0

Source: U.S. Government Printing Office (2000a). *Health, United States.* Washington, DC: Author, 327.

The average monthly charge for nursing home care paid by the resident or family was $3,643 in 1997 ($3,081 if paid by Medicaid, and $6,037 when paid by Medicare), with considerable variation across geographic regions of the United States and across facility size (U.S. Government Printing Office, 2000a:335, Table 124). Thus, it does not take long for most elderly people to exhaust their life savings and become eligible for welfare assistance via Medicaid. For many elderly people, admission to a nursing home is viewed as close to death itself in terms of negative life events. If the elderly also must "go on welfare" to pay for nursing home care, the impact on self-respect and ego integrity can be tremendously eroding. Little wonder that many elderly nursing home patients have been found to be suffering from emotional depression.

If, as is widely contended, personal empowerment is essential for maximizing health status, nursing home care, as presently provided in the United States, is a major force defeating that objective. For-profit nursing homes have one overriding objective—to make as much profit as possible—and are therefore operated to meet the needs of administrators and stockholders rather than those of the residents or their families (Olson, 1994:32).

However, the Balanced Budget Act of 1997 markedly reduced Medicare reimbursement to skilled nursing facilities (SNFs) through the introduction of a prospective payment system (PPS). For a while, this resulted in many nursing homes refusing to accept Medicare patients, with the claim that they could not "afford" to do so with such reductions in reimbursement. In 1999 the regulations were modified with the passage of the Balanced Budget Refinement Act (BBRA), which increased reimbursements for certain classifications of nursing home patients with more medically complex needs. The PPS introduced in nursing homes is comparable to the diagnosis related group (DRG) system, which was introduced in hospitals in 1983 in an effort to establish a "rational" basis for per diem charges for patient care, and which is the first change in reimbursement to skilled nursing facilities since Title XVIII of the Social Security Act that introduced the Medicare system in the United States. In nursing homes, DRGs were replaced with RUGs (resource utilization groups), which employ a scale to assess the level of acute care needed, requiring skilled professional services (Society for Social Work Leadership in Health Care, 2000).

In 1997, there were about 17,000 nursing homes in the United States. Of this total, 11,400, or about 67 percent, were for-profit nursing homes; 4,400, or 26 percent, were private nonprofit organizations; and the remaining 1,200, or 7 percent, were public tax-supported facilities (U.S. Government Printing Office, 2000b:133).

Nursing homes are "big business" in America. If, in 1997, 67 percent of nursing homes outside of hospitals were for-profit enterprises and about $87.8 billion was expended in the United States for nursing home care, presumably about $59 billion of the total went to the for-profit sector in revenues.

The nursing home industry is rapidly being consolidated into the hands of a few huge corporations (Karger and Stoesz, 1994:224-225). Furthermore, conglomerates unrelated to health care, such as Avon Products and Marriott Corporation, have entered the market as well (Margolis, 1990:157, cited in Olson, 1994:32). In 1996, ninety-four U.S. corporations were operating skilled nursing home chains. Four of these had combined revenues of $6.701 billion, as depicted in Table 6.2.

The Quality of Nursing Home Care

A recent thorough study of nursing home state inspection reports for 1998 (Harrington et al., 2001) found that investor-owned nursing homes averaged 46.5 percent more deficiency citations overall than nonprofits and 43.0 percent more than public facilities. Investor-owned nursing homes also averaged 40.5 percent more "severe deficiency" citations overall than nonprofits and 35.8 percent more than public facilities, and one-fourth of all deficiencies were "severe." The authors conclude in their "discussion" section:

> Our results suggest that investor-owned nursing homes deliver lower quality care than do nonprofit or public facilities. Moreover, investor-owned facilities are usually part of a chain, and chain ownership *per se* is associated with a further decrement in quality. (1454)

TABLE 6.2. Top Four Revenue-Producing Nursing Home Corporations, 1996

Company Name	1996 Revenues (in Billions)	Number of Employees (in Thousands)
1. Beverly Enterprises	3.243	82
2. Manor Care, Inc.	1.322	31
3. Sun Healthcare Group, Inc.	1.136	28
4. Continental Medical Systems, Inc.	1.000*	14
Total	6.701	155

Source: Gale Publishing Company (1997). *Wards Business Directory of U.S. Private and Public Companies,* Volume 5. Detroit, MI: Author, 115-116.

*Indicates estimated financial figure. Note that this fourth corporation is a subsidiary of Horizon/CMS Healthcare, which was eighth on the list of skilled nursing home corporations, with revenues the same year of another $639 million.

Of the 13,693 nursing homes, 65.8 percent were investor owned, 27.7 percent were nonprofit, and 6.5 percent were public.

In general, nursing homes in the United States are sterile environments modeled after the interior appearance of a hospital but without the quality of care provided in most hospitals. Instead, many nursing homes lack adequate rehabilitative services, mental health assessment and treatment services, meaningful social activities, or efforts to encourage decision making by the residents (Olson, 1994:34).

Most of the care is provided by laypersons with little or no training, such as certified nursing assistants (CNAs). Anecdotal reports from CNAs and family members indicate that state regulations concerning the ratio of CNA staff to patients per shift are frequently violated, especially when fewer visitors are expected. According to Ellen Flaherty (2001), project director for the GITT Center of New York University Division of Nursing, "Very few nurses in the nursing home have any formal training in geriatrics at all" (49).

Since the Omnibus Budget Reconciliation Act (OMBRA) of 1987, nursing assistants in nursing homes must have at least seventy-five hours of training that addresses the nursing, psychosocial, physical, and environmental needs of residents, as well as medical needs, although many would agree that less than two weeks of training is not much preparation for the heavy responsibilities of the job (Kane and Caplan, 1990:277).

Use of chemical and physical restraints has been common in nursing homes. Although OMBRA, effective January 1989, was a major effort to reduce such abuses, mandating that restraints can only be used in emergencies and only with the consent of the patient or family or by physician order, regulations have not resulted in major changes in institutional practices (Olson, 1994:35). The Health Care Financing Administration (2000) summarized the actions, difficulties, and successes that have arisen regarding efforts to reduce the use of restraints in nursing homes. The state of Pennsylvania was cited for outstanding progress in reducing the use of restraints, both physical and chemical, and in training programs for health care facility staff regarding behavioral management, fall prevention, and individualized assessment procedure. Some remarkable and moving success stories citing imaginative innovations were presented. The newsletter noted that some nursing home staff still think that a particular device is not a restraint if it is used to prevent the patient from falling, such as "lap buddies" or side rails, and such devices are often used without first having done a thorough assessment of the person's strengths and weaknesses. Resident assessment protocols exist and should be used for such assessments (6).

THEORETICAL PERSPECTIVES

An Alternative to Hospital Care or Home Care

Presumably, the basic rationale for having nursing homes at all is that some persons have health problems and accompanying functional impairments such that they do not require hospital care but are unable to be cared for at home. They may be incapable of self-care, they may not have family or other volunteers who are willing and able to provide the needed care, or they may not have the financial resources to pay for round-the-clock formal home care services.

Because health problems, functional disabilities, and loss of family supports tend to increase with advancing age, most nursing home residents are elderly. However, only an estimated 5 percent of all persons age sixty-five and over and 20 percent of the disabled elderly reside in nursing homes at any given time (Pepper Commission, 1990:92, cited in Olson, 1994:27). Thus, most elderly people, with or without disability, live outside of nursing homes or other institutions, indicating that the decision whether to remain at home or to enter a nursing home is probably more a function of social and economic supports than of health status. In fact, most (nearly 58 percent) nursing home residents in 1997 were transferred from a hospital or another nursing home and about one-third came from private homes in the community. About 60 percent of those who entered from private homes had been living with a family member, while the remaining 40 percent had been living alone. Most entering residents were widowed when they were moved to a nursing home (Sahyoun et al., 2001).

Cost Savings

Another rationale for nursing home care is that it is less costly than hospital care. Total personal health care expenditures for hospital care in 1998 reached $382.8 billion, or 37.5 percent of the total $1,019.347 billion expended that year for personal health care (U.S. Government Printing Office, 2000b: Table 156), compared to 8.6 percent for nursing home care ($87.835 billion). Skilled nursing home care cost an average of $523 per day in 1998, compared with $2,401 per day in a hospital (U.S. Government Printing Office, 1999:2).

The PPS and DRG system meant that hospitals could no longer keep patients as long as they saw fit and expect to be accordingly reimbursed. Instead they needed to discharge patients within a set number of days or not be reimbursed either by Medicare or the patient for the overstay days. Furthermore, discharge prior to the expiration deadline meant that the Medicare reimbursement for any unused days could be realized by the hospital as pure profit.

The Concept of Caring

Theoretically, nursing homes provide extensive supportive assistance to maximize the comfort and function (physical, emotional, and social) of residents with chronic and/or terminal health conditions. This is caring at the third stage of health care. This type of caring means providing the patient with the tools, equipment, services, environmental supports, income supports, and supportive interpersonal interactions they require to maximize their comfort and function.

Surely a basic service of caring is to provide pain relief. Currently, much concern is being expressed in the health professional literature concerning alleged lack of adequate pain relief in the U.S. health care system generally. Dr. Joan Teno, associate director of the Brown University Center for Gerontology and Health Care Research, and some colleagues conducted a study, funded by the Robert Wood Johnson Foundation, of inadequately treated pain among nursing home residents. Teno (2001:50) reported that untreated pain "is an important national public health problem" among this population.

Teno and colleagues (2001) recommend that patients and family members ask a nursing home about its pain policy and whether the staff assess pain. The reported data reflect what nursing home staff ascertain, and they have a reputation for underestimating patient pain. Nonetheless, the nursing home staff reported, in the minimum data set required by the Center for Medicare and Medicaid, that 41.2 percent of patients who were in pain around April 1, 1999, still experienced moderate daily pain or excruciating pain 60-90 days later. Of individuals in a nursing home between 2 and 6 months, one in seven had persistent pain. Nationwide, pain rates in nursing homes varied between 39.5 and 49.5.

A new standard of the Joint Commission on the Accreditation of Healthcare Organizations (JCAHO) is that hospitals and nursing homes must now monitor and document pain as a fifth vital sign along with blood pressure, pulse, respiration, and temperature.

The new JCAHO standards to assess and manage pain are as follows:

- Assess the nature and intensity of pain in all patients.
- Establish safe medication prescription and ordering procedures.
- Ensure staff competency and orient new staff in pain assessment and management.
- Monitor patients post-procedurally and reassess patient problems appropriately.
- Educate patients on the role of pain management in treatment.
- Address patient's needs for symptom management in the discharge planning process.
- Collect data to monitor performance. (Solovy, 2000)

Subacute Care

To some extent, nursing homes are expected to provide caring at the secondary level of health care as well. Since the prospective payment system began, acute-care patients are released from hospitals as soon as possible, and many are transferred as subacute cases to nursing homes to convalesce before returning home. These are not necessarily elderly people. In addition, many elderly people are transferred to nursing homes following episodes such as a stroke or hip fracture, not only because they need assistance to function, but also because they need physical therapy and/or speech therapy to be rehabilitated and return home. Such therapies or treatments are forms of curing, whereas interventions to facilitate and encourage the accessibility and effectiveness of these therapies may be called caring or supportive interventions.

JCAHO Standards for Pain Assessment and Management

- Assess the nature and intensity of pain in all patients.
- Establish safe medication prescription and ordering procedures.
- Ensure staff competency and orient new staff in pain assessment and management.
- Monitor patients postprocedurely and reassess patient problems appropriately.
- Educate patients on the role of pain management in treatment.
- Address patients' needs for symptom management in the discharge planning process.
- Collect data to monitor performance. (Solovy, 2000)

Two-thirds of the people admitted to nursing homes stay less than three months (U.S. Senate Special Committee on Aging, 1990). According to Sahyoun et al. (2001), in 1997, 30 percent of nursing home residents recuperated enough to return to the community, and their average length of stay in the nursing home was forty-five days; another 36 percent of residents were transferred to a hospital or other nursing home, and their average length of stay was 284 days; another 25 percent died, and their average length of stay had been 562 days (or about one and one-half years); the outcome for the remaining 9 percent was "unknown." According to Sahyoun et al. (2001), in 1997, the average nursing home resident stayed 903 days, or about two and one-half years (3).

The Medical Model

Although Medicare regulations require interdisciplinary teamwork to help implement a biopsychosocial perspective, neither the physical environment nor the daily activities, schedule, or services of most nursing homes is conducive to a "whole person" focus.

Presumably, the sterile atmosphere in many nursing homes reflects an attempt to resemble a place where people are not merely warehoused, but instead treated, that is, to present a hospital-like atmosphere. Patient rooms are generally furnished with the same type of beds, bedside tables, and chairs commonly found in hospitals. Floors are bare tile. Rooms usually are lined up along narrow halls, leading to the nurses station, and so on. In short, the atmosphere in most nursing homes is not homey, and it is not conducive to social interaction or personal empowerment.

In 1991, a nursing home resident, then age ninety-three, with a bachelor's degree in architecture, wrote an article (Mead, 1991) about his perception of the discrepancy between the type of atmosphere he had earlier enjoyed in a home for the aged, which had since been closed, and that of the nursing home facility to which he was moved and in which he was now residing. He wrote:

> If we recognize that the primal nature of human beings is to seek fellowship, human understanding and inward comprehension, fostered by mutual inspiration and concern, then the nursing home becomes a very pernicious and inappropriate form of confinement (12) . . . while concentrating on the medical and habitational aspects of such facilities, the *in corpore* [physical] items mentioned earlier, we often overlook the *mens sana* [mental health] portion of the equation (14). . . . Maintenance of normal physical functioning can well be considered as primary, but without the assurance of being happy, competent and fully alive, to what degree can we appreciate good health? (15)

These remarks imply that the mental and emotional and spiritual needs of people have to be addressed, as well as their physical needs. These needs all affect one another.

Caplan (1990) argues that most nursing home patients do not enter nursing homes to receive acute medical care, "yet the daily life of the nursing home is permeated by a model of staff-resident relationships that is firmly rooted in an ethic drawn from acute-care medical settings" (41).

HUMAN DIVERSITY RELEVANCE

In the better quality nursing homes, homes for the aged, and so forth, due regard is given to the characteristics of the population being served. For example, Jewish elder care facilities have always tended to provide high-quality care, with well-trained professional staff, appropriate ethnic diet, and other types of consideration for ethnic-related preferences and traditions. Such consideration is more likely to be found in large cities where there are concentrations of specific ethnic groups, often with distinct languages, diets, and customs.

Unfortunately, where the population is predominately of white European background, and ethnic diversity is rare, members of such ethnically diverse groups are likely to encounter relative insensitivity to their preferences in the society in general, as well as in health care facilities, such as nursing homes.

Race and Ethnicity

Both hospitals and nursing homes were racially segregated in the United States until relatively recent years, and there is some evidence that this trend continues. Technically, racial discrimination in health care facilities ended in the mid-1960s with the passage of Medicare and Medicaid. However, in practice most continue to be racially segregated, as do public schools. This health care facility segregation was largely accomplished by the exclusion of black physicians from membership in the AMA, resulting in their exclusion from practicing in hospitals that required such membership (Smith, 1990). This situation continued for many years, even after the Hill-Burton Act of 1946 was passed, providing federal funds for hospital and nursing home construction, stipulating nondiscrimination but providing exception to this if "separate but equal" facilities were provided. Racial segregation in hospitals in both the South and North continued until the mid-1960s (Smith, 1990:564).

The NAACP (National Association for the Advancement of Colored People) and the NMA (National Medical Association), the professional organization of black physicians, led the fight against racial discrimination in health care facilities (Smith, 1990:567). It was not until 1963, however, that the U.S. Court of Appeals issued a majority opinion that hospitals were sufficiently involved with the state and federal governments to fall within the constitutional prohibition against racial discrimination. The surgeon general immediately issued new strict nondiscrimination regulations for those facilities applying for Hill-Burton funds (Smith, 1990:574).

These events were followed by passage of the Civil Rights Act of 1964, Title IV of which stated the following:

> No persons in the United States shall, on the grounds of race, color or national origin, be excluded from participation in or be denied the benefits of, or be subjected to discrimination under any program or activity receiving federal financial assistance. (U.S. Civil Rights Commission, 1963)

Finally, in 1965, Medicare and Medicaid were enacted, which raised the stakes further for hospital compliance with antidiscrimination laws. Noncompliance would have meant that patients could not use their Medicare or Medicaid coverage in the noncompliant hospitals, meaning both physicians and hospitals would have lost income (Smith, 1990:575).

However, the impact on nursing homes was not the same. These facilities were not eager to have poor patients covered by minimal Medicaid reimbursement, and they did not expect Medicare, with its restrictive eligibility, to amount to a very substantial part of their revenues (Smith, 1990:576). As it turned out, Medicaid expenditures to state governments spiraled much faster than expected, and since heightened efforts to ensure blacks had equal access to nursing home care would have meant even greater Medicaid expenditures, little was done to enforce nondiscrimination (577).

Although hospitals soon became subject to Medicare-compliance reviews, which further served to enforce racial integration in hospitals, nursing homes were not subject to such reviews. In 1989, the Health Care Financing Administration (HCFA) of the United States observed that

> Although in 1985 blacks constituted 31 percent of the Medicaid recipients and accounted for 21.8 percent of Medicaid expenditures nationally, they comprised [only] 8 percent of the recipients and accounted for [only] 8.9 percent of the expenditures for skilled nursing facilities. (HCFA, 1989:85)

In 1981, the Institute of Medicine noted that "most persons who have studied and written about black use of nursing homes believe that racial discrimination is a major explanatory factor" (Institute of Medicine, 1981:98).

It has been argued that black families are more likely to prefer providing home care supportive assistance over nursing home care (Morrow-Howell et al., 1996). The Institute of Medicine noted that blacks are overrepresented in government psychiatric and chronic care facilities—which suggests that blacks will utilize services where they feel they will be accepted and respected (Smith, 1990:585-586).

Morrison (1995) reported similar findings among both blacks and Hispanics in New York City: "Blacks represented 32 percent of residents in public facilities, 13 percent in proprietary facilities, and 11 percent in voluntary facilities. For Hispanics, the percentages were 8 percent, 1.5 percent, and 4.5 percent respectively" (Morrison, 1995:19).

Morrison (1995) asks whether America may continue to have a dual system of nursing homes: public ones for ethnic minorities and private ones for the white elderly. Although these ethnic groups are represented in proportion to their percentage of the total population, there is much evidence that their elderly populations have higher rates of disease and disability than their white counterparts (24).

Salive and colleagues (1993) reported a large longitudinal study to compare white and African-American elderlys' use of nursing homes, and found that African-American elderly were admitted to nursing homes only about one-half as often as white elderly. The main risk factors for nursing home admission among whites were urban residence and mental health problems of a cognitive nature, whereas these were not found to be significant risk factors among African-American elderly. In fact, the study was not successful in identifying the determinants of the ethnic difference in nursing home admission rates.

Morrison (1995) proposed that the United States explore the feasibility of minority owned and operated nursing homes, home care agencies, and other health care services for the respective ethnic groups as an alternative to the current unsatisfactory situation.

Although areas of the United States with sizable Jewish, Japanese, Native American, Hispanic, and other ethnic populations sometimes have ethnic-specific residential care facilities for the elderly, the difference in proposing separate facilities for African-American elderly is that other groups have done it to more appropriately meet the culture-specific needs of their elderly, who often speak a language other than English and have distinct foods and customs. With black Americans, the rationale is more to try to ensure quality care services in face of racial discrimination in the mainstream sector.

Social workers in health care need to recognize that even when a culture traditionally places great importance on family responsibility to care for the elderly, as cultures change the family members designated as caregivers may experience considerable conflict between traditional expectations and present circumstances (Freed, 1990). For example, in Japan, one study closely explored the attitudes, feelings, and behaviors of a set of families engaged in home care of an elderly family member and found that (as in the United States) wives, daughters, or daughters-in-law were the main caregivers, and in most cases, they admitted that they filled the role reluctantly and resented having to do so (Freed, 1990).

As in the United States, many Japanese women are now employed outside the home and are better educated than before. Although Japan has nursing homes, they are largely used for brief respite stays, and nursing home placement of an aged family member is viewed as a disgrace. Since hospitalization is not so regarded, many families leave the elder in a hospital much longer than necessary to avoid the conflict between home care and nursing home care (Freed, 1990).

Given that the family is now recognized as a social system, the assumption of responsibility for taking in and giving care to an aged parent is often disruptive to the family system.

Another ethnic population in the United States that lacks access to appropriate nursing home care is the Native American elderly (Mercer, 1994). According to Mercer, 71 percent of Native Americans over age sixty have ADL functional impairments, yet there are few nursing homes designed for them, and currently, most Indian elders who require nursing home care must leave the reservation and live away from home and family. Unfortunately, most facilities have no Indian staff who speak the residents' languages, nor do they serve traditional foods or encourage traditional customs and needs, which can lead to social isolation and depression and an erosion of health status and quality of life (4).

One notable exception is the Navajo nursing home at Chinle, Arizona, on the Navajo reservation, described in the Mercer (1994) study. The elderly Navajo residents are addressed by titles that they regard as endearing and respectful, are served Navajo foods, and are permitted to sleep on the floor in native fashion if they prefer. All but two of the staff are Navajo. Although it is an intermediate care facility, residents appear comfortable and content. According to Mercer (1994), Native Americans have a particular need for more quality nursing homes that are culturally appropriate because many live on remote reservations where formal home health care services are not available, and where family members are often unable to care for them (Mercer, 1994). In this and another article, Mercer describes a variety of fascinating cultural characteristics of the Navajo elders she observed (Mercer, 1994, 1996).

The AIDS Stigma

Nursing home social workers also need to be sensitive to the problem of providing appropriate care for persons with AIDS, since the social worker often is responsible for admissions. Linsk and Marder (1992) found that hospital social workers rarely pursued nursing home placement for hospitalized AIDS patients upon discharge because previous efforts had met with universal failure. Yet many of these patients lack the financial resources or informal supports to allow for home health care (106). This dilemma results in unusually long stays in hospitals, which is the most costly alternative in the health care system.

Linsk and Marder (1992) later found that new hospital social workers made extensive efforts to obtain nursing home placements for AIDS patients and were unsuccessful, while experienced social workers called upon lesser-known alternative resources in the community, such as specialized AIDS residences that could contract with HHC agencies. The authors report that the solutions obtained were usually less than were needed and lament the continued refusal of most nursing homes to accept AIDS patients. They also point out that nursing homes ought to be aware that the chances are that, unknowingly, they already have some patients with the HIV virus, and should therefore currently be enforcing the use of universal precautions by their staff. Meanwhile, there is a need for specialized facilities for AIDS patients (Linsk and Marder, 1992:114).

In a letter to *Health and Social Work,* the president of the National Foundation for Long Term Care argued that, indeed, specialized facilities for AIDS patients were needed, in the same way that not all facilities can provide all services, whether the service required is for AIDS, Alzheimer's disease, or ventilator-dependent children (Freeman, 1988).

This type of situation is one of many potential ethical dilemmas that nursing home social workers can encounter.

Sex and Sexuality

Since at least the late 1970s, the issue of sexual expression in nursing homes has been acknowledged (Kaas, 1978; Wasow and Loeb, 1979; Brown, 1989). A survey was recently conducted of social workers employed in twenty-nine randomly selected nursing homes in New York (Fairchild, Carrino, and Ramirez, 1996) concerning their perceptions of staff attitudes toward resident sexuality. The social workers reported that all twenty-nine of the nursing homes studied allowed married couples to share rooms if both agreed; masturbation is thought to be the most common form of sexual expression among nursing home residents; and over one-half thought that the nursing home managers would not tolerate homosexual activities among residents. In addition, many respondents said they made no effort to ascertain the residents' sexual orientation. All but one of the nursing home social workers reported no formal policy or staff orientation regarding resident rights in the area of sexual expression, although about one-half indicated that the issue had come up in staff meetings. Fairchild, Carrino, and Ramirez (1996) offer some suggestions for development of in-service training directed toward clarifying specific resident rights in the area of sexual expression.

Although it is generally held that elderly nursing home residents need more privacy for sexual activities, a thought-provoking study of men with an average age of seventy, living in a VA medical center long-term care facility, found that when asked to rate the importance of intimate social, intellectual, emotional, or physical interactions, the men rated physical sexual intimacy as least important and social intimacy as most important. This was found among both married and unmarried men (Bullard-Poe, Powell, and Mulligan, 1994).

More research is needed about the adequacy of nursing home policy and practice concerning residents' sexuality.

INTERDISCIPLINARY TEAMWORK

Nursing home regulations issued by both Medicare (Health Care Financing Administration, now called the Centers for Medicare and Medicaid

Services <http://www.cms.gov>) and the Joint Commission on the Accreditation of Healthcare Organizations (JCAHO) (1993) require that each patient has an individualized interdisciplinary plan of care based on a comprehensive assessment of patient health and psychosocial status. Social services are delineated as essential to the multidisciplinary care team and as having fundamental responsibility for the psychosocial assessment and for sharing in the meeting of patients' psychosocial needs.

All nursing homes that receive funds through Medicare or Medicaid are required to hold regular interdisciplinary team meetings within a few days of patient admission and periodically thereafter. The idea is that each key team member will conduct an assessment of patient status and needs in his or her own professional skill area and identify tentative objectives and associated interventions for that resident's care. This information is then shared among team members so that understanding and intervention are coordinated.

Nursing homes that expect to accept Medicare patients must be Medicare certified and undergo a survey by the Health Care Financing Administration (HCFA), the federal umbrella agency responsible for Medicare and Medicaid programs, at least once every ten months (Williams, 1997). However, the Joint Commission on the Accreditation of Healthcare Organizations is an independent, nonprofit organization and the oldest and largest standard-setting and accrediting body in health care, but nursing homes are not required to be accredited by JCAHO, and only about 10 percent of nursing homes have JCAHO accreditation (Williams, 1997).

Furthermore, JCAHO allows a variety of options in the provision of social services: a social worker who has completed the course work for an MSW from a CSWE-accredited school of social work, one who has the documented equivalent in education, training, and/or experience ("a qualified social worker"), or someone with a bachelor's degree, preferably with a social work sequence and additional on-the-job training ("a social services assistant") (JCAHO, 1993). A social services assistant must consult with a qualified social worker on a monthly basis. If none of these options are selected, an alternative is to contract with an outside organization, such as a school of social work or community agency, that uses the direct services of a qualified social worker (JCAHO, 1993:53). Obviously, cost-conscious facilities under pressure to reduce overhead will tend to opt for the least-expensive alternative.

Finally, I have observed considerable variation across nursing homes in the quality of interdisciplinary (ID) teamwork. In some nursing homes, regular and frequent ID team meetings are held with a full spectrum of professional staff, who attend the meetings well-prepared to share with one another the results of their assessments of patients and their helping intervention plans. Sometimes a concerned family member and/or the patient is present and included. At the other extreme are nursing homes whose ID teamwork practice is a farce. These are characterized by irregular and infrequent team meetings, attended by few representatives of professional staff, who sometimes appear to regard the team meetings as a necessary, but annoying, government requirement and give little indication that they have developed, or intend to develop, thoughtful care plans.

ORGANIZATIONAL CONSIDERATIONS

Essentially, the extent to which interdisciplinary teamwork is a reality in nursing homes depends greatly on the extent to which the nursing home management values it as ideal and takes appropriate action to facilitate its working.

All health care settings are secondary or "host" settings for social work, and so the organizational mission is defined and dominated by persons other than social workers (Dane and Simon, 1991, cited in Kruzich and Powell, 1995).

Bureaucratization

Brannon (1992) wrote:

> From the viewpoint of the student of organizations, nursing homes are paradoxes. Although organizational size is usually positively associated with levels of bureaucratization, nursing homes are small organizations that exhibit decidedly bureaucratic structures. Families and residents experience bureaucracy in a variety of ways including: the routinized, sometimes "assembly line" nature of care routines; the highly regulated hierarchy of information exchange and authority within the staff; and the prominence of rules and procedures over negotiated relationships as guides for behavior. . . . Yet some nursing homes feel less bureaucratic than others. Examples of autonomy-enhancing organizational strategies have been cited (Kane and Caplan, 1990) and innovations within the industry are apparent. The challenge is for second-generation nursing home researchers to simultaneously look within and across facilities to identify patterns of organizational design, work design, and human resource strategies that enhance resident well-being. This will require cross disciplinary thinking, which results in studies of individual behavior framed in organizational context

variables and studies of institutions attending to individual differences. (294) Copyright © The Gerontological Society of America. Reproduced by permission of the publisher.

Organizational Priorities and Objectives

Presumably, if the facility is managed by a business administrator, as for-profit facilities are likely to be, the organizational objectives and priorities will tend to diverge from those of a voluntary or public facility often managed by a health care professional, such as a registered nurse or MSW social worker. The organizational objectives of such health care professionals will tend to revolve around a greater commitment to a biopsychosocial and inter-disciplinary perspective directed toward a high quality of life and care of the residents.

The less priority placed on financial profit, the more likely the facility is to employ well-trained professional staff who are dedicated to high-quality care and sensitivity to human diversity, who value the relationship between patient empowerment and patient health status, and who understand the need for nursing assistants to have a low enough patient care load that they can provide sensitive, individualized, quality caregiving that is rewarding for both patient and caregiver.

Authority Structure/Decision-Making Style and Sense of Empowerment

Some evidence suggests that the less a nursing home relies on a bureaucratic authority structure and the more the organization functions as a participatory democracy, the greater the sense of empowerment of the staff, including social workers. One nursing home study (Kruzich, 1995) compared perceived control of directors of nursing, directors of social services, activity directors, charge nurses, and nursing assistants over various areas of decision making. The study showed that the greater the perceived influence of the nursing director, the less the perceived influence of the charge nurse; the greater the perceived influence of the charge nurse, the greater the perceived influence of the nursing assistants; and the greater the perceived control of the activity directors over resident care decisions, the greater the perceived influence of the social service directors over resident care decisions (210).

The three *structural variables* most associated with increased perceived influence of all staff combined were nonprofit organizational status, larger size facilities, and nonunionized facilities, while the *process variables* most associated with increased perceived influence were nursing assistant participation in shift report, more frequent staff meetings, and less rotation of nursing assistant staff among residents and units (Kruzich, 1995:213).

A study of nursing home social workers in Wisconsin found that of five broad areas of potential social worker influence in the nursing home, both the line social workers and directors of social work in the nursing homes studied agreed that the two areas of greatest social work influence were (1) care planning, including making changes in care plans and planning residents' care, and (2) resident transfer, specifically deciding if residents are transferred in or out of the facility (Kruzich and Powell, 1995:218).

The same study also found that social work directors in nursing homes perceived themselves as having more influence in publicly owned and non-profit facilities than in for-profit facilities. Also, such facilities employed more full-time social workers (Kruzich and Powell, 1995:218).

Curiously, social workers employed in nursing homes with a resident council perceived themselves as having more influence than social workers in homes without a resident council, and the extent of perceived social worker influence was positively correlated with the degree of resident autonomy and resident satisfaction in the home (Kruzich and Powell, 1995: 221).

Although it is not clear whether social worker influence is the cause or result of organizational flexibility and shared decision making, the findings indicate that the lone social worker in a for-profit facility is likely to be in a relatively powerless position (Kruzich and Powell, 1995). The significance of these study findings is that they provide some clues as to the impact of organizational variables on staff and resident satisfaction, which is believed to be correlated with level of perceived autonomy or influence, which is, in turn, associated with well-being and health status (Kruzich, 1995).

Use of Proprietary Nursing Homes As Settings of Social Work Student Practicums

A 1991 survey (Hancock, 1992) of MSW educational programs in universities explored their use of for-profit organizational settings for field placements and found that health care organizations were most commonly used, and the universities were fairly evenly split between whether they do or do not use such settings without restrictions or criteria. Over one-half, or 55.4 percent, reported using for-profit nursing homes for placements, and about 61.8 percent did so without restriction (334). Use of for-profit settings for social work student field placement was found to vary by geographic region, with the highest percent (57.1 percent) in the Southwest, followed by the Southeast (43.7 percent), Mid-Atlantic (33.0 percent), West (28.6 percent), and Midwest (26.7 percent), with the lowest percentage in the Northeast (18.2 percent). Furthermore, the programs in the Southwest were least restrictive, while those in the Northeast were the most restrictive (335). In short, although most MSW programs in universities use for-profit settings for field placements, they vary considerably in their level of comfort with such placements (337).

Role Conflict and Staff Burnout

Another study (Barber and Iwai, 1996) examined the relative influence of (1) staff characteristics, (2) workload and caregiving involvement (emotional closeness with patients, number of patients cared for, and number of hours worked per week), (3) work environment characteristics (role ambiguity and role conflict), and (4) social support in predicting burnout among caregiving staff of Alzheimer's patients in nursing homes.

Role conflict, defined as two or more simultaneous expectations that are incompatible, such that performance of one makes it difficult to comply with the other, was found to account for most (56.5 percent) of the variance in likelihood of burnout. This implies that organizational strategies that minimize role conflict should effectively reduce burnout (Barber and Iwai, 1996:113). In addition, the findings underscore the developing conviction that both staff and patients/residents function better when they feel empowered and that a sense of powerlessness or helplessness is destructive to humans.

CLIENT PROBLEMS AND SOCIAL WORKER FUNCTIONS

Client Problems

As previously suggested, it may be useful to conceptualize client problems in health care settings as the following:

1. Barriers to admission to the facility or service
2. Problems of adjustment to the facility or service
3. Problems of adjustment to the diagnosis, prognosis, or care plan
4. Lack of information to make informed decisions and take control
5. Lack of resources to meet needs
6. Barriers to discharge from the facility or service

In 1992, Vourlekis, Gelfand, and Greene provided a list of twenty-eight psychosocial needs of nursing home residents and families which "was generated through a reiterated process of experiential and intuitive identification of issues on the part of a diverse group of nursing home experts, literature review in the psychosocial domain . . . and critique and revision by the expert group" (114). Thus, their list is presented in Box 6.1 as a legitimate list of psychosocial needs of nursing home residents and their families that nursing home social workers should address.

BOX 6.1.
Psychosocial Needs of Nursing Home Residents and Their Families

1. Emotional support in coping with the transition to the home
2. Help with feelings of loss throughout the stay in the home
3. Help with fears/anxieties . . . throughout the stay in the home
4. Specific help in preparing for and coping with death
5. Recognition by staff that "difficult behavior," including aggressiveness and withdrawal/apathy, may signify emotional distress, and need for interventions based on a specific understanding of that distress
6. Help with financial planning and decision making prior to coming to the home, and assistance in locating and accessing financial resources at any point during the stay in the home
7. Opportunity and assistance as needed with access to activities and events within the home which are diverse enough to match each resident's capabilities and interests
8. Opportunities and needed assistance with access to outside activities and events
9. Help with acquiring or replacing needed personal belongings or other practical transactions
10. Choice concerning important daily routines
11. Choice and control over decisions affecting care
12. Recognition of need and opportunity to express religious, ethnic, cultural identity
13. Recognition of status and wholeness of one's life history
14. Ongoing relatedness and intimacy with family and loved ones
15. Specific emotional support to family members/significant others in response to their needs or reactions
16. Family collaboration in care planning and decision making
17. Informal social opportunities with other residents
18. Independence in functioning and opportunity to do for oneself whenever possible, whatever the level of functioning

(continued)

(continued)

19. Structured social and group interaction opportunities both inside and outside the home
20. Maintaining contact with friends/associates/community ties outside home
21. Contributing to the life and functioning of the nursing home community
22. In-depth orientation to the home, staff, policies, procedures
23. Orientation to resident/family rights/obligations, and grievances process
24. Family/resident input to survey/certification and accreditation process
25. Opportunity for formal feedback to home personnel on level of satisfaction with aspects of home care
26. Opportunity for structured dialogue between families, residents, and home personnel concerning care management
27. Security that appropriate care will be in place at points of transition whether into, within, or out of the home
28. Assurance that care/resources which are supposed to be provided, are provided

Source: Vourlekis, Betsy S., Gelfand, Donald E., and Greene, Roberta R. (1992). Psychosocial Needs and Care in Nursing Homes: Comparison of Views of Social Workers and Home Administrators. *The Gerontologist,* 32(1):115. Copyright © The Gerontological Society of America. Reproduced by permission of the publisher.

Social Worker Functions

Vourlekis, Gelfand, and Greene (1992) also have provided a list of twenty-three nursing home social worker functions that was developed from 1988 to 1989 by NASW's Nursing Home Clinical Indicator Work Group (114) (see Box 6.2).

The Vourlekis, Gelfand, and Greene (1992) study comparing the expectations of a sample of NASW member social workers and nursing home administrators for the social worker role in the nursing home setting found the following:

1. Nursing home administrators rated higher than social workers the importance of all but one of the listed needs of residents, family, and staff; they also rated higher than social workers the expected frequency of performance of the functions.

2. Some differences were seen in ranking of functions between the staff social workers and consultant social workers, with staff social workers focused more on direct services to residents and consultant social workers more involved in training and otherwise working with staff.

3. Administrators expected social workers to spend more time working with resident discharges than social workers reported doing.

4. Of twenty-eight psychosocial needs of nursing home residents, three of the five that both administrators and social workers rated most important were the same: (1) transitional support, (2) help with loss, and (3) relatedness and intimacy.

BOX 6.2.
Nursing Home Social Worker Functions

1. Review appropriateness of admission applications and provide information and referral as needed.
2. Promote applicant's participation in the decision to enter the home.
3. Perform comprehensive social psychological assessment, including resident's preferences.
4. Help residents and their families cope with the immediate effects of the decision to move to the nursing home.
5. Orient residents and families to the facility.
6. Assist resident and family with financial planning.
7. Involve residents and families in care planning including their attendance at care conference if they desire.
8. Work with relevant staff to implement each resident's care plan, addressing especially issues that express and reinforce individuality and identity.
9. Enable social functioning using varied treatment interventions (group, individual, family).
10. Assist residents to adapt to living in an institutional environment.
11. Mediate issues that arise between and among residents, family, and staff.
12. Ameliorate emotional distress of resident and family.
13. Provide linkage with community resources by maintaining knowledge of other systems, making referrals/contacts, and identifying unmet needs.
14. Empower residents and enable maximum choice in matters affecting them.
15. Provide crisis intervention.
16. Help resident, family, and staff prepare for and cope with death.

---

17. Monitor the effect of governmental and facility rules and regulations and their interpretation on the everyday life of residents/ families.
18. Affect facility policy/practice to promote choice in schedule and lifestyle.
19. Train, and consult with, other staff and volunteers regarding psychosocial needs of both individual residents and the resident group as a whole.
20. Advocate on a case level.
21. Advocate on a policy and program level.
22. Participate in policy decision making which affects resident care and family involvement.
23. Plan discharges with resident and family participation to assure continuity of care for transfers in and out and discharges from the nursing home.

Source: Vourlekis, Betsy S., Gelfand, Donald E., and Greene, Roberta A. (1992). Psychosocial Needs and Care in Nursing Homes: Comparison of Views of Social Workers and Home Administrators. *The Gerontologist,* 32(1):115. Copyright © The Gerontological Society of America. Reproduced by permission of the publisher.

Social Work Functions According to NASW Standards

According to Standard 4 of NASW Standards for Social Work Services in Long-Term Care Facilities:

> The functions of the social work program should include but not be limited to *direct services* to individuals, families, and significant others; *health education* for residents and families; *advocacy; discharge planning; community liaison* and services; participation in *policy and program planning; quality assurance; development of a therapeutic environment* in the facility; and *consultation* to other members of the long-term care team.

Interpretation

The social work program is directed toward providing services designed to identify and meet the social and emotional needs of each resident; to assist each resident and family to adjust to the effects of the illness or disability, treatment, and stay in the facility; and to assure adequate discharge planning and the appropriate use of community and social and health resources.* (NASW, 1981:5) (emphasis added)

Specific social work service functions include the following:

- Preadmission services, including psychosocial assessment and participation in interdisciplinary evaluation of the individual's need for institutional care and preparation of the incoming resident.
- Development of individual social services plans designed to meet the needs of the resident, the family, and significant others. The initial goals of the individual plan should be to promote adjustment and lessen the trauma of relocation to the new environment.
- Assistance to residents, potential residents, and families and significant others in finding and utilizing financial, legal, mental health, and other community resources.
- Provision of individual, family, and group services focused on the enhancement of psychosocial functioning and on social and emotional problems, such as adjustment to illness or disability, institutional living, inter- or intra-institutional transfers, interpersonal relationships, reestablishing community living, and coping with separation, loss, dying, and death.
- Participation in the interdisciplinary care team comprehensive resident treatment planning and evaluation and coordination of patient care services.
- Advocacy of the rights of residents through the development and implementation of policies for the facility and self-governing councils, and assurance that guardianship, conservatorship, and case management services be made available to residents in need.
- Facilitation of the resident's integration into the community through discharge planning and follow-up services.
- Orientation and supervision of volunteers when appropriate.
- Participation in planning and policy development for the facility as a whole, including collaboration with other members of the staff in the identification of social, psychological, and cultural factors essential to the enhancement of the therapeutic and physical environment.
- Participation in orientation and in-services training of other facility personnel.

---

*Copyright 1981, National Association of Social Workers, Inc., NASW Standards for Social Work Services in Long-Term Facilities.

- Contribution to the development of community resources by participating with community groups to initiate, plan, and carry out programs concerned with the health and welfare needs of the target population.
- Supervision of fieldwork in affiliation with an accredited school of social work.
- Participation in research and demonstration projects that may be conducted either independently or collaboratively.* (NASW, 1981:5-6)

To assist social workers and reviewers in monitoring and evaluating the adequacy of social services in the nursing home setting, the NASW has developed several indicators, or benchmarks, for such measurement. Four of these indicators concern the *process* of social work services, and an additional two concern the *outcome* of such services.

===

The Functions of Social Work in Nursing Homes

"The functions of the social work program should include but not be limited to direct services to individuals, families, and significant others; health education for residents and families; advocacy; discharge planning; community liaison and services; participation in policy and program planning; quality assurance; development of a therapeutic environment in the facility; and consultation to other members of the long-term care team.

Interpretation

The social work program is directed toward providing services designed to identify and meet the social and emotional needs of each resident; to assist each resident and family to adjust to the effects of the illness or disability, treatment, and stay in the facility; and to assure adequate discharge planning and the appropriate use of community and social and health resources." (NASW, 1981:5)

===

According to NASW Clinical Indicators for Social Work and Psychosocial Services in Nursing Homes (NASW, 1993:1-12) the four essential indicators of the quality of the *process* of social work services in nursing homes are the following:

---

*Copyright 1981, National Association of Social Workers, Inc., NASW Standards for Social Work Services in Long-Term Facilities.

1. Timely psychosocial assessment (Comprehensive resident evaluation occurs soon after admission to the home.)
2. Comprehensive psychosocial assessment (Resident's psychological and social circumstances are assessed adequately.)
3. Resident involvement in care planning (The resident is included in care planning and decision making.)
4. Family involvement in care planning (The wishes and thoughts of the resident's family are explored with sensitivity to cultural factors and lifestyle, and the family is aware of the care plan and decisions made by the care planning team.)*

The two essential indicators of the quality of the *outcome* of social work services in nursing homes are as follows:

1. Resident satisfaction with choice (Residents are satisfied with the degree of choice available in everyday matters in the home.)
2. Problem resolution (Residents' psychosocial problems are ameliorated.)

The rationales for these six indicators of the quality of social work services in nursing homes follow, in order:

Rationale 1: Information and conclusions of a comprehensive social history and social and psychological assessment that includes racial, cultural, ethnic, and religious information and sexual orientation must be available on a timely basis to guide care planning and ongoing care provision.

Rationale 2: To adequately guide planning and decision making the psychosocial history and assessment addresses both needs and strengths (for example, assets and resources) in the resident and in his or her situation and spells out the implications of this information for care planning.

Rationale 3: The resident's plan covers matters that define the parameters of everyday life. It must reflect his or her preferences and choices, including cultural, ethnic, and religious background and sexual orientation. Residents or their surrogates must be aware of what is embodied in the care plan and must have the right to refuse aspects of care.

Rationale 4: Family input into care planning provides important information to guide decision making. Once a care plan is in place the family should be fully informed to enhance positive collaboration. The social worker facilitates communication between the family and the care team before and after the care-planning conference.

Rationale 5: Greater control over one's life is presumed to contribute to social and psychological well-being. Though social work is not solely responsible for positive or negative outcomes on this dimension, one function of social work is to identify preferences and individuality in the psychosocial assessment and to facilitate choices through working directly with residents and their families, educating and sensitizing staff, developing mechanisms for choice, and working at policy levels in the home.

Rationale 6: The intent of social work intervention is to help residents meet psychosocial needs and improve and solve problems related to nursing home life and care. Problem resolution is an indicator of whether the intervention has achieved its goal.* (NASW, 1993:6-8)

KNOWLEDGE REQUIREMENTS

Client Population

Age

In 1997 about 4.5 percent of the age sixty-five and over population of the United States were residing in nursing homes. As age increases, the percentage of older people residing in nursing homes also increases. For example, for males, only 3.2 percent age sixty-five and over versus 11.9 percent age eighty-five and over, compared to, for females, only 5.4 percent versus 22.2 percent, respectively, were residing in nursing homes in 1997 (U.S. Government Printing Office, 2000a:298, Table 96).

The average age at admission to a nursing home in 1997 among persons sixty-five and older was 82.6 years, and slightly over one-half (51 percent) of nursing home residents in 1997 were age eighty-five and older (Sahyoun et al., 2001).

---

*Copyright 1993, National Association of Social Workers, Inc., NASW Clinical Indicators for Social Work and Psychosocial Services in Nursing Homes.

Race

The percentage of the U.S. population age sixty-five and over residing in nursing homes significantly decreased among the white population between 1985 and 1997 but significantly increased among the black population, from 6 to 10 percent (Sahyoun et al., 2001). These trends are especially notable among the eighty-five and over age group, the explanation for which is not clear, although it may reflect the general increase in life expectancy among this group (U.S. Government Printing Office, 2000a:298, Table 96).

However, the racial distribution of nursing home residents in the United States continues to be disproportionately white. Based on the National Nursing Home Survey in 1997, 88.4 percent of nursing home residents were white, while 9.4 percent were black. The survey also classified the remaining 2.2 percent of nursing home residents as of Hispanic ethnicity, though not included as a racial category (U.S. Government Printing Office, 2000b: 134, Table 209).

Sex

The same National Nursing Home Survey in 1997 found that 25.4 percent of nursing home residents were male, while the remaining 74.6 percent were female (U.S. Government Printing Office, 2000b:134, Table 209). Presumably, this reflects the greater average longevity of females, as well as the tendency for a higher percentage of elderly males to be married, often to younger women who may serve as their husbands' caregivers, when needed.

What Nursing Home Social Workers Say They Need to Know More About

The Omnibus Budget Reconciliation Act of 1987 (PL 100-203) placed renewed emphasis on the importance of psychosocial care in nursing homes, theoretically strengthening the position of social services in nursing homes (Greene et al., 1992). Technically, medically related social and emotional needs of patients must now be identified, and a clear plan is required to assist each patient in adjusting to the social and emotional aspects of his or her illness, treatment, and stay in the facility (40). Every nursing home facility of 120 or more beds must provide the services of a social worker (40).

However, the reality of the situation is that the federal statutes only require a "qualified social worker" if the facility has more than 120 beds. As a result, many nursing home social workers have no more than a bachelor's degree in social work or a "related field" (Quam and Whitford, 1992) and may be expected to assume responsibility for functions for which they are ill prepared. When 301 nursing home social workers were asked to rate a variety of subject areas by level of interest, relevance to job, and level of present competence, *they generally indicated a need to know more about behavior problems of the elderly, medical terminology and prescription information, mental health issues, cognitive changes in aging, and how to work with families* (Quam and Whitford, 1992:151).

However, even a survey (Greene et al., 1992) of 152 professional social worker members of NASW who were employed by nursing homes, many as consultants, concerning the nursing home characteristics, perceptions of their work, and perceived knowledge needed for the work, reported a less than rosy picture. Of these social workers, 87 percent had MSW degrees and 11 percent had BSW degrees (Greene et al., 1992:43). Over one-half (54 percent) reported their facility employed only one social worker (44). Staff social workers were more likely to be found in nonprofit agencies, while the consultant (part-time, contracted) social workers were more often found in proprietary facilities.

Greene and colleagues (1992) found that at least one-fourth of social workers responding to their study viewed the nursing home in which they worked as no better than minimally adequate. They rated as no better than marginal the effectiveness of their own efforts to mediate conflicts between organizational policy and resident preferences; they rated as "marginal or below" the effectiveness of the interdisciplinary team functioning. Of responding social workers, 18 percent rated their own overall effectiveness in the facility as "marginal or below" (44).

The main areas of educational/training needs identified by the social workers were categorized by Greene and colleagues (1992:48) as follows:

1. *Human behavior*—for example, knowledge of the aging process, pharmacology, neurological deficits, biopsychosocial processes, life cycle development, management of behavior of disoriented and/or aggressive patients
2. *Methods*—for example, communication, interviewing, intervention (especially crisis intervention, stress management, and family and group treatment interventions), time management, and data management
3. *Policy and services*—for example, entitlement programs, programs for the elderly, and OMBRA legislation
4. *Research*—for example, statistical techniques, program evaluation, and current research findings

Interdisciplinary Teamwork

That 25 percent of social worker respondents felt they were relatively ineffective on the interdisciplinary team suggests a need for improved educational preparation of health care social workers for interdisciplinary teamwork (Greene et al., 1992:52).

Cohen-Mansfield and colleagues (1991), following their study, that found some discrepancies in perceptions by nurses and social workers of patients in nursing homes, concluded that the educational programs of both professions must provide their students with better understanding of each other's professions (146). They also concluded that the differences in professional perceptions of the status of nursing home residents' cognitive functioning, social functioning, and level of depression probably reflected differences in the skills and responsibilities of each discipline (1991:143).

Social Work Consultant Role

Social workers who wish to become employed as social work consultants to nursing homes are advised to become familiar with the state regulations (via state nursing home associations), federal guidelines, and survey procedures for nursing homes (state health departments) (Horejsi, 1987). Workshops on long-term care are also recommended, and there are books compiling examples of typical contracts and forms used (155). An assessment of the social worker designee's educational background and skills also helps to determine the kinds of help the consultant can best offer (155).

The Importance of Patient Transitioning

Because feeling in control of one's life is positively associated with health status and sense of well-being, social workers in health care are encouraged to support the principle of client self-determination and to avoid situations and events that serve to impose unwanted, unplanned experiences on people. Thus, it is important for social workers to be aware of the types of situations or events that are at high risk for trauma to nursing home clients.

One area of needed knowledge concerns transitioning in and out of the nursing home. It is well established that nursing home residents often do not adapt well to sudden, forced relocation (Beirne et al., 1995). When one facility was abruptly closed because of a temporary loss of certification for Medicaid reimbursement, a follow-up study a year later, following recertification, compared the outcome for patients who were returned within three months with those who remained elsewhere. The study found that 65 percent of those who did not return deteriorated or died, compared with 19 percent of those who returned (116). In addition, a significant difference was found in the outcomes of those who had social supports and those who did not (119).

Another follow-up study (Reinardy, 1995) of elderly patients recently admitted to nursing homes found a significant positive correlation between the extent to which residents perceived that they had participated in the decision to move into the facility and their satisfaction with the facility. There was also a positive correlation between the extent to which they had wanted to move into the facility and their satisfaction with it and their level of participation in nursing home activity (36).

Scharlach (1988) found that the use of trained peer counselors, that is, other residents who reach out to newly admitted residents and provide needed information and social support, had a significant and positive effect on new residents' adaptation to the facility.

Preadmission Screening for Mental Illness and Mental Retardation

Nursing home social workers responsible for resident admissions and discharges need to be aware of the following legal requirement of OMBRA 1987. One of its many provisions concerning nursing home reform is that patients residing in a nursing home prior to January 1, 1989, and those currently being considered for nursing home admission must undergo preadmission screening by a physician, hospital discharge planner (registered nurse or licensed social worker), or a qualified mental health and mental retardation professional. Such screenings determine whether patients have a major mental disorder, are mentally retarded, or have a "related disorder," essentially another severe developmental disability (Mosher-Ashley, Turner, and O'Neill, 1991). Each state provides a standard form for this preadmission screening and resident review.

The major mental disorders of concern include schizophrenia, paranoia, major affective, schizoaffective disorders, and atypical psychoses as defined in the DSM-III and now the DSM-IV-TR (Mosher-Ashley, Turner, and O'Neill, 1991:250). The reason for the required screening is to determine which patients need professional assessment of treatment needs.

This concern over mental disorders arose as a result of the deinstitutionalization movement since the 1950s, which resulted in large numbers of transfers of institutionalized mentally ill and developmentally disabled persons from state hospitals into Medicaid-certified nursing homes, where, for the most part, the services they needed were not available. OMBRA requires that any such patients who do not need nursing home care must be relocated to a more appropriate setting, unless they have resided in the facility for thirty months or more and wish to stay (Mosher-Ashley, Turner, and O'Neill, 1991:250).

Nursing Home Ombudsman Program

Nursing home social workers should be aware that since Congress created the Long-Term Care Ombudsman Program in 1978 under the Older Americans Act, most states have such a program. States have the option of employing people to fill these positions or using volunteers. The effectiveness of these programs varies considerably, but reviewers have generally agreed that the best ombudsman programs attract, train, and retain volunteers (Nelson, 1995). The 1987 Older Americans Act strengthened the authority and responsibility of ombudsmen, assuring them access to nursing home facilities, and many states specify responsibilities such as complaint investigation, technical assistance and training, advocacy in coordination with other state agencies, public education, and program management and development (Nelson, 1995:32). Some of the features of more effective ombudsman programs include high visibility, rapid handling of complaints, legal support, independent status, and strong enabling legislation (36). As one ombudsman reported:

> when we walk in, the staff starts hopping. They are very aware of who we are and why we're there. It's hard to know for sure, but they feel my presence there. The administration and staff are much more attentive to the care and dignity of the residents. (Nelson, 1995:39)

VALUES AND ETHICS CONSIDERATIONS

Legitimate Sources of Patient Information

There are multiple and complex values and ethics issues of which nursing home social workers ought to be cognizant. One of these is that using family or staff proxies for information concerning residents is hazardous because some evidence suggests that these alternate informants may not know as much about the residents as is sometimes assumed (Tennstedt et al., 1992).

Residents' Rights and Proactive Care Preferences

Since the Patient Self-Determination Act of 1990, which became effective in 1991, one of the many functions usually assigned to the social worker in a nursing home is to inform each resident soon after admission, or a family member if the patient appears incompetent, of the *patient rights* in the facility. Then the social worker should explore with residents their specific wishes concerning medical decisions and determine whether they have, or are interested in having, a durable power of attorney and a living will. Most nursing homes have written documents to assist in this process and usually try to obtain a *living will* (signed statement, witnessed by two people, clarifying the resident's wishes about the circumstances under which they do or do not wish to be provided with medical treatment, nutrition and hydration, and pain medication). A *durable power of attorney* is a legal document that must be completed while the person is still mentally competent. This document allocates responsibility to a specified person to make specific kinds of decisions on the patient's behalf should he or she become incompetent to act alone. The patient is expected to discuss with the designee or agent what he or she wishes done in the future, given certain circumstances, and the agent is expected to honor those wishes.

Needless to say, discussing issues of future disability and death with nursing home residents and their families requires considerable sensitivity to their feelings. Newly admitted patients and their families are understandably anxious and often overwhelmed with simply adjusting to all the change and uncertainty associated with nursing home admission. Thus, the social worker ought to individualize each situation in terms of deciding on the most opportune and appropriate occasion to attempt to engage residents and/or families in considering these serious issues.

Nonetheless, they need to be discussed as quickly as possible, for the following reason: "The absence of advance directives can lead to stress, confusion, painful introspection, and expenditure of time and emotional and financial resources by both family members and health care providers who are forced to exert a substituted judgment" (Spears, Drinka, and Voeks, 1993:409).

In cases in which the client is already too incompetent to either select a power of attorney or to make advance directives, legal action to appoint a guardian may be necessary (Spears, Drinka, and Voeks, 1993:409). State laws may vary concerning these alternate procedures, so social workers need to become familiar with those in their particular states.

The Issue of Resident Autonomy

Social workers who wish to work in nursing home-type settings would do well to obtain a copy of the excellent book *Everyday Ethics: Resolving Dilemmas in Nursing Home Life,* edited by Kane and Caplan (1990). It could serve as an ongoing reference source in helping to resolve ethical issues and be used for in-service training with nursing home staff. An underlying position in this book is as follows:

> The mission of the nursing home must be to assist residents in their attempts to exercise their autonomous will rather than to manage their behavior. Resident autonomy for all residents capable of asserting it must replace institutional efficiency as the central goal. (Foldes, 1990:35)

The issue of autonomy or self-determination is closely related to quality of life. It is not enough that nursing home patients are allowed to designate a durable power of attorney or complete a living will; it is all of the little decisions of everyday life that make the difference in an individual's sense of control, which is vital to happiness, health, and well-being. People need to decide for themselves when they will get up in the morning and go to bed at night, when they will eat and what they will eat, when they need to go to the toilet, what they will wear, and which activities they will engage in (Caplan, 1990:39-41).

The principle of respect for autonomy implies *individualized care* in the nursing home setting (Kane and Caplan, 1990:81) and requires that staff really know their residents' likes and dislikes, values, beliefs, habits, behavioral patterns, and so forth.

The Death and Dying of Residents

Another area of nursing home care that is often dealt with poorly is the death of a resident. Most residents and their families need and want to know what is going on and to have death and dying dealt with honestly and respectfully. The dying resident, his or her family, other residents, and nursing home staff do not benefit from either socially isolating the dying resident or acting as if nothing has happened. Other residents need to express what feelings they have and to be able to sense that their own future deaths will be met by those around them with loving kindness, warmth, and reverence.

The Nursing Home's Mission

"The mission of the nursing home must be to assist residents in their attempts to exercise their autonomous will rather than to manage their behavior. Resident autonomy for all residents capable of asserting it must replace institutional efficiency as the central goal." (Foldes, 1990:35)

Social workers in the nursing home can often be helpful to staff, families, and residents in promoting such an environment, as well as providing opportunities for everyone concerned to talk about their feelings and receive mutual support. In addition, it is important to be aware of and respect family and ethnic traditions concerning death and dying (Kane and Caplan, 1990: 209-221).

HELPING INTERVENTIONS

Treating Resident Depression with Group Work

One of the common problems of nursing home residents is emotional depression associated with multiple losses, ageism in the society, medication side effects, and feelings of helplessness arising from functional dependency and loss of customary social supports (Dhooper et al., 1993).

Three MSW-level social workers were hired by a research project to experiment with group work with depressed elderly residents in a nursing home (Dhooper et al., 1993). The intervention was an eclectic combination of approaches derived from reminiscence therapy/life review, problem solving, cognitive therapy, communications theory, and feelings exploration and ventilation. The objectives were to help the group members regain or develop a sense of ego integrity, feel more empowered, experience social support and social intimacy, and maintain cognitive function and social skills.

Patients selected were diagnosed with mild to moderate depression and were randomly assigned to experimental and control groups. The treatment group participated in nine one-hour sessions, the objectives of which Dhooper and colleagues include in an appendix to their article (Dhooper et al., 1993:99). Subjects measured very much the same on level of depression on the pretest, but on the posttest the treatment group scored significantly lower on mean level of depression, compared with both pretest and the control group posttest.

The findings suggest that an eclectic approach to social group work, which allows residents to share their life histories, to identify and express their feelings, and to acquire problem-solving skills, may be a more effective intervention in treating emotional depression in nursing home residents than a more limited approach (Dhooper et al., 1993:97).

Helping Family Members Through a Family Council

The importance of the social worker in the nursing home working closely with family members from the time of receipt of a request for admission to the facility cannot be overemphasized (Bogo, 1987). Engagement and assessment of the family situation and perspective as they relate to the potential resident's needs are essential, partly because consideration of admission of an elderly parent to a nursing home is often a signal of a family crisis, which may or may not be best resolved through such a placement (Bogo, 1987). The application of systems theory to the family unit becomes clear to nursing home social workers, and Bogo (1987) has detailed the process and potential outcomes of involving the family early on.

Another social worker intervention in nursing homes can be organizing and leading a family council, whose purposes include helping the resident's family to adjust to the placement, facilitating positive relationships with staff, and enhancing relationships with other residents (Palmer, 1991:122).

A family council is a mechanism for involved members of the resident's family to share with one another their expectations and concerns, to obtain information to clarify their questions, to problem solve together, and to feel their suggestions are being heard by administration (Palmer, 1991:124). In the group reported (Palmer, 1991), the social worker and a family member cofacilitated the group. The details of the process and experience of this group are provided by Palmer (1991).

The distress experienced by family members when a close relative is admitted to a nursing home has been described by Judith Weisberg, a nursing home social worker whose own mother became a patient (Weisberg, 1991). It is a tender and moving story that should help other nursing home social workers to better understand and more effectively respond to other families' experiences.

Resident Empowerment Through the Resident Council

Silverstone and Burack-Weiss (1982) wrote:

> Ways must be found in the nursing home environment wherein residents can regain or feel they have regained some control over their lives. The less restrictive the nursing home the better. . . . A tried and tested method is the establishment of resident councils. (30)

Silverstone and Burack-Weiss (1982) recommend that to make a resident council work effectively, the nursing home administration must declare the council's establishment and support its function; specific tasks with meaning should be assigned to council members (such as planning an activity schedule or menus); and opportunity for resident feedback should be provided (30). Care must be taken to avoid such a council from being powerless, or it will soon dissolve, leaving behind bitter feelings.

Getzel (1983) believes that a resident council should perform a "mediating function," that is, provide an opportunity for conflict resolution, based on the idea that all the players in a nursing home need one another to function well. Therefore, it is of mutual benefit to establish mechanisms by which conflicts can be aired, addressed, and resolved as soon as possible.

Getzel (1983) conceptualizes eight phases in the development of such a resident council:

Phase 1: Introduction of the concept of the resident council and identification of natural leaders among the residents

Phase 2: Formalization of structure

Phase 3: Engagement of isolated residents

Phase 4: Expression of felt concerns and problem solving

Phase 5: Engagement of key institutional personnel

Phase 6: Enhancement of resident solidarity

Phase 7: Support and mutual aid during member crises

Phase 8: Community linkages and social action (formation of coalitions of resident councils in a geographic area)

Getzel (1983) comments:

> An honest approach to Resident Councils opens the opportunity for expanded activities despite the aged's frailty and limited mobility. Faith in a human being's capacity for democratic participation and growth should not end when she or he enters a nursing home. (185)

Pet Therapy with Nursing Home Residents

There is considerable evidence that the availability of pets to nursing home residents who enjoy animals, who are not allergic to them, and who are not likely to fall over them can have a variety of positive effects on the residents, such as relieving their sense of isolation, stabilizing their heart rhythms, providing the joy of caring for another and feelings of being loved, and fulfilling the need for touching (Hoffman, 1991). In addition, sometimes pets can induce greater physical activity or exercise, enhance self-esteem, provide something to look forward to, and stimulate memories that can be an aid to reminiscence therapy.

Nursing homes more often permit outside organizations to bring well-behaved pets into the facility periodically, but all states now allow pets to actually reside in nursing homes as "mascots" (Hoffman, 1991:202). The more sustained availability of live-in pets allows residents to enjoy more enduring comfort and pleasure.

The potential importance of pets in nursing homes is suggested by another study that found that nursing home residents generally do not form close interpersonal relationships among themselves and thus may lack opportunities for a sense of intimacy (Gutheil, 1991). The findings suggested that residents use friendships within the nursing home as a way of coping with living there, but rarely talk about anything very personal or emotional, especially if it is sad. It is as if they are so "defended"—in a state of being defensive—in order to tolerate life in a nursing home that they cannot expose their vulnerability enough to share their innermost feelings of sadness.

Addressing the Hostile-Aggressive Nursing Home Resident

Cox (1993) reminds us that the primary goal of social work is to improve the functioning of the person in his or her environmental context. Therefore, it is inappropriate to assume that the cause of the hostile or aggressive behavior of a nursing home resident is entirely intrapsychic and to attempt to deal with it through chemical and/or physical restraints. Instead, Cox (1993) recommends a behavioral assessment to search for underlying contributing conditions, such as hearing or speech impairments; organic brain syndrome; interpersonal relationships with staff, roommate, and family; recent history of losses; and impact of nursing home rules, regulations, activities, and restrictions on resident autonomy.

Cox (1993) points out that aggressive behavior is often a natural response to feeling threatened and, in some ways, may be a healthier alternative to giving up and subsequent withdrawal and depression, however dysfunctional for the facility. Thus, the social worker is expected to mediate between the needs of the resident and those of the nursing home operation.

Depending on the identified causes of the disruptive behavior, interventions may include supportive therapy and counseling, behavioral approaches, environmental change, operant conditioning, reality orientation, physical restraints, and medications (Cox, 1993:186). Cox (1993) discusses each type of intervention and cites examples of appropriate circumstances of their use (186-190):

1. *Supportive therapy*—including group therapy, can help with problems associated with adjusting to the nursing home placement. The focus is on expression of feelings and receiving emotional support from others to build a sense of competency to cope.

2. *Behavioral approaches*—involve identifying the antecedents of the behavior that need changing and learning a new response to it, such as relaxation techniques or assertiveness training to express thoughts and feelings without provoking the other person.

3. *Environmental change*—may involve changing roommates, advocating for more staff accommodation to resident preferences, inducing involvement in activities and/or social interaction, and in-service training to improve staff understanding of, and sensitivity to, resident needs.

4. *Operant conditioning*—involves the use of positive responses (rewards) or negative responses (loss of enjoyed things) to induce desired behavior. The behavior and the response must be consistently and immediately combined so that the person is reconditioned or retaught. Positive reinforcement is generally preferred, both for humanitarian reasons and because it has the advantage of reinforcing the desired behavior rather than simply discouraging the undesirable behavior.

5. *Reality orientation*—is used with residents who are temporarily confused and agitated because of too much environmental change and stimuli, sometimes combined with early cognitive frailty. This approach can involve maintaining a calm, consistent routine with a lack of stimulation; reminders of the date, day, and time from family and staff; and a constantly warm and reassuring manner that both models the desired behavior and calms the resident. Calendars, clocks, photographs, and familiar objects can be helpful with this approach.

6. *Physical and chemical restraints*—are generally discouraged, having been found to be both physically and psychologically damaging. Since OMBRA 1987, severe restrictions are placed on nursing homes in their ability to use either form of restraint. Social workers should never be party to their use and are required to take action to prevent their use, except temporarily, in a dire emergency, and with the order of a physician. Physical restraints are now believed to be associated with increased risk of injury from

falls out of bed (Evans and Strumpf, 1989, cited in Bruno, 1994:139), abnormal changes in body chemistry, increased basal metabolic rate and blood volume, orthostatic hypotension, contractures, lower extremity edema and decubitus ulcers (bed or pressure sores), decreased muscle mass, tone, and strength, bone demineralization, overgrowth of opportunistic organisms, and EEG (electroencephalogram) changes (Evans and Strumpf, 1989, cited in Bruno, 1994:132).

In addition, restraints can lead to disorganized behavior, emotional desolation, fear of abandonment, feelings of being punished, sensory deprivation, and loss of self-esteem (Bruno, 1994:132). Bruno (1994), citing Williams (1989:385), wrote:

> The key to restraint free care . . . is to practice "individualized care," centered on the person, and his or her particular needs . . . staff must get to know the resident, not merely as a "patient" . . . and they need to continue to work together to exchange information and ideas. (141)

Another social worker (Lerer, 1995) employed in a veterans' extended care facility reported on her experience working with the "irascible" patient. She observed that most of the facility's patients, the majority of whom are male, "have a strong sense of entitlement" (171) as veterans and tend to be cognitively intact, but are severely impaired physically, often non-ambulatory, and incontinent. In addition, they often have a lack of impulse control and a history of few lasting social relationships. Lerer (1995) expressed her belief that the physical dependency of these patients produces low self-esteem and acting-out behavior (172), which reflects a sort of regression to an earlier developmental stage (173).

Lerer (1995) has described her counseling activities with these patients, which involves an "initial stage" of attentive listening to ventilation of complaints, offering support and acceptance, and modeling patient, calm behavior. In a "middle stage," she explored with the patient his history, interests, and hobbies, as well as his ideas about what would constitute ideal care from the staff. The understanding and acceptance from the worker gradually calms the patient, who begins to get in touch with his innermost feelings of loneliness and despair. He remembers who he was, before physical impairment and adult dependency, and this helps to restore his self-esteem. In the "sustaining stage," the patient begins to grieve his losses, to improve his self-esteem, and to be less depressed. Relationships with other staff improve, and the social worker provides less frequent, but ongoing, emotional and social support. The worker lets the nursing staff know how they have helped the social worker to better understand that the patient's abusive behavior is his response to fear and sense of loss of control (Lerer, 1995:178).

In-service training by the social worker with line staff is an important supplement to more effectively dealing with irascible patients, through a combination of teaching, opportunity for ventilation, exchange of concerns and ideas, and mutual support.

Managing Agitation in Nursing Home Patients

The majority of nursing home patients today have some form of dementia (Ouslander, Osterweil, and Morley, 1997, cited in Nasr and Osterweil, 1999). Many nursing home residents with dementia, as well as some nursing home residents without dementia, at times manifest agitated behavior. Since OMBRA 1987 and the subsequent HCFA recommendations concerning the act, care facilities are expected to avoid pharmacological interventions and instead use forms of behavioral management.

Agitation may be expressed verbally, vocally, or with movements that are seen as inappropriate and are repetitive. Examples of such behaviors include pacing, making peculiar noises, undressing, verbal pleas for help (e.g., "Come here please"), or verbal expressions of anxiety (e.g., "Oh dear, oh dear . . ."). Agitation symptoms may or may not be aggressive. Practical results of agitated behavior may include injuries to oneself or others. Most important to understand is this:

> Agitation is not a random behavior. It results from underlying distress experienced by the elderly person. This distress can stem from cognitive impairment, psychiatric and medical disorders, and functional impairments. (7) Hearing, vision, and mobility impairments can increase the sense of isolation experienced by cognitively impaired residents. . . . Hunger, thirst, or need for toileting may result in agitation if the patient is unable to fulfill or express these needs because of functional impairment. (Nasr and Osterweil, 1999:8)

Prior to involving a physician for a thorough history and physical examination considering possible "physical, medical, functional, and psychiatric causes, a variety of basic information is needed concerning the resident, including a description of the behavior, its antecedents and consequences, a medical history, social history, and physical signs" (Nasr and Osterweil, 1999:4). The point is that every effort should be made to identify and appropriately treat any treatable underlying conditions, whether medical, psychiatric, or functional. A variety of rating scales are available to assess agitated behavior, and these "can be invaluable for determining the predominant type of behavioral disturbance, the appropriate therapeutic approach, and the response to treatment" (9). The Nasr and Osterweil piece cited identifies eight of these rating scales that are useful tools in the assessment and treatment of agitated behavior.

Although cognitive deficits are most often associated with agitated behavior, there are other possible causes, such as other psychiatric disorders or endocrine and neurological disorders, and appropriate intervention depends on accurate diagnostic assessment. The range of possible interventions, depending on the assessment findings, include music therapy, pet therapy, white noise (such as tapes of forest, ocean, or bird sounds), touch, bright light treatment, increased activity level or exercise, increased social interaction or recreational activity, play objects, reduction in noise and other stimuli, increased personal space, and use of specially designed and staffed physical units for care of persons with special needs, such as Alzheimer's units. In addition, some forms of behavioral therapy can sometimes be effective, in spite of memory impairment, such as modifying either the antecedent stimulus to the agitated behavior or the response to the consequent behavior, or using positive response to reinforce desirable behavior. Reminiscence and life review are also sometimes helpful. In any case, "pharmacologic agents should be used only as a last resort or in acute situations and for the shortest period possible" (Nasr and Osterweil, 1999:15).

Dealing with Aggressive Members of Residents' Families

A less familiar problem in nursing homes is that of family members who reportedly are rude and otherwise verbally abusive toward staff, largely in reaction to what they perceive as poor care of their resident loved ones. A survey (Vinton and Mazza, 1994) of seventy nursing homes in Florida obtained reports of more than one thousand acts of verbal aggression and thirteen acts of physical aggression on the part of residents' family members toward nursing home care staff during a six-month period.

Daughters (31 percent) and wives (28 percent) were more often reported as the aggressors than were husbands (14 percent) or sons (11 percent), and the rest (16 percent) were perpetrated by a variety of other relatives (Vinton and Mazza, 1994:530). Social work staff were reported to be the ones most often asked to resolve such conflicts, and Vinton and Mazza (1994) comment that since most of the conflicts concerned an issue related to the quality of nursing service, one wonders why they were not most often resolved by the nursing directors.

The strategies most often used to resolve such conflicts were reported to be (1) discussing the situation with the staff person, (2) discussing the situation with the aggressive family member, and (3) discussing the situation with the staff person and family member together. Vinton and Mazza (1994) note that since other possible alternative approaches listed on the questionnaire—such as in-service training, using the resident's care plan for care criteria, establishing policy, and contracting with family members—were not used, many potential avenues for conflict resolution are not being explored by nursing home social workers and others who are asked to address such problem situations.

A nationwide survey of family caregivers who were members of caregiver support groups found that those whose care recipient relative was now in a nursing home had the highest measured level of anxiety about their own anticipated aging. It was not clear whether this resulted from a fear of deterioration or from fear of themselves becoming recipients of poor-quality care in such facilities. However, the reportedly heightened anxiety about their own future aging may help to explain some of the aggressive behavior of family members toward nursing home staff, as reported in other studies (Wullschleger et al., 1996).

Helping Former Family Caregivers

As the previous paragraph suggests, family members who were home care caregivers of the nursing home resident before the placement may have special difficulty adjusting to the placement (Montgomery and Kosloski, 1994; Riddick et al., 1992).

According to Riddick and colleagues (1992):

> While admission to a nursing home may diminish the amount of time a (family) caregiver needs to devote daily to his/her loved one, other concerns apparently arise and consume the attention of the caregiver. More specifically, the caregiver still experiences burdens surrounding the caregiver role, and emotional conflicts over his/her relative's placement in the nursing home. (70-71)

In addition, family caregivers often have devoted a significant period of their lives in the caregiving role prior to their loved ones' placement. Riddick and colleagues (1992) found the average length of time was seven years (58), and satisfaction with the nursing home was inversely related to the family caregiver's ongoing sense of burden following the placement.

Caregiver burden refers to the family caregiver's sense of internal conflict concerning such emotions as unhappiness, guilt, anger, depression, and anxiety over one's future (Riddick et al., 1992:52). Monahan (1995) called it "felt stress" and pointed out that some observers have suggested that it may even increase after institutional placement. Riddick and colleagues (1992) report what one daughter said of her feelings about placing her parent with dementia in a nursing home: "[I realize that] I must somehow 'learn' I must be responsible for myself first or I'll die. Intellectually, I know the answer, but it is very difficult to carry out. How do you abandon those you love?" (72).

According to Riddick and colleagues (1992), the practice implications are that social workers must (1) provide family caregivers with counseling that addresses the emotions they tend to experience both before and following the placement; (2) educate them concerning nursing home life; (3) sensitize nursing home staff to what the family caregivers experience; and (4) teach nursing home staff behaviors that facilitate the residents' and families' adjustment and acceptance of the nursing home—especially spouses of residents, who have greater difficulty relinquishing their former role to the staff (72).

That former family caregivers continue to feel responsible for monitoring the nursing home care of their loved ones is suggested by the finding of Dempsey and Pruchno (1993) that the tasks assumed by family caregivers after the placement reflect the "principle of substitution." That is, family caregivers tend to assume whatever tasks they perceive the residents need done that the staff have not covered, especially nontechnical ones (141).

Dempsey and Pruchno (1993) recommend the following: (1) family caregivers need to understand which tasks the nursing home should be responsible for providing (mostly technical tasks, such as toileting, bathing, dressing, feeding, administering medicines and treatments); (2) nursing home staff should be encouraged to view the family caregivers as competent to assist in the residents' care, especially in the provision of nontechnical services (such as managing their money, shopping, providing plants and other "extras" in the room, marking the residents' identification on their clothing and other possessions, giving or withholding consent for procedures, and writing letters); and (3) staff should help family caregivers to find activities they can share during visits to relieve family members' sense of helplessness (143).

Monahan (1995) reported the findings of a survey of former family caregivers of patients admitted to a dementia unit in a nursing home in New York in an effort to identify variables associated with the level of caregiver burden. The variables that best explained the variance in caregiver burden were caregiver health (poorer health equaled greater burden); age and gender (older and male caregivers felt more burdened); race, marital status, and educational level (nonwhites, married, and those with higher educational levels had more burden); and caregiver perception of the quality of nursing home care (the poorer the perceived quality, the greater the burden). Monahan (1995) also recommends that social workers in nursing homes help family caregivers and staff to develop "partnerships for care planning and provision" to avoid staff interpretations of family "overinvolvement" and help reduce family caregiver burden.

Kramer (2000) conducted a longitudinal study of husbands who were caregivers of wives with dementia, both during the time they were caring for their wives at home and one year later when some of them had placed their wives in a care facility. The purpose of the Kramer study was to compare the patterns of change in the husbands before and after institutional placement of their wives. Various instruments were used to measure the wives' level of functional impairment, according to the husbands' judgment, the wives' memory and behavior problems, and the husbands' level of financial strain from caregiving self-reported health status. The husbands rated the stress on themselves of their wives' functional limitations and the level of their own psychological well-being. In summary, the aim was to compare "time 1" with "time 2" in terms of stressors, resources, appraisals, and psychological well-being.

The most curious finding was that the husbands who had placed their wives in a care facility reported *greater* levels of perceived stress than the husbands who continued taking care of their demented wives at home, even though the objective level of stressors was higher among the latter. Although some of the husbands who had placed their wives expressed considerable worry about the financial strain of paying for nursing home care, it is not clear that this was the only variable involved. Instead of, or in addition to, financial concerns, other variables may have been at work suggesting that family caregiving is a complex phenomenon relative to, for example, motivation, sources of satisfaction, sense of control, companionship, and conscience.

As Kramer (2000) noted, one implication is that health care social workers should probably help family caregivers to explore these facets carefully and weigh them accordingly in order to decide whether to undertake nursing home placement or instead seek alternative supplemental resources in home care or day care.

COMMENTARY

Clearly, there is a need to design a system for nursing home care reimbursement that serves to promote a higher quality of care, both in terms of medical services and personal care services, with an overriding incentive to rehabilitate rather than merely "warehouse." Nursing home care needs to be designed to fulfill, in practice, the theoretical concept of caring at the third stage of the care continuum, i.e., rehabilitation and maximization of comfort and function.

People should not have to impoverish themselves to be able to pay for nursing home care through Medicaid. Long-term care needs to be a Medicare provision, regardless of care level, so that people who need the services are not humiliated by economic dependency in addition to dealing with care dependency.

Health and social services must be nonprofit if they are to have quality care as their primary objective. It is obscene to reduce nursing home care, or any other health or social service, to a business enterprise. Of course, if home care were made more feasible, economically and otherwise, nursing home care could be reduced.

Quality nonprofit facilities could doubtlessly use some of the savings from what formerly went to stockholders to provide better training, pay, and benefits to the certified nursing assistant (CNA) staff, thereby improving the quality of services and reducing line staff turnover. In addition, CNA staff need to be included in ID team meetings, since they are the ones who work most closely with the patients.

Patients themselves need to be engaged in redesigning the structure and program of nursing homes. This would not only help to empower the residents, thereby facilitating their potential well-being, but also provide for adapting the environment to residents' cultural needs, health condition needs, and personal preferences. Presumably, any organization in which the "customers" are satisfied and truly like the service is likely to be a happier place for staff as well. As the data indicate, in nursing homes, this apparently is a function of staff and resident empowerment.

Clearly, many nursing home facilities do not employ enough social workers with the needed training and skills to adequately address residents' needs or meet NASW standards for social work services in nursing homes. This is due, to a great extent, to both the for-profit status of most nursing homes in the United States, which tend to do no more than is legally required, and the lack of consistency in relevant federal statutes dealing with expectations of nursing home care coupled with appropriate requirements for service providers. As we have seen in our presentation of social work services in other health care settings, the numbers and degree level of social work staff tend to be inversely associated with the profit orientation of the facility. After all, it is far cheaper to employ someone "on call" than full-time, to hire one person when two or three are needed, and to select someone with a BSW rather than an MSW. The problem is that if the facility actually needs one or more MSWs full-time, and the problems they must address are not something those with BSWs are qualified to do, questions arise about the adequacy of the care provided.

Finally, hopefully, everyone would agree that family caregivers and other loved ones should not have to feel that they are sending their relatives to a "house of horrors," if not to their deaths, when they finally realize that they simply must admit their loved ones to a nursing home, nor should anyone live their later lives with the fear that this may be their own end.

Chapter 7

Social Work in Hospice Care

HISTORICAL BACKGROUND

The terms *hospice, hospital, hotel,* and *hostel* imply hosting or providing hospitality, that is, warmly receiving and taking care of the needs of fellow human beings. Hospice care emerged in the 300s A.D. in the region of the Holy Land through the efforts of the Eastern Orthodox Christian Church, as a means of offering aid to needy travelers, often going to or coming from religious sites (Kerr, 1993:13). A well-to-do Roman woman, Fabiola, witnessed such care by the Eastern Church and carried the idea back to Italy, where she and a Roman senator, Pammachius, began a similar program in Ostia, a Mediterranean port city (Phipps, 1988).

In the fifth century, St. Bridget of Ireland established what amounted to a hospice for ill or dying people (Richman, 1995:1358). During the Middle Ages, religious orders often opened their doors to travelers in need—such as poor, ill, disabled, and dying persons—and called their service a hospice or hostel (Proffitt, 1987:813).

In 1846, a Catholic Mother and founder of the Irish Sisters of Charity, Sister Mary Aikenhead, opened her home in Dublin, Ireland, to care for the dying. After her death, her Daughters in Christ, in response to her example and inspiration, established Our Lady's Hospice (Richman, 1995:1359-1364; Kerr, 1993:13).

In the late 1800s, in the United States, the Dominican Sisters began to provide inpatient care of dying persons, following the English pattern, and their programs continue today (Proffitt, 1987:813). In 1905, the idea of hospice care caught hold in London, and St. Joseph's Hospice was established. A medical social worker and nurse, Cicely Saunders, later worked there and eventually became a physician (Richman, 1995:1359). In 1967, at age fifty-seven, Saunders opened another hospice, called St. Christopher's of London, which became a famous center for research and teaching concerning the care of dying people, as well as a model for quality hospice care services, both inpatient and at home (Richman, 1995:1359; Kron, 1978). St. Christopher's Hospice was the site of great advances in pain management through the work of Saunders, and her work ignited the modern hospice movement (Proffitt, 1987:813).

Modeled after St. Christopher's, the Hospice of Connecticut, in New Haven, was established in the United States in 1974 (Hayslip and Leon, 1992; McNulty and Holderby, 1983; Paradis, 1985; Saunders, 1982). However, in the United States, the concept of hospice care soon developed into a specific care philosophy, with its associated program of services, apart from a particular place. Whereas the European hospice model revolved around palliative care in a facility known as a hospice, in America, hospice care became a home care-based program. In October 1983, hospice programs were approved by Medicare to provide continued care, whatever setting the patient entered (National Association for Home Care, 1996).

Growth and Cost of Hospice Care

As of January 2001, the Medicare program identified 2,273 participating hospices, that is, Medicare-certified ones. In addition, there are an estimated 200 volunteer hospices in the United States (National Association for Home Care, 2001:2).

Medicare

In 1985, the first year when Medicare payments were made for hospice services, $34 million were spent, but during 1998 a total of $2,800 million in Medicare payments was expended for hospice care. Although this represents about a sixty-one-fold increase during the first fourteen years of the hospice benefit through Medicare, still, in 1998, only about 1 percent of total Medicare benefit payments for all types of health care services was for hospice care (U.S. Government Printing Office, 2000:114, Table 168).

One way to gain perspective of the relative extent to which hospice care is currently utilized is to consider the number of people who die in the United States each year in comparison to the number of people who used hospice care programs. According to the National Hospice and Palliative Care Organization (NHPCO), nearly 2.4 million people died in 1999 in the United States (2000:3), but only 600,000, or 25 percent of them, died in hospice care, while another 25 percent died in a nursing home, and about 50 percent died in a hospital (NHPCO, 2000:4). Variation across the United States in where people die largely reflects the availability of hospital beds. The more availability, the more they are used (Bern-Klug, Gessert, and Forbes, 2001).

According to Naomi Naierman (2001), president and CEO of the American Hospice Foundation, eligibility for the Medicare hospice benefit requires that

1. the patient be a Medicare (Part A) beneficiary,
2. the patient's primary care physician and the hospice medical director confirm a life expectancy of less than six months (note that this may be renewed every six months), and
3. the patient agrees in writing not to pursue curative treatments.

According to the National Association for Home Care (2001:2), "a hospice may contract with an approved hospital or skilled nursing facility to provide inpatient hospice care. Hospices provide routine home care services to residents of nursing and assisted living facilities." Medicare per diem reimbursement rates to hospice programs vary as follows:

Effective April 1, 2001, the Health Care Financing Administration (now known as the Centers for Medicare and Medicaid Services) provided an increase of 5 percent in the payment rates for hospice care services. The current national Medicare rate for routine home care is $106.93; continuous care 625.13; respite care $110.62; and for general inpatient care $475.69 (adjusted for regional wage differences). . . . In 1999, 95 percent of the days of service were routine home care, 3 percent of the days were inpatient care, 1 percent was respite care, and 1 percent was continuous home care. (NHPCO, 2000:3)

Medicaid

Hospice is an optional Medicaid benefit that in 2001 was offered by forty-four states and the District of Columbia. Medicaid payments for hospice services in 1998 were estimated at $325 million. This amount represented only two-tenths of 1 percent of total Medicaid expenditures (National Association for Home Care, 2001:8).

Other Payers

The following represents the distribution of hospice primary payment sources for 1998 (U.S. Department of Health and Human Services, Centers for Disease Control and Prevention, National Center for Health Statistics, 1998, cited in National Association for Home Care, 2001:4):

Medicare: 72.4 percent
Medicaid/MediCal: 4.9 percent
Private insurance: 14.2 percent
Indigent care: 3.4 percent
Other: 5.1 percent
Total: 100.0 percent

The Medicare program, the largest payer of hospice care, provided payment for a record number of 401,140 hospice patients in 1998 (National Association for Home Care, 2001:6). Presumably, additional hospice care is paid out of pocket, since some hospice care provider organizations are not certified by any standard-setting organization.

THEORETICAL PERSPECTIVES

The Concept of Caring

As its history suggests, hospice care is a moral imperative, rooted in the value of concern about human suffering and the ethical sense of responsibility to help relieve that suffering. As Eric Cassell (1982) pointed out, suffering is caused not only by physical pain but also by the sense that personal integrity is endangered.

As the medical profession developed a curative technology and associated value system during the twentieth century, physicians grew to regard chronic and terminal health problems as their own personal failures, withdrawing from such situations with the attitude, and sometimes the remark, that "nothing more can be done" (Preston, 1979). Such a stance reflects a lack of recognition that even when people are terminally ill, they still have other needs while they are alive—such as relief from suffering—whether biological, psychological, social, or spiritual. Relief of suffering is referred to as *palliative care,* meaning "comfort care."

The difference between the medical model and the hospice model and the difficulties of introducing a hospice service within a traditional health care setting are elaborated by Wade Smith (1994). He notes that the adjustment is not only a shift away from the focus on curing but also a shift from technology to the use of interpersonal relationships as the principle healing force, something in which physicians are not as well trained (204-206). Freund and McGuire (1991) add that contemporary biomedicine is essentially directed toward the conquest of death, and even though it cannot always cure disease it, unfortunately, often can prolong life. This reflects the *technological imperative,* that is, the compulsion to employ a technology if it is available (253-254).

The objective of hospice care is to maximize the quality of a patient's remaining life and to facilitate his or her "safe passage." According to Corbett and Hai (1979), the objective of hospice care is *euthanatos,* or a "good death," that is, a death preceded by intensive *caring* rather than intensive care. Hospice care does not substitute for family care, but rather supplements and supports family care as needed. The units of care and attention in the hospice philosophy are the patient, family, and caregiving staff (Rusnack, Schaefer, and Moxley, 1988), and hospice care is conceptualized as escorting the patient in his or her transition to death, during which caregivers keep company with the dying to ensure a safe passage (Corr and Corr, 1985).

Essentially, the hospice perspective is one of *caring* at the tertiary level of health services, that is, giving supportive assistance to maximize comfort and function and to prevent secondary disabilities from lack of appropriate societal responses to a primary impairment. This can be accomplished through providing needed services, tools and equipment, income supports, environmental modifications, and supportive interpersonal interactions. Caring, in whatever form, revolves around *empowering* the person, that is, strengthening his or her sense of wholeness, intactness, and control. Thus, the patient must be personalized and individualized with a strong supportive relationship.

Biopsychosocial and Holistic Perspectives

The motivation to provide hospice care is essentially an ethical one. The interventions provided by hospice workers emerge from a developing body of theory and knowledge about such issues as the nature of suffering and the control of pain; healthy and unhealthy grief and bereavement; the interaction and interdependence of mind, body, social and cultural environments, and spiritual needs; the family as a system; and the etiology and modification of a person's sense of *locus of control.*

Hospice care has a *holistic* perspective in that it directs attention to the needs of the whole person. In an inspirational keynote address, Balfour Mount (1993), physician and director of Palliative Care at McGill University in Montreal, talked about whole-person care as involving interaction with the spiritual person of the patient as well as attending to his or her physical needs. Mount describes *spiritual* as that part of a person capable of transcendence (34).

Hospice care has a *biopsychosocial* perspective, recognizing that the biological, psychological, and social spheres of our lives interact and affect one another. We use the term *social* to include not only relationships and interactions with other people through family, groups, organizations, community, and society but also cultural influences, such as ethnicity, language, values and beliefs, customs and traditions, social status, and religion or spirituality. Hospice health care professionals know that the experience of physical pain is greater when the patient is feeling hungry, lonely, guilty, remorseful, afraid, powerless, ashamed, unfit, misunderstood, rejected, or abandoned (Strang, 1992; Mount, 1993:28).

Continuity of Care

Because terminally ill people often reside in a variety of settings during their passage from assessment of terminal status to death—including hospital, home, and nursing home—the hospice philosophy also includes the importance of ensuring continuity of care. As a program rather than a place, hospice care can follow the patient from setting to setting, and hospice philosophy holds that it is necessary to do so to ensure ongoing quality of comfort care.

Primary Prevention

In a sense, hospice care is not only a form of tertiary care but also a form of primary preventive care. Its inclusion of bereavement care for the family, which continues after the patient's death, serves to help reduce the potential impact of the stress of unresolved grief on family members' health and life expectancy (Stubblefield, 1990). Hospice philosophy recognizes that loved ones who will be left behind need to have time and opportunity to express their grief so they can go on with their own lives afterward with maximum well-being. In fact, stress research indicates that unresolved grief is a significant factor in predicting health status and life expectancy (Weiner, 1984: 258).

Systems Perspective

Hospice programs, and social work performed within them, also have a *systems perspective* in the sense of recognizing the interdependence of biological, psychological, and social systems as well as that of the various levels of social organization: individual, family, small group, organization, community, and society. That is, the effectiveness of the hospice program itself depends in part on the patient's family; the hospice organization's structure, auspice, and philosophy; the resources available from other community organizations; and the social welfare policies and programs enabled by the society's economic and political systems. In short, how we live and how we die are not entirely up to us but are influenced by all the social structures in our environment with which we are interdependent.

HUMAN DIVERSITY RELEVANCE

In discussing the social worker's psychosocial assessment of the hospice patient and family, Lusk (1983) wrote: "To be responsive to the uniqueness of each patient-family system, the social history must be cognizant of ethnic and cultural considerations" (213). This is especially necessary given the significant variations across nationalities, religions, ethnicities, sexual orientation, and gender regarding attitudes and practices relating to death and dying. It is important for hospice workers to be aware of these variations and to know where to look to learn about clients' cultures. A major and recent resource for this type of information is the text edited by Parry and Ryan (1995). A list of other related resources may be found at the end of this chapter.

As indicated earlier in this book, variation exists both between groups and within groups, so one cannot assume that because a person is a member of a certain group that he or she holds a certain set of values, beliefs, customs, and so on. Again, social workers need to be familiar with the client's general group culture but also should explore with the individual and family how their own convictions do or do not conform to those of the group.

Some of the ways in which cultural variations can influence appropriate hospice care include the following:

- Customs concerning whether to tell the person (and his or her family) that the condition is terminal
- Attitudes toward the use of various types of medicines, both traditional and folk medicines (for example, many cultures have prohibitions against the extensive use of opiates to control pain)
- Perceptions of what sort of physical environment would be peaceful, beautiful, comfortable, and so on
- Religious implications for encouraging the client and/or family to express anxieties, concerns, questions, feelings of guilt, and so forth
- Attitudes concerning efforts to prolong life and/or to facilitate death when a person is in severe pain and death is inevitable

In short, human diversity variables may affect perspectives on practically everything: appropriate clothing, food, conversation, and pain relief; the meaning of death and the allocation of roles; disposition of the deceased's body; bereavement practices; the significance of certain colors; dying at home; and the extent to which patient, family, and health care providers should be involved in decision making (Parry and Ryan, 1995; Storey, 1993).

INTERDISCIPLINARY TEAMWORK

Concept of Interdisciplinary Teamwork

Interdisciplinary teamwork differs from multidisciplinary teamwork in that team members are not simply all attending to the same case, but are cooperating in and coordinating their work, that is, operating together toward the same end.

Rationale for Interdisciplinary Teamwork

Because hospice care recognizes the interaction of biological, psychological, and social factors, it adopts a team approach. The team can include the family, supervising physician, nurses, nursing assistants, social worker, chaplain, physical therapist, occupational therapist, and so forth, as needed, with members cooperating in a type of group practice. Hospice benefits via Medicare include the following:

- Physician visits
- Skilled nursing services
- Physical, speech, and occupational therapy
- Home health aide visits
- Social work and supportive services
- Medical equipment and supplies
- Spiritual counseling
- Nutritional counseling
- Volunteer services
- Prescription pain medications
- Inpatient respite care
- Bereavement support for the family for at least a year after the death (Naierman, 2001)

Medicare Standards for Hospice Team Composition

Medicare standards for hospice programs name the core members of the interdisciplinary team as including at least "a doctor of medicine or osteopathy, registered nurse, social worker, and a pastoral or other counselor," with other professionals added as needed (U.S. Government Printing Office, 1994:26).

The National Hospice Organization Recommendation for Hospice Team Composition

The National Hospice Organization suggests that the core group needed to provide quality hospice service should include the patient's attending physician, registered nurses, clergy or other spiritual counselor, master's-level social workers, and trained volunteers (Richman, 1995:1360-1361). Note that this differs from the Medicare standard by specifying the need for both MSWs and trained volunteers.

The Effect of Per Diem Reimbursement on Team Composition

A current problem with Medicare's per diem reimbursement for hospice care is that the hospice organization, whether public, proprietary, or voluntary, must decide which services it can afford to provide for the per diem rate. This may require settling for less than optimum team composition and services.

The Dilemma of Role Flexibility Without Role Subsumption

Because not all team members are with the patient all of the time, roles need to be flexible. This can be not only a strength of hospice teamwork but also a source of tension and role ambiguity (McDonald, 1991:276; Kulys and Davis, 1986; Donovan, 1984).

According to Fish (1994:411), role overlap or blurring is inevitable. A potential problem is that those professionals who are required to be with the patient the most, such as the nurses, may be inclined to assume the functions of other team members, for example, providing psychosocial assessment and counseling or acting as a liaison with other community agencies, which are the responsibilities of the social worker. This can lead to the latter being used less and less often and eventually being excluded from the core team altogether (Dush, 1988a). At the same time, the staff person who assumes the functions of others becomes burdened with excessive demands, and the patient and family receive lower-quality service because of the difference in training and experience in that particular function.

Rodway and Blythe (1994) commented, "While there are many advantages to a team approach to palliative care, the lack of a clearly delineated model of palliative care may well be the result of its interdisciplinary nature" (421).

Reece and Sontag (2001) reviewed and summarized the literature dealing with problems affecting social work role and function on interdisciplinary teams in health care and offered suggestions for addressing each of these sources of difficulty. For example:

- ID teams should adopt a norm of "respect for each other's knowledge and expertise" (168) and be oriented to each other's knowledge and expertise by making a joint home visit with each professional on the team (168-169).
- The problem of role overlap could be addressed by establishing some protocol for determining to which professional to refer cases, depending on given criteria (169).
- Since research indicates that physician-social worker teams are effective in increasing advance directives, and social workers are more likely to discuss death anxiety and social support with hospice clients, other team members should make such referrals to social workers, although they themselves may respond to any topics the clients raise (169).
- Alleged differences in value and theory bases, such as whether the professional-client relationship is more authoritarian or client empowering, or differences in perceptions of client confidentiality in the context of team sharing, or where the boundary is drawn between a client-professional relationship and a person-person one, could be resolved by sustaining a client-centered focus in team interaction (169-170).
- Differences in theoretical perspectives, such as a person-in-environment versus individual centered, or a preoccupation with medical versus biopsychosocial-spiritual issues, should be accepted nonjudgmentally (171).
- Other sources of team conflict, or at least unfulfilled potential, such as barriers to teamwork due to differences in status, may be addressed by orientation of new members to positive group norms (171).
- Since the general public often misunderstands contemporary social work and instead associates it with welfare, it may be useful to orient new hospice patients and their families to the team together, or for the representative having the initial contact with the hospice clients to introduce each person on the team and explain his or her role and functions (173).
- Last, increased use of social workers by hospice agencies may result from presentation of the evidence that social workers tend not only to reduce hospice provider costs by linking the clients with the appropriate funding sources but also to stabilize the functioning of the patient and family by addressing psychosocial issues, thereby avoiding somatized reactions to unresolved stresses (173).

ORGANIZATIONAL CONSIDERATIONS

The same kinds of organizational considerations affecting social work practice in other health service settings also influence hospice social work.

Organizational Ownership

For example, whether the organization is public, private nonprofit, or private for profit will be a determinant of organizational goals and objectives. According to the most recent national home and hospice care survey, 73.0 percent of hospice organizations were voluntary nonprofit, 23.0 percent were proprietary, and 4.1 percent were government and other types of organizations (U.S. Government Printing Office, 2000:132, Table 205). Since only 7.3 percent of hospices were proprietary in 1994, this represents more than a threefold increase.

When the major goal of the health service organization is financial profit for shareholders rather than delivering the highest possible quality of human health services to its clients, and unless specific quantities and qualities of services are mandated by standard-setting organizations, the incentive is to reduce service quality and quantity to whatever level will enhance profit margins. Often, this results in the employment of too few staff, with minimal rather than optimal qualifications, to do the work. "Soft" services whose impact is apt to be measurable only qualitatively, such as social work and clergy, are likely to be minimally provided. Reductions in staff size and qualifications imply a reduction in the amount and quality of client care services.

Sectarian or Secular

Whether the organization is sectarian or secular and the nature of the religious beliefs of a sectarian organization will influence professional practice in the hospice setting.

Governing Standards

The rules and regulations of the funding sources concerning client eligibility for service also make a difference, such as whether a family caregiver must be present or whether reimbursement for services is per diem, per capita, or fee for service. Again, per diem or per capita structures reduce costs through reducing services.

Certification Status

As of January 2001, the Medicare program identified 2,273 participating hospices, that is, Medicare-certified ones. In addition, there are an estimated 200 volunteer hospices in the United States. Of the 2,273 hospices, 960 (42.2 percent) are freestanding (not attached to a nursing home, hospital, or other health care organization), 739 (32.5 percent) are home health agency based, 554 (24.4 percent) are hospital based, and the remaining 20 (0.9 percent) are skilled nursing facility based. Little is known about those which do not participate in Medicare or Medicaid programs and are licensed by their states, whose regulations vary (National Association for Home Care, 2001).

According to *Statistical Abstracts of the United States* (U.S. Government Printing Office, 2000:132), in 1998, 96.6 percent of hospice-providing organizations were Medicare certified and 92.3 percent were Medicaid certified. These data are also derived from the national home and hospice care survey.

In late 1993 and early 1994, Sontag (1996) studied a stratified random sample of U.S. hospice programs and found, among other things, that the Medicare-certified programs sought certification primarily to enhance their credibility, and hence income, and were more likely than non-Medicare-certified hospices to focus on the medical problems of patients and to use more professional and fewer volunteer staff. In addition, a higher percentage of staff of noncertified hospice programs reported high staff morale. Finally, Medicare-certified hospices were more likely to require patients to sign a do not resuscitate (DNR) order and less likely to require a family primary caregiver (PCG) before accepting patients into their programs (37-40).

Sontag (1996) also found that Medicare-certified hospices were more likely to be affiliated with a medical service organization, such as a hospital or home care agency, and thus may be more entrapped in the traditional medical model. If so, there may be less attention to psychosocial needs of patients and families, generally provided by MSWs with training in assessment and counseling of such needs, and other staff may sense the negative effects of such a lack on the patients and their families, thereby eroding employee morale.

With the increase in certification by Medicare and in affiliation with medical care organizations rather than freestanding voluntary organizations, hospice programs also have begun to employ a variety of technologies (Kaye and Davitt, 1995:263). Some of this technology raises a question about whether the pure philosophy of hospice care is being contaminated by the traditional health care sector—and its medical model.

CLIENT PROBLEMS AND SOCIAL WORKER FUNCTIONS

Introduction

As has been pointed out, hospice is a program and a philosophy rather than a particular place or setting. However, although most hospice care is provided in the home, hospice agencies sometimes follow former home care patients into nursing homes to provide continuity of appropriate care. In addition, acute care hospitals sometimes provide hospice care service on the hospital site—partly as a result of the trend in hospitals toward vertical integration of health care services other than acute care, since acute care stays are shortened by cost-saving government measures. Furthermore, there are some freestanding hospice facilities in the United States especially for AIDS patients. Thus, client problems and social worker functions relating to hospice care are made more complex by the variation in type of organizational setting.

Client Problems

From the perspective of social worker functions, the problems of patients in hospice care may be classified as those associated with

1. admission to the hospice service;
2. adjustment to the service or facility;
3. adjustment to the diagnosis, prognosis, or care plan;
4. the lack of information to make informed decisions and take control;
5. the lack of needed supportive resources, such as supportive tools and equipment, support services, income supports, supportive environmental adaptations, and interpersonal supports; and
6. barriers to discharge from the service or setting.

Barriers to Admission

Terminally ill patients and their families often need someone to help assess their financial resources and eligibility for coverage under the various available sources of funding for hospice care. In addition, they may need help in coming to terms with the diagnosis, prognosis, and recommended care plan; for example, acceptance of Medicare coverage for hospice care requires an agreement that all curative efforts will cease in favor of palliative care. This coming-to-terms process often involves working through questions patients and families may have and providing information to help address those issues, as well as addressing their associated emotions. Finally, terminally ill patients and/or their families may have practical issues—such as how family members will manage financially if they take a leave of absence from their employment to help care for the patient, or who will stay with the patient while the family caregiver goes shopping or simply gets away every now and then.

An additional problem concerning access to hospice care can sometimes be that physicians have the mistaken idea that they must be sure the patient has less than six months to live for fear they may be investigated by Medicare, and so they tend to postpone recommending hospice care. According to the National Hospice and Palliative Care Organization (2001), "Currently there are two initial 90 day benefit periods followed by an unlimited number of 60 day periods. A physician must re-certify that a patient has six months or less to live before each benefit period" (3). This tendency for physicians to be overly cautious in making hospice referral is suggested by the following data provided by NHPCO: "In 1999, 32 percent of those served by hospice died in seven days or less, and 11 percent died in 180 days or more. The average length of service was 45 days" (2).

Another related barrier to patient and family access to hospice care is that, next to cancer, congestive heart failure and chronic obstructive pulmonary disease are the second and third major causes of death, but there are more chronic conditions that can be quite impairing in terms of independent comfort and function, so they usually do not fit the time limitation for use of hospice care. As a result, Haiden Huskamp, a health economist, and her colleagues at Harvard Medical School have recommended that Medicare incorporate exceptions for cases when the patient prefers to adopt a palliative care approach but the disease course is unpredictable (American Society on Aging, 2001:15). An additional barrier to admission to hospice care is that, currently, about 75 percent of surveyed members of the U.S. public did not know that hospice care can be provided at home, and 90 percent did not know that such care can be fully covered by Medicare (NHPCO, 2000:6).

Adjustment to the Service or Facility

Much hospice care is provided in the patient's home by a home care agency. Having "outsiders" coming and going is a major adjustment for most people. Some concerns may be about staff stealing from the home, failing to secure locks on doors when they leave, or simply invading the family's privacy. Most people are accustomed to feeling relatively independent, especially in their own home. Consequently, home hospice care can produce conflicting feelings of both gratitude for the help and resentment regarding the sense of helplessness and dependency. However, the impression I have received from hospice social workers is that they become so close to the patients and families that, before long, they are received as if they are part of the families.

If patients are to be admitted to a hospice facility, whether freestanding or within a nursing home or hospital unit, the idea of being in "a place to die" can seem threatening. Most people feel more vulnerable in such a facility than they would in their own homes. On the other hand, the social worker can help by pointing out the advantages of such places. For example, some hospice sites may offer the assurance of more effective pain control, supervision by qualified professionals, ready access to oxygen to ease breathing distress, high standards of cleanliness, and ever-present staff to assist when needed. Further, some terminally ill patients may find it comforting to interact with other terminally ill people and to share with others a common experience, especially if the facility promotes a homey atmosphere, one, for example, that permits patients to keep pets or to have wine with their dinner if they wish. Still, in 1999, 61 percent of persons who died while receiving hospice care did so at home, and within three months, a survey of a sample of their family members which asked, "Would you recommend hospice services to others?" received a 99 percent "yes" response rate (NHPCO, 2000:5).

Most hospice patients do die at home, and acceptance of the hospice service is likely to be related to acceptance of the prognosis. The well-trained and well-informed social worker can be most helpful to the patient and family in coming to terms with and feeling that they have some control over the prognosis.

Adjustment to the Diagnosis, Prognosis, or Care Plan

Coming to terms with a serious diagnosis, especially one that is imminently terminal, is usually experienced as gravely threatening. This process involves dealing with many complex feelings and questions. Aside from the terminal prognosis, the diagnosis itself sometimes raises issues concerning the expected effect on physical attractiveness, the possible judgments of other people regarding the etiology of the disorder and the patient's previous lifestyle, preconceptions about pain and suffering, and how loved ones will cope with the diagnosis.

As is now well known, awareness of impending death, either one's own or a loved one's, is experienced as a loss to be grieved. The grief experience passes through a series of stages, varying in order among different people, but generally including such responses as denial, anger, bargaining, depression, and acceptance or resignation (Kübler-Ross, 1969).

Adjustment to the recommended care plan concerns issues such as trading further curative efforts for comfort care and coming to terms with site and/or provider selection among the available options. According to Bern-Klug, Gessert, and Forbes (2001), "Social workers can strive to be 'context interpreters' by providing individuals and families with the information they need to understand the natural course of the illness, the likely dying trajectory, and the medical decisions they are likely to face" (44).

Lack of Information to Make Informed Decisions and Feel in Control

Terminally ill patients are particularly prone to a sense of diminished control. The social worker, with other team members, plays a vital role in helping patients and their families to counteract this tendency by providing them with honest and accurate answers to their questions, as well as relevant information to assist them in thinking through their decisions. As Bern-Klug, Gessert, and Forbes (2001) noted, "most people who are dying value awareness and control at the end of life, especially in light of the possibility of being confronted with medical decisions" (43).

Lack of Resources to Meet Needs

In the role of case manager, the social worker is often responsible for, and best suited to, ascertaining the clients' resource needs from talking with them, family members, and other team staff and to assist them in obtaining resources. Resource needs vary, not only with client and family situation but also with the hospice care setting. However, most patients are cared for at home and are not likely to own equipment such as a hospital bed, bedside commode, suction machine, Hoyer lift, portable oxygen, and so on. Needed resources can include medical aids and appliances/tools and equipment, supplemental services, income supports, environmental adaptations, and interpersonal supports.

Barriers to Discharge

Discharge planning refers to assisting the patient and family in making arrangements for termination of one service and transfer to another setting and/or service. In the case of hospice care, patient service is usually terminated upon death. However, most hospice programs provide varying amounts of bereavement care service to the family following a patient's death. Medicare hospice programs fund at least a year of postdeath bereavement care for the family. Presumably, some family members may become quite attached to hospice staff and may find it difficult to terminate their relationship. Social workers, with their training and skill in the process of service termination, are particularly qualified to facilitate the timely termination of hospice services to the family.

Sometimes, however, hospice services provided to a patient in one type of setting may need to be terminated when the patient is transferred to another setting. For example, a hospitalized patient in an inpatient hospice unit may be released to home hospice care; a home hospice patient may decide to enter a freestanding hospice; or a patient who has been receiving non-certified home hospice services on an out-of-pocket basis may decide to enter a nursing home and apply for hospice services there through a Medicaid-certified hospice agency to become eligible for Medicaid coverage. In such situations, there may be financial, psychological, informational, or practical barriers to resolve.

Client Health Problems and Their Effects

Diagnoses. According to the *Statistical Abstracts of the United States* (U.S. Government Printing Office, 2000:132, Table 206), in 1998, 57.5 percent of hospice patients had a primary diagnosis of neoplasms when admitted to hospice care; an additional 12.6 percent had a primary diagnosis of circulatory system disease; 10.6 percent had a respiratory system health problem; and 9.5 percent had a disease of the nervous system or a sense organ. The remaining 9.8 percent of the diagnoses were not given due to lack of precision or reliability.

Physical suffering. People who have terminal health conditions often experience a variety of associated physical discomforts, such as pain, breathing difficulty, physical weakness, eating and sleeping problems, digestion and excretion problems, and sometimes sensory impairment, paralysis, skin problems, or swallowing difficulty (Fish, 1994; Germain, 1984:183). Effective pain control is central to hospice care and is a highly technical subject (Doyle, 1994). According to Buckingham (1996), physicians sometimes write *PRN,* or "as needed," orders for pain medication. This can result in ineffective pain control because hospice staff may wait until the patient is having pain before administering medication to relieve it (69).

Janet Abrahm (2001), oncologist and director of the pain and palliative care programs at the Dana-Farber Cancer Institute and Brigham and Women's Hospital, both in Boston, developed a classification of "barriers to assessing and treating pain":

Health Care Professionals

- May not believe the patient's report of the intensity of the pain
- May not know the difference between the manifestations of acute and chronic pain
- May not use validated pain-assessment tools
- May not involve families in pain assessment
- May mistake the changes of aging for treatable problems
- May perform incomplete or incorrect assessments in patients who are cognitively impaired
- May not know the common cancer-related pain syndromes

Older Patients

- May assume pain is a natural, unmodifiable consequence of aging
- May not use the word *pain* to describe symptoms
- May not or cannot use pain-assessment tools due to cognitive, visual, auditory, or motor impairments
- May be reluctant to take pain medications

Family Caregivers

- May not know what chronic pain looks like
- May not know how to assess side effects
- May deny the intensity of the older person's pain for fear that it means the disease is worsening
- May be afraid of giving potent medications to the patient

Emotional and spiritual distress. With or without physical discomfort and functional impairments, hospice patients also often experience considerable emotional distress—such as fear of dying, losing control, being alone, being socially rejected, and feeling helpless, as well as apprehensions regarding "unfinished business," regrets about the past, or the distress of having family members burdened because of them (Germain, 1984:184; Allison, Gripton, and Rodway, 1990:207).

Van Loon (1999) explored the issue of what it may mean when a terminally ill person expresses a wish to die. She concluded that it could mean the person is seriously depressed, is considering suicide, or has come to terms with his or her condition and life and is ready to die. However, because of the first two possibilities, such expressions should be assessed so that appropriate intervention is identified and offered. Van Loon suggests that cognitive therapy may often be helpful in assisting the depressed client to sort through his or her thoughts and feelings and examine them, while those who are suicidal may need antidepressant medication and/or hospitalization. In any case, all terminally ill clients need considerable social support.

Barriers to Assessing and Treating Pain

Health care professionals
- May not believe the patient's report of the intensity of the pain
- May not know the difference between the manifestations of acute and chronic pain
- May not use validated pain-assessment tools
- May not involve families in pain assessment
- May mistake the changes of aging for treatable problems
- May perform incomplete or incorrect assessments in patients who are cognitively impaired
- May not know the common cancer-related pain syndromes

Older patients
- May assume pain is a natural, unmodifiable consequence of aging
- May not use the word "pain" to describe symptoms
- May not or cannot use pain-assessment tools due to cognitive, visual, auditory, or motor impairments
- May be reluctant to take pain medications

Family caregivers
- May not know what chronic pain looks like
- May not know how to assess side effects
- May deny the intensity of the older person's pain for fear that it means the disease is worsening
- May be afraid of giving potent medications to the patient (Abrahm, 2001)

Van Loon cites a position statement of the NASW (1997) on the issue of social workers' options if their clients should express a desire for assisted suicide and request the presence of a social worker. All social workers should be familiar with this position.

Family Member Problems and Needs

Family members are regarded as part of the client system, with their own problems and needs, such as the following:

- Lack of respite (mental and physical)
- Mental and physical exhaustion
- Social isolation or loss of external social life
- Financial needs

- Loss of employment income due to caregiving
- Anticipatory grief
- Unresolved conflicted relationships with the patient
- Generalized feelings of stress from all of these, in addition to the helpless sense that the patient cannot be saved
- Grief after the patient dies

As Fish (1994) wrote, "It is in these areas of psychosocial and emotional problems that social workers can have an impact on the lives of patients and families" (408).

Social Worker Functions and Interventions

Objectives of Hospice Care

One approach to conceptualizing social worker functions and interventions is to think about the objectives of hospice care as follows:

- Relief of suffering
- Preservation of important relationships
- Facilitation of anticipatory grief
- Resolution of residual conflicts
- Supporting the clients' sense of integrity and control over decisions of importance to them (Weisman, 1972, cited in Moore, 1984:269)

Hospice Social Worker Functions

Thus, the broad function of social work in hospice care is to maximize the adjustment of hospice patients and their families to the challenges they face (Richman, 1995:1361).

Hospice Social Worker Roles

This broad function is performed through roles that Richman (1995) describes as broker, liaison, administrator, counselor, educator, lobbyist, and program planner, that is:

1. providing information and financial assistance [broker],
2. interfacing with the community [liaison],
3. administering and managing [hospice] agencies [administrator],

4. doing clinical work with individuals and families [counselor], and
5. promoting the acceptance of hospice philosophy and care by patients, the health care system, and society as a whole [educator, program planner, lobbyist]. (1361)

Fish (1994:410) cites some main tasks of social workers in hospice care as named by Pilsecker (1979):

1. Help patients and families to
   a. get in touch with their feelings and understand their options;
   b. develop or maintain meaningful communication; and
   c. locate and use needed community resources.
2. Help other involved health professionals to
   a. get in touch with and acknowledge their own feelings;
   b. understand and respect patient and family needs; and
   c. meet patient and family needs in a sensitive manner.

Bern-Klug, Gessert, and Forbes (2001) have identified four clinical social worker roles and associated tasks, as follows:

1. *Counselor*—works with individuals who are dying and their loved ones on issues related to values clarification, emotional assessment, crisis intervention, goal setting, decision making, dealing with transition and loss, active pursuit of interpersonal growth, and the pursuit of peace of mind
2. *Context interpreter*—works with other health professionals to ensure that the medical prognosis is understood (by the client, family, and team) within the client's social context; facilitates consensus building among all parties to define goals for a meaningful end of life experience; assists with advance care planning
3. *Advocate*—helps client gain access to medical care in the location of their preference; advocates for aggressive pain relief; advocates for financial relief; helps with negotiations with authority figures; helps clients gain access to mental health services and care for spiritual concerns
4. *Team member*—coaches clients and loved ones to identify and communicate physical pain, symptoms, and suffering; assists clients in achieving a good dying process; helps fellow team members with their emotional concerns related to providing end-of-life care

Selected Roles and Tasks of Clinical Social Workers in Hospice Programs

1. *Counselor*—works with individuals who are dying and their loved ones on issues related to values clarification, emotional assessment, crisis intervention, goal setting, decision making, dealing with transition and loss, active pursuit of interpersonal growth, and the pursuit of peace of mind
2. *Context interpreter*—works with other health professionals to ensure that the medical prognosis is understood (by the client, family, and team) within the client's social context; facilitates consensus building among all parties to define goals for a meaningful end of life experience; assists with advance care planning
3. *Advocate*—helps client gain access to medical care in the location of their preference; advocates for aggressive pain relief; advocates for financial relief; helps with negotiations with authority figures; helps clients gain access to mental health services and care for spiritual concerns
4. *Team member*—coaches clients and loved ones to identify and communicate physical pain, symptoms, and suffering; assists clients in achieving a good dying process; helps fellow team members with their emotional concerns related to providing end-of-life care (Bern-Klug, Gessert, and Forbes, 2001)

Hospice Social Worker Roles in an Acute Hospital Setting

Stark and Johnson (1983) explored social worker roles with terminally ill patients, families, staff, and students in an oncology unit of an acute care hospital, which may be summarized as follows:

1. Roles with patients and families:
   - Counseling
   - Advocacy
   - Liaison to community resources
   - Informant to facilitate informed decisions
   - Mediating as needed between patient, family, and staff
2. Roles with staff and students:
   - Collaboration, coordination, facilitation of team effort
   - Educating new staff/students about hospice concepts
   - Educating new staff/students about relevant community resources
   - Supportive counseling as needed

Effects of a hospice experience on acute care staff. Stark and Johnson (1983) report a number of serendipitous effects of their efforts to develop a hospice service within the teaching hospital oncology service where they were employed:

1. Increased attention to symptom control by all disciplines in the hospital as they developed understanding of the hospice philosophy
2. Increased comfort in shifting goals from curing to caring
3. More awareness of the need for patient and family to have options clearly presented, time allowed for them to process the information, and support and assistance if needed in making decisions
4. Increased appreciation of the advantages to staff of being involved in work with a variety of patients at all stages of disease, allowing them the feeling of having fulfilled a commitment to help the person live well until he or she dies, and providing an opportunity to work with the person's family
5. A growing awareness of the advantage of having the experience of working with dying patients and their families, available to students of all disciplines, an experience they can take with them into their professional lives (68)

Hospice Social Worker Roles in a Nursing Home Setting

Amar (1994) explored the difference between social work with hospice patients and families in a nursing home setting compared to a home care setting. Amar found nursing home patients to be older and more frail, with more chronic health problems and poorer mental health status, and thus less amenable to talk therapies (18-19); also, with less family support available, patients were more vulnerable to the organizational environment, culture, and competence of the nursing home and its staff. Thus, person-in-environment "fit" between nursing home patient and nursing home environment becomes crucial to provide effective social work with hospice patients in such a setting.

Amar (1994) argues that the hospice social worker attending nursing home patients has entered a more complex organizational situation. The hospice program, affiliated with an outside organization, the patient and his or her family, and the nursing home organization—all have things the others want, and the social worker needs to mediate fairly among them. The hospice and nursing home organizations have economic interests at stake. Hospice social work in a nursing home calls for more group work, negotiation, education, and advocacy, and the focus of attention is expanded from patient and family to also include nursing home and hospice staff (Amar, 1994:22).

Psychosocial Assessment in Hospice Social Work

Presumably, most hospice social workers would agree with Quig (1989: 22-23), who saw that the essence of social work in hospice care ought to revolve around *psychosocial assessment* and *supportive counseling* with the patient and family—by working with patients and families and their interactions, using a systems or ecological perspective.

Fish (1994) places fundamental importance on skilled psychosocial assessment by the social worker as the key to appropriate hospice team services to the patient and family:

> Assessing for strengths and weaknesses, coping strategies and defenses, communication patterns, availability of social support beyond the nuclear and extended families, the need for legal or financial assistance and interpreting these issues to other team members helps the entire team to better understand the overall situation and to plan care within the appropriate framework. (408)

Lusk (1983) has presented a psychosocial history outline adapted to social work in hospice care (see Box 7.1). However, readers who wish to use this psychosocial assessment tool are urged to read Lusk's (1983) article, in which he elaborates a rationale for each part of the outline in a way that will facilitate and maximize the utility of the outline as a social work tool. Lusk (1983) reminds us:

> A psychosocial evaluation of a patient is an important first step in the provision of care to hospice patients and their families. It serves as a guide for intervention . . . hospice recognizes the uniqueness of each individual as he or she confronts life's final challenge. An adequate psychosocial evaluation brings that uniqueness into focus. (217)

Another potential function of such a psychosocial history is that it can serve as a *life review* or *oral history* for the patient and be instrumental in helping elderly people, especially, to achieve a sense of ego integrity. However, an interesting question for further research is how such a life review affects a terminally ill person who is not expected to reach old age.

The Issue of a Unique Function for Hospice Social Work

According to McDonald (1991:274-275), a wide variety of roles, functions, and activities have been allocated to hospice social workers in the social work literature. These include referral, brokerage, generic problem-solving services, supportive and bereavement counseling, psychosocial assessment, case management, client advocacy, staff training and support, crisis intervention, hospice legislation reform, research, and community education.

BOX 7.1.
Psychosocial Assessment of the Hospice Care Client

I.   Basic Information (name, marital status, diagnosis, etc.)
II. Social History
    A. Developmental History
        1. Family system background
        2. Educational and occupational history
        3. Significant losses and crises
        4. Ethnic and cultural considerations
    B. Current Family System
        1. Size and structure
        2. Stability
        3. Caregivers and supporters
        4. Possible problem areas
III. Physical Resources
    A. Source and adequacy of income
    B. Medical insurance
    C. Need for services or referrals
        1. Financial services
        2. Medical equipment
        3. Social services
    D. Postmortem arrangements
IV. Psychosocial Functioning
    A. Mental Status
        1. Level of consciousness
        2. Orientation
        3. Memory and cognitive functions
        4. Appearance and expression
        5. Mood and affect
        6. Appropriateness of behavior
    B. Patient's Reaction to Illness
        1. Stage of grief
        2. Defense mechanisms
        3. Reactions to increased dependence
    C. Family's Reaction to Illness
        1. Stages of grief
        2. Defense mechanisms
        3. Reactions to patient's increased dependence
        4. Relationship between primary caregiver and patient
    D. Role impairment
        1. Patient's role in family
        2. Roles affected by illness
        3. Responsibilities reallocated to others

Source: Lusk, Mark (1983). The psychosocial evaluation of the hospice patient. *Health and Social Work,* 8(3): 211.

Potential Areas for Development of Hospice
Social Worker Function

However, what little research has been done on what social workers actually do in hospice programs suggests a general lack of unique role or function and considerable role overlap with other disciplines, especially nursing (McDonald, 1991:275). McDonald reports that his own observations from interactions with social workers and other hospice workers at meetings of the New York State Hospice Association concur with the findings of the Kulys and Davis study in 1986: "non-social workers regularly provide psychosocial care in hospice and that financial and civil-legal assistance are the only functions that nurses and other team members unambiguously attribute to hospice social work" (McDonald, 1991:276).

Research, political activism, and community organization. Still, McDonald argues that hospice social workers may need to think more about other hospice needs, such as research, political activism, and community organization (1991:279), since a glance at the demographics of hospice clients reveals underrepresentation of people of color, the poor, and the uninsured. Also, funding is often inadequate to provide all the services needed by the patient and family; in addition to which, hospice programs have tended toward increased client load and paperwork while sacrificing quality of patient and family services.

Psychosocial pain control techniques. Rodway and Blythe (1994) report from the findings of a study they conducted in 1988 that few hospice social workers were engaged in such potentially useful pain control interventions as relaxation therapy, hypnosis, or meditation (424).

Facilitating a pleasant physical environment. Another area of potential development for social work includes attending to the physical environment of the patient, such as facilitating the provision of a room that is pleasantly decorated and comfortable to the patient.

Improving the adequacy of bereavement and other psychosocial services. Rodway and Blythe (1994) also express concern that hospice programs tend to give considerable lip service to the value of bereavement counseling and psychosocial services to patient and family, but in practice often fail to demonstrate understanding of the need for organized, consistent, psychosocial services provided by qualified professionals (426). According to Buckingham (1996), hospice programs generally provide bereavement services only to families at 90 and 180 days after the death, with some variation across programs (74).

Bereavement service to grieving children. It is important to remember that often those grieving the loss of the relative are children. Sontag, Nadig, and Henry (1994) have reported a very useful description of imaginative ways to help children to express and work through their grief. The therapeutic medium was group work, and the social worker employed techniques such as helping the children

1. share with the group their stories of the person who died and the circumstances of the death;
2. share a photograph and biography of the deceased with the group;
3. express their feelings about their loss at a special time set aside in the group;
4. learn relaxation and physical health exercises; and
5. talk about their conceptions of death and afterlife.

Each child also compiles a memory book of the deceased to keep, and the social worker helps the parents individually with their own grief and with knowing how to help with their children's grief.

Outreach to grieving others. Social workers need to remember that it is not only children who have difficulty dealing with death and their feelings of grief; we all do, to varying degrees. Certainly men, in particular, tend to have more difficulty expressing their feelings, and thus are likely to be burdened with unresolved grief for a longer time.

Perhaps hospice organizations someday will assume responsibility for recruiting volunteers to read daily the obituary page of the local newspapers and reach out to every family who has had a recent death among them—to explore how they are doing and inform them of local resources for assistance, such as grief support groups. This would likely serve also as a form of primary prevention of health problems and premature death of the bereaved.

KNOWLEDGE REQUIREMENTS

In addition to generic social work knowledge, hospice social workers need to have hospice-specific knowledge concerning

1. the client population and client problem(s),
2. the organizational setting,
3. the community and its resources,
4. intervention modalities, and
5. needed research, evaluation, and documentation.

Kovacs and Bronstein (1999) conducted a study of social worker members of the National Hospice Organization to obtain their views of the adequacy of their social work education in terms of preparation for hospice work. On a scale of 1 to 5 (most helpful to least helpful), the four courses whose weights averaged less than 3 were practice, medical social work, family treatment, and crisis intervention. Respondents generally indicated that although interdisciplinary teamwork preparation was very important, it was best obtained through both classroom information and practicum or on-the-job training. In addition, the hospice social workers noted a need for learning more about medical aspects of care, such as the medical process, terminology, and paperwork. Respondents also felt it would be helpful to have more social work education dealing with grief and loss.

The Client Population

Demographic Characteristics

Age. The following represents the age distribution of hospice patients (U.S. Government Printing Office, 2000:132, Table 206):

Under forty-five years:	4.6 percent
Forty-five to fifty-four:	6.4 percent
Fifty-five to sixty-four:	10.6 percent
Sixty-five and over:	78.4 percent
Total:	100.0 percent

Although more than three-fourths of hospice patients are over age sixty-five, it is nonetheless important to remember that not all fatal illness strikes in later life, and all hospice care must be individualized accordingly.

Sex. The sex distribution of hospice patients is as follows (U.S. Government Printing Office, 2000:132, Table 206):

Male:	42.7 percent
Female:	57.3 percent
Total:	100.0 percent

Obviously, a somewhat higher percentage of females than males receive hospice care. It may be noted that the sex distribution of hospice patients is more equal than it is among home health patients, where only 33.6 percent are male.

Marital status. Finally, the marital status of hospice patients was reported as follows (U.S. Government Printing Office, 2000:132, Table 206):

Married:	44.6 percent
Widowed:	35.8 percent
Divorced/Separated:	8.5 percent
Never Married:	7.5 percent
N/A:	3.6 percent
Total:	100.0 percent

Even though over 78 percent of hospice patients are age sixty-five and over, about 45 percent are still married, thus in nearly one-half of cases the social worker may be working with the spouse as well as with the patient.

Health Condition

The essence of the patients' health condition in hospice care is that they are dying. The nature of death and dying has changed from what it was a century ago. Bern-Klug, Gessert, and Forbes (2001) have highlighted the characteristics of death and dying at the beginning of the twenty-first century as follows:

- Most deaths occur with or because of chronic illness.
- Most deaths occur in old age.
- High-technology medical interventions can interrupt, postpone, prolong, or deform the dying process.
- Death has many different trajectories; most deaths are not preceded by a time in which the person is recognized as dying.
- A gulf separates people with medical knowledge from people who lack it, especially in regard to trajectory of illness, effects of treatments, and the dying process.
- Pain and uncomfortable symptoms can be relieved in most cases but often are not identified and managed.
- Dying is often regarded as a medical event; movement to recognize dying as a psychosocial, spiritual, and personal process is under way.
- An advance planning process with a series of structured planning decisions is becoming more common.
- One-third of families face financial impoverishment during the dying of their loved ones.

Perhaps the one common denominator within the hospice patient population is that all patients are facing fairly imminent death, usually estimated as within six months. For this reason, hospice social workers need to come to terms with their own feelings and attitudes toward death before they can hope to help others with their grief and bereavement (Moore, 1984). In this instance, knowledge cannot be reduced to familiarity with facts and theories, but must include some experiences that help to develop empathy. Moore reported a sensitivity training program for hospice social workers that involved the following kinds of exercises:

1. Complete a multiple choice questionnaire concerning your past experiences, present beliefs, and personal perceptions relating to death.
2. Write down what you would want to accomplish if you had ten years to live. Then repeat the task for the different intervals of five years, one year, one month, and, finally, one week.
3. Make up your own obituary as it would be written today, and as it would be written in your old age.
4. Imagine yourself arriving at a cemetery, spotting your own tombstone, and seeing what was written on the stone in memoriam.
5. Write a letter to someone deceased, addressing "unfinished business" and unresolved feelings, sign it, and share it with someone else if you wish.
6. Imagine you have received a telegram informing you of the imminent death (within minutes) of a significant other. You have five minutes to say your last words to that person. (Moore, 1984:270)

Moore (1984:271) also describes a series of concluding exercises that helps to counteract the participants' sense of emotional exhaustion. Moore implies that the previously described exercises can be quite traumatic to persons with compromised coping capacity and are not to be engaged in indiscriminately.

End-of-Life Characteristics at the Beginning of the Twenty-First Century

- Most deaths occur with or because of chronic illness.
- Most deaths occur in old age.
- High-technology medical interventions can interrupt, postpone, prolong, or deform the dying process.
- Death has many different trajectories; most deaths are not preceded by a time in which the person is recognized as dying.
- A gulf separates people with medical knowledge from people who lack it, especially in regard to trajectory of illness, effects of treatments, and the dying process.
- Pain and uncomfortable symptoms can be relieved in most cases but often are not identified and managed.
- Dying is often regarded as a medical event; movement to recognize dying as a psychosocial, spiritual, and personal process is under way.

- An advance planning process with a series of structured planning decisions is becoming more common.
- One-third of families face financial impoverishment during the dying of their loved ones. (Bern-Klug, Gessert, and Forbes, 2001)

To work effectively in a hospice setting, the social worker must understand who the patients are and the significance of their characteristics, both in terms of health and demographics. Thus, it is important to understand how, for example, young women with terminal breast cancer differ from children with terminal leukemia, or from young gay men with AIDS, or from older people with congestive heart failure.

The Organizational Setting

As indicated earlier, it is important to understand the nature of the hospice organization—whether affiliated with a hospital, home care agency, nursing home, hospice inpatient facility, or a freestanding organization. It is also important to know how it may differ from other hospice organizations, due to affiliation with a religious group, the personality of the current director, the policy of its funding sources, or other influence such as community or regional attitudes and values.

It is necessary to realize that hospice philosophy and values tend to represent an alternative paradigm to the rest of the health care system, in that the focus is on process more than product, on a qualitative service rather than a quantitative outcome. According to Gummer (1988), hospice programs are based on the alternative paradigm that function follows form, and so they emphasize three functions of organizational form: (1) the primacy of process over product, (2) power equalization with participatory decision making, and (3) small size to encourage intimacy.

In short, what matters most is the quality of the interaction of hospice workers with patients and families, the empowerment of patients and families through influencing decision making, and the maintenance of relationships among them all that are characterized by mutual support and affection. Hospice objectives are achieved as a result of these structural patterns.

The Community and Its Resources

The hospice social worker needs to know what policies and programs are available to assist hospice clients. Most hospice patients are in home care situations, where they not only often need Medicare or Medicaid financing to pay for their care but also such resources as home-delivered meals, tool and equipment rentals, support groups for family caregivers, and visits from friends and neighbors.

The culture of a community can impact on attitudes and readiness to help victims of certain types of problems. For example, some communities may be ignorant and fearful or superstitious about certain health conditions, such as cancer or AIDS.

The more rural the community, the less specialized or "high tech" the resources it is likely to have. In such areas, alternative resources often need to be explored.

Intervention Modalities

The hospice social worker requires a repertoire of effective interventions to address particular needs of clients. The psychosocial assessment of the patient and family determines which approaches are selected. For example, choice of intervention depends on the extent to which they need information and referral, pain control, skill development, supportive counseling, behavioral change, cognitive change, improved intrafamily communication and understanding, environmental modification, social support networking, empowerment and development of coping skills, or advocacy. Hospice social worker functions and interventions were discussed earlier in this chapter under Social Worker Functions and Interventions.

Needed Research, Evaluation, and Documentation

Dush (1988a,b) points out that although nurses and other hospice care workers have tended to assume social worker responsibilities in the area of psychosocial assessment and treatment, little research has been done to develop knowledge about which particular intervention modalities work best with particular types of clients or client problems.

What was said about home health care research and evaluation applies to social work in hospice care as well (see Chapter 5), and, as always, the social worker needs to know the documentation requirements of the service provider and funding source and take care to accurately and completely comply with these requirements to ensure continued support for social work services. In the past, errors in documentation have sometimes resulted in reimbursement losses and reductions in use of that discipline by the service provider.

VALUES AND ETHICS CONSIDERATIONS

The values and ethics of the social work profession are remarkably compatible with those of hospice care. Above all, anyone working with a hospice program must be able to value every human individual, the principle of client confidentiality, human diversity, social justice and commitment to serve vulnerable populations, and client self-determination.

Stark and Johnson (1983) described the efforts of the teaching hospital in which they worked as social workers to incorporate a hospice service within the oncology inpatient service. They noted some ethical issues that were raised:

- What constitutes ordinary versus extraordinary means?
- How should the social worker be involved in this decision?
- To whom should the social worker be responsible when there is an irreconcilable conflict concerning patient care decisions between patient and family or between patient/family and physicians? (68-69)

Since most hospice care is provided in the home, much of what was said about values and ethics in home health care also applies to hospice care (see Chapter 5). In addition, some of the more obvious social worker values and ethics challenges to which hospice social work is most vulnerable include the following hypothetical examples:

- The social worker perceives an important unmet need of the patient and/or family that the hospice organization and/or funding source is unwilling or unable to meet.
- The patient or family tells the social worker something in confidence that other team members ought to know.
- The social worker learns that the hospice agency is charging for services that were not provided.
- The social worker finds that the hospice agency is violating some rule or failing to meet some standard of the funding or certifying organization.
- The social worker is offered an exciting employment opportunity elsewhere, but one or more hospice patients and their families have grown exceedingly dependent on the social worker for understanding and emotional support and indicate that they "couldn't make it" if the social worker left.

SKILL REQUIREMENTS

Professional skill is the ability to perform well whatever activity is involved in one's work and must reflect the integration of relevant knowledge as well as values and ethics. Such skill is used while interacting with a complex set of variable conditions; therefore, true professional skill is conscious, purposeful, disciplined, and responsible.

It is not enough to "care about" people; one also needs to know how to help them and how to "take care" of them. Unfortunately, failure to understand this results in much wasted effort, as well as actual harm, by well-meaning but unqualified helpers in the name of "caring."

One skill recommended by Bern-Klug, Gessert, and Forbes (2001), which some readers may see as more of a medical or nursing function, is that of pain assessment. Bern-Klug, Gessert, and Forbes (2001) recognize that hospice patients are not always able to precisely describe their physical discomfort to others nor to realize that they have every right to expect intervention to relieve it, and that the issue of resultant addiction to pain medication at this stage is irrelevant. The issue of discomfort is not limited to pain, however, but includes many other potential manifestations, such as cramping, itching, nausea, shortness of breath, and so on (46). This can be seen as a clinical social worker function insofar as the dynamics involved revolve around emotion and cognition. In addition, helping clients to acknowledge and describe their discomfort in detail and to have the social workers focus on its illumination and advocating for its relief becomes a form of validation of the clients' worth.

COMMENTARY

Hospice social work is not for every social worker or other health professional. However, anecdotal reports from people who do hospice work often claim that it is the most rewarding experience of their lives, even if they were not immediately attracted to it. Thus, the reader is urged not to rule it out without a closer look through a practicum experience.

CROSS-CULTURAL RESOURCES

Ford, Gillian (1993). Hospice in England—A palliative care system: The Marie Curie model. *The American Journal of Hospice and Palliative Care* (July/August): 27-29.

Johanson, Gary A. (1993). Palliative care in Argentina: A gringo's perspective. *The American Journal of Hospice and Palliative Care* (July/August): 11-12.

Kerr, Derek (1993). Lin zhong guan huai: Terminal care in China. *The American Journal of Hospice and Palliative Care* (July/August): 18-26.

Parry, Joan K. and Ryan, Angela Shen (Eds.) (1995). *A cross-cultural look at death, dying, and religion.* Chicago: Nelson-Hall.

Rosner, Fred (1993). Hospice, medical ethics, and Jewish customs. *The American Journal of Hospice and Palliative Care* (July/August): 6-10.

Storey, Porter (1993). Hospice settings around the world. *The American Journal of Hospice and Palliative Care* (July/August): 4-5.

Suzuki, Shizue, Kirsschling, Jane Marie, and Inoue, Iku (1993). Hospice care in Japan. *The American Journal of Hospice and Palliative Care* (July/August): 35-40.

Zylicz, Zbigniew (1993). Hospice in Holland: The story behind the blank spot. *The American Journal of Hospice and Palliative Care* (July/August): 30-34.

SECTION III:
HEALTH SERVICE DELIVERY
AND FINANCING

Chapter 8

U.S. Health Care System
Strengths and Problems

DESCRIPTION AND ASSESSMENT OF THE SYSTEM

Economic Access to Health Services

The U.S. "nonsystem" of economic access to health care services represents a mixed model with the following features: (1) *Medicare,* which amounts to national health insurance for selected groups (elderly and disabled who are eligible for Social Security, as well as persons who are medically dependent upon expensive renal dialysis treatments for survival as a result of end-stage renal disease), financed from employee payroll taxes; (2) *Medicaid,* a public assistance program financed from state and federal general revenues for persons who qualify for subsistence income assistance from government programs, in addition to low-income pregnant women and children, with types of coverage and benefit levels varying across state programs; and (3) *private health insurance* coverage for most employed persons, financed, in full or in part, by their employers.

The Uninsured Population

Unfortunately, these three basic sources of health insurance coverage do not fit together in such a way that all Americans are included; rather, they leave gaps that cause a substantial portion of the population to go without any coverage. In 1998, 16.3 percent of the U.S. population, or 44.281 million persons, were without any health insurance—Medicaid, Medicare, or private health insurance (U.S. Government Printing Office, 2000b:118, Table 178).

Recent increase in uninsured. The size of the uninsured population has increased in recent years. The percentage of Americans without health insurance coverage increased from 12.9 percent in 1987 to 15.4 percent in 1995 (U.S. Government Printing Office, 1997b:120) and to 16.3 percent in 1998 (U.S. Government Printing Office, 2000b:118, Table 177).

Geographical variation. The size of the uninsured population varies across states within the United States. In 1998 the uninsured population percentage ranged from a low of 9.0 percent in Nebraska to a high of 24.5 percent in Texas (U.S. Government Printing Office, 2000b:118, Table 178). As of 1997, the percentage of the U.S. population without any form of health insurance was highest in the South (20.7 percent), next highest in the West (20.4 percent), second from lowest in the Northeast (13.4 percent), and lowest in the Midwest (13.1 percent) (U.S. Government Printing Office, 2000a: 341, Table 128).

Ethnic variation. As is the case with most advantages in the United States, racial and ethnic minority group members tend to fare worse than the white majority. In the United States, in 1998, 15.0 percent of whites, 22.2 percent of blacks, and 35.3 percent of Hispanics had no health insurance (U.S. Government Printing Office, 2000b:118, Table 177).

Age variation. Across age groups, the elderly are most advantaged in terms of health insurance coverage; only 1.1 percent of persons age sixty-five and over were without health insurance in 1998, while 30.0 percent of young adults ages eighteen to twenty-four, 23.7 percent of adults ages twenty-five to thirty-four, and 15.4 percent of children under age eighteen had no health coverage (U.S. Government Printing Office, 2000b:118, Table 177).

Employment status. According to Billings (1999), "the profile of the typical uninsured person might be a young adult in a low-wage job working for a small employer in the retail/service sector of the economy . . . more than half of the uninsured earn less than $10,000 per year, and 85 percent earn less than $20,000" (406).

Firm size. Another variable affecting the worker's access to health insurance is the number of employees. Clearly, as firm size increases, the likelihood of the employer offering health insurance as a fringe benefit also increases. Only slightly more than one-half (52.4 percent) of all private firms offered health insurance in 1997; only 32.9 percent of those with fewer than ten employees offered health insurance to their employees, but 93.8 percent of those with 100 or more employees did so (U.S. Government Printing Office, 2000b:119, Table 179).

The Underinsured Population

In addition to the uninsured population, a large segment of the U.S. population has only partial health insurance coverage, requiring out-of-pocket contributions in the form of deductibles, coinsurance, and uncovered services. In 1998, Americans' out-of-pocket expenses were 3.4 percent of total costs of hospital care, 32.5 percent of nursing home care costs, 15.6 percent of total physicians' services, and 38.4 percent of all other *personal health care expenditures*—or about 19.6 percent of all personal health care expenditures of $1,019.3 billion (U.S. Government Printing Office, 2000a:327, Table 119). In 1998, Americans expended out-of-pocket payments totaling $574.6 billion, or about 17.7 percent of all *national health expenditures* of $1,149.1 billion (U.S. Government Printing Office, 2000b:108, Table 152). Note that national health expenditures include not only personal health care expenditures (such as health services and supplies and insurance premiums) but also such expenses as medical research and medical facilities construction.

The Original Intent and Current Outcomes of the Medicare and Medicaid Programs

Reflecting perhaps the disadvantages of a residual approach to social welfare policy and programs, neither Medicare nor Medicaid has developed as their authors intended. In an interesting piece about the history of Medicare (Title XVIII of the Social Security Act), passed by Congress in 1965, Robert M. Ball (1996), consultant on Social Security who was instrumental in getting the Medicare policy enacted and who is a past commissioner of Social Security and a current member of the Social Security Advisory Council, laid out the history of efforts to pass national health insurance legislation in the United States. He explained that he and all the others who developed and fought for the passage of Medicare saw it as a "last ditch" effort to obtain national health insurance for all Americans. It was never intended to be permanently limited to health insurance for the elderly only. Instead, targeting the elderly was a planned political strategy based on the following assumptions: the public would be most sympathetic to this group; the American Medical Association (AMA) would have a harder time opposing a program to help older people; and hospitals would tend to favor having a means for being reimbursed for care of older patients, who in the past were often unable to pay their hospital bills because they were retired and without employer-provided private health insurance.

On the other hand, Medicaid (Title XIX of the Social Security Act), also passed in 1965, was originally intended to provide health insurance for public assistance recipients, such as AFDC (Aid to Families with Dependent Children) families (Lyons, Rowland, and Hanson, 1996). However, due to the long-term care limitations of Medicare coverage for the elderly and the lack of other insurance coverage for many indigent and disabled persons, by 1993 only 27 percent of Medicaid funds were used for health care for welfare recipients, while 28 percent of Medicaid spending paid for nursing home and home care for the elderly (most of which is not covered under Medicare), 31 percent for health care for disabled people, and the other 14 percent went to DPS (disproportionate share) hospitals—that is, hospitals providing extensive health care services to the poor and uninsured (Lyons, Rowland, and Hanson, 1996).

Although Medicaid was originally intended to provide economic access to health care for the poor population, as of 1998 only 50.6 percent of the U.S. population with income below the government poverty line were covered by Medicaid (U.S. Government Printing Office, 2000b:115, Table 170).

Types of Health Service Organizations

A mixed model form also characterizes the health services themselves, in that the hospitals, nursing homes, home care agencies, outpatient clinics, and other organizational settings of such services are sometimes public tax-supported, sometimes private nonprofit, and sometimes private for-profit. The current trend is toward domination by the for-profit sector, except for hospitals and hospice organizations, where, despite an increase in for-profit hospital and hospice organizations, the nonprofit sector continues to predominate. As of 1998, only about 31.7 percent of U.S. hospitals were operated for profit (U.S. Government Printing Office, 2000b:127, Table 194), and only 23.0 percent of hospice-providing organizations were proprietary (U.S. Government Printing Office, 2000b:132, Table 206).

Health Service Payer Trends

However, although a growing percentage of organizations providing health services are proprietary, an increasing percentage of health care costs, about 44 percent (43.6 percent), are covered through public tax-supported programs, such as Medicare, Medicaid, and the VA (U.S. Government Printing Office, 2000a:327, Table 119). The share of hospital care paid by government health insurance and other government health programs increased from 42.5 percent in 1960 to 60.8 percent in 1998; for nursing home care, it rose from 15.7 percent in 1960 to 60.4 percent in 1998; for physicians' services, it rose from 7.1 percent in 1960 to 31.9 percent in 1998; and for all other personal health care, it increased from 8.1 percent in 1960 to 26.8 percent in 1998 (U.S. Government Printing Office, 2000a:328, Table 119).

The Quality of Health Care

If one can afford it, almost any desired health care service or procedure is available in America, and often of a very high quality—including not only routine interventions but also cosmetic surgeries, organ transplants, and joint replacements. Overall, most Americans are very satisfied with the health care services they receive (Zis, Jacobs, and Shapiro, 1996), and professional health care providers, such as physicians, nurses, and allied health care professionals (social workers, physical therapists, occupational therapists, and speech therapists) are generally well trained, with high legal and professional practice standards.

It is common to hear Americans exclaim that "the United States has the best health care in the world; that's why people who can afford to come here from all over the world for health services they can't get in their own countries!" or "If the Canadian health care system is so great, why do so many Canadians come to the United States for services they can't get in their own country?" (The second comment is generally made in reference to Canadians who pay for elective, nonurgent procedures in the United States rather than waiting for them to be scheduled and covered by national health insurance in Canada.)

The first remark may reflect our high technology for "repair" work, or what has been coined "the proliferation of technology" in U.S. health care. Joseph Newhouse (1996), director of the Division of Health Policy Research and Education at Harvard University, has asserted that the major cause of increased health care costs probably is the tremendous increase in medical capability, that is, technology.

Yet Harry E. Simmons (1996), president of the National Leadership Coalition on Health Care, has said that "the three serious and interrelated problems facing our health care system . . . are rising costs, decreasing coverage, and problems in quality" (57). Simmons attributes the fact that "our *per capita* health care costs are almost double those of other developed nations" (57) to excessive use of technology, in that we tend to use it even when the resultant benefits are not established. In fact, many medical and surgical interventions employed by U.S. physicians are not well grounded in outcomes research; both the quantity of medical care and the types of interventions vary widely across geographical regions, with a lack of evidence regarding variance in outcomes (Simmons, 1996; Kane, 1995:13, 15).

All of this reflects a greater lack of scientific knowledge in medicine than we tend to assume (Simmons, 1996). In addition, technology is sometimes knowingly misused, for example, due to pressure from patients to give antibiotics for a cold; pressure from hospitals to use expensive equipment, such as an MRI machine (magnetic resonance imaging), to help pay for it; or pressure from patients or families, or physicians' own internal pressure, to "do something," even when curative interventions for the problem are not known.

Furthermore, the error rate in medical interventions may well exceed the annual rate of fatal auto accidents, indicating a serious lack of quality control and challenging the use of patient satisfaction surveys as a measure of the quality of our health care system (Simmons, 1996). In short, improvement in the quality of health care through better knowledge of comparative outcomes of interventions, fewer medical errors, and proper use of interventions could significantly reduce health care costs (Simmons, 1996).

In 1999, the Institute of Medicine (IOM) released a report on medical errors titled "To Err Is Human" that provided alarming statistics on injuries and deaths in our health care system that could have been avoided. In 2001, the IOM released a follow-up report on medical error titled "Crossing the Quality Chasm: A New Health System for the 21st Century," calling for a total overhaul of our health care system (Sarudi, 2001a).

A private watchdog group, the Leapfrog Group, has demanded that three main standards be met: (1) implement a computerized physician order entry system; (2) meet certain volume thresholds for certain complex procedures, such as coronary bypass and esophageal surgery; and (3) hire intensive care specialists (Sarudi, 2001b).

Many Americans no doubt watched the four-part public television video documentary series titled *Critical Condition: How Good Is Your Health Care?* during the spring of 2001. One part of the series, "The Quality Gap: Medicine's Secret Killer," reported on the estimated 90,000 deaths annually in the United States as a result of medical errors (the series is obtainable through Films for the Humanities and Sciences:<http://www.films.com>). This series cited actual examples of the problem of medical error and its causes and also reported on some outstanding and successful programs at various health centers for addressing it.

Shi (2000) reported the results of a recent study to examine the relationship between the quality of primary care received and whether one has private or public (Medicaid) health insurance. The study found that the privately insured are able to obtain better primary care than the publicly insured, and those in fee-for-service plans obtain better quality primary care than those in HMO plans and are more likely to have a "usual source of primary care." Shi questioned whether the findings implied that the United States has a two-tiered health care system, according to economic status.

Health Care Costs

Interestingly, Medicare recipients have been found to be more satisfied with their health insurance plan than employed people, Medicaid recipients, or unemployed people, and Medicare has lower administrative costs than private health insurance programs (Lave, 1996). According to Lave (1996), the causes of the high costs of clinical services covered by Medicare include a combination of technology changes, the focus of Medicare coverage on acute care rather than both preventive and long-term supportive care services, as well as the general tendency to try to control costs through price controls, deductibles, and coinsurance rather than by changing utilization incentives.

Reviewing trends in health care reforms worldwide, all of which appear directed at controlling health care costs, Kirkman-Liff (1996) lists the common features of these directions as follows:

1. Use of a national global health care budget to achieve cost control.
2. Shifting management responsibility from government to private/ quasi-private institutions.
3. Capitation paid to primary group-medical practices.
4. Use of primary care physicians as gatekeepers to the rest of the health care system.
5. Encouragement of medical practice in group or health center settings.
6. Financial incentives to physicians to focus on health maintenance.
7. Prospective payments to hospitals (e.g., DRGs), or risk-based contracts with hospitals to cover a population, often paid by primary care physician groups (e.g., HMOs) from capitated budgets.
8. Integration of specialists with hospitals.
9. Consumer choice of provider-integrated networks (managed care organizations) under contract with a primary care physician group budget-holder or health insurer budget-holder.
10. A guaranteed minimal set of services assured to all citizens.
11. Individual freedom to purchase supplemental health service insurance. (69)

One of the issues in health care is whether nonprofit or for-profit health care organizations are better. One side of this issue concerns the quality of care, while the other side of the coin is relative cost/benefit.

Two relevant tendencies in public opinion in America today include (1) confusing a free market economic system with freedom and democracy in the political system and (2) an assumption that market principles will make health or social welfare programs more efficient for the same reasons they tend to produce efficiency in other business and industrial operations.

Worldwide Trends in Health Care Reform

1. Use of a national global health care budget to achieve cost control
2. Shifting management responsibility from government to private/quasi-private institutions
3. Capitation paid to primary group-medical practices
4. Use of primary care physicians as gatekeepers to the rest of the health care system
5. Encouragement of medical practice in group or health center settings
6. Financial incentives to physicians to focus on health maintenance
7. Prospective payments to hospitals (e.g., DRGs), or risk-based contracts with hospitals to cover a population, often paid by primary care physician groups (e.g., HMOs) from capitated budgets
8. Integration of specialists with hospitals
9. Consumer choice of provider-integrated networks (managed care organizations) under contract with a primary care physician group budget-holder or health insurer budget-holder
10. A guaranteed minimal set of services assured to all citizens
11. Individual freedom to purchase supplemental health service insurance (Kirkman-Liff, 1996:69)

However, some evidence is beginning to emerge that challenges these assumptions. For example, a large study (Woolhandler and Himmelstein, 1997) was recently reported that compared the costs during 1994, according to Medicare reports submitted by hospitals, of the three organizational types of hospitals. The study found that the for-profit hospitals cost significantly more than nonprofit or public hospitals in terms of (1) the average percentage of the hospital's budget devoted to administration, (2) the average cost per inpatient day, and (3) the average cost per discharge/inpatient stay. On the other hand, for-profit hospitals also had lower costs/overhead for employee wages, salaries, and benefits (raising issues of the quality of services). Administrative costs of for-profit psychiatric and rehabilitation hospitals, which are exempt from DRGs, were found to be especially higher.

Rachlis (1995), among the "lessons for Americans from Canada's health care system," noted:

> The cost savings from a single-payer plan are real. Canada's system is approximately 3 percent [2.7 percent in 1997] of Gross Domestic Product less expensive than that of the U.S. The savings are due to factors associated with a single-payer plan, including lower administrative costs, and reduced hospital and physician costs [related to less paperwork]. Canadians have better access to almost all health services than do Americans. [In fact] Canadians use more physicians' services and hospital services than do Americans. (151)

Given the evidence that for-profit hospitals are not cost-effective, in addition to the fact that multiple private health insurance companies such as we have in the United States involve monumental administrative costs in comparison to a national health insurance system, such as Canada's single-payer system, it is particularly relevant to heed what Woolhandler and Himmelstein (1997) noted:

> Even before these recent rises in expenditure for administration, the U.S. General Accounting Office calculated that the administrative savings that would result from a shift to national health insurance would fully fund universal coverage (Woolhandler, Steffie, and Himmelstein, David U. [1997]. Costs of care and administration at for-profit and other hospitals in the United States. *New England Journal of Medicine*, 336(11):769-799. Copyright 1997 Massachusetts Medical Society. All rights reserved.)

Given this, it is amazing to hear leaders of health care professions or organizations publicly assert that, in spite of rising health care costs in the United States, the solution is not to shift to a system of national health insurance, such as in Canada, because it would only increase costs further.

It is a curious fact that Canadians utilize more physician and hospital services than Americans do, yet administrative costs in the Canadian health care system are significantly less than those in the United States (Rachlis, 1995:144, 146). Surely, it is not coincidental that the United States is the only industrial nation in the world, besides South Africa, without a national system for ensuring universal economic access to basic health care, yet the United States also spends considerably more, both per capita and in terms of GDP, on health care than any of these other industrial societies, all of which have national health insurance, a national health service, or other system of universal economic access to basic health care.

The U.S. Government Printing Office (2000a:321, Table 114) provides some comparative data on health expenditures in the United States and twenty-nine other industrial nations, according to both percentage of GDP and per capita (see Table 8.1). The data show that in 1997, the United States expended 13.4 percent of its GDP on health care, compared with Germany, the next highest at 10.7 percent, while twenty-four of the twenty-nine countries spent less than 9 percent.

In addition, the United States spent $3,912 per capita for health care during 1997, and Switzerland was the next highest in terms of per capita health care costs that year, at $2,611. Canada, whose health care system Americans

TABLE 8.1. Health Care Expenditures, Life Expectancy, and Infant Mortality, United States and Selected Countries, 1995-1997

Country	1997 Expenditures		1995 Life expectancy at birth (years)***	1996 Infant mortality per 1,000 births*
	% GDP**	$ per capita		
United States	13.4	3,912	72.5 m 78.9 f	7.3
Switzerland	10.0	2,611	75.1 m 81.9 f	4.7
Germany	10.7	2,364	73.3 m 79.8 f	5.0
Canada	9.2	2,175	75.2 m 81.2 f	6.1
France	9.6	2,047	74.2 m 82.6 f	4.9
Denmark	8.0	2,042	72.8 m 77.9 f	5.7
Sweden	8.6	1,762	76.2 m 81.6 f	4.0
Japan	7.2	1,760	76.4 m 82.9 f	3.8
Finland	7.4	1,525	72.8 m 80.3 f	4.0
United Kingdom	6.8	1,391	74.3 m 79.6 f	6.1

Note: Countries listed in order by per capita health care expenditures.
*U.S. Government Printing Office (2000a). *Health, United States*. Washington, DC: Author, 157, Table 26.
**U.S. Government Printing Office (2000a). *Health, United States*. Washington, DC: Author, 321, Table 114.
***U.S. Government Printing Office (2000a). *Health, United States*. Washington, DC: Author, 158, Table 27.

often claim they could not afford, expended $2,175 per capita for health care in 1997, a mere 55.6 percent of U.S. expenditures for health care, while both Sweden, Denmark, and Finland, which are known for their very generous universal health and social welfare systems, each expended a fraction of the U.S. health care costs per capita, 45 percent, 52 percent, and 39 percent respectively (see Table 8.1).

Cost-Benefit Issues

Americans like to assert that the United States has the best health care system in the world—in spite of the fact that the United States ranks lower than many other nations in terms of basic indicators of population health status, such as life expectancy and infant mortality rate. In 1996, the infant mortality rate in the United States was 7.3 deaths of infants under one year out of every 1,000 live births; this is higher than twenty-five other industrial nations and almost twice as high as Japan's infant mortality rate of 3.8 the same year (U.S. Government Printing Office, 2000a:157); this was despite the fact that Japan spends less than one-half of what the United States does on health care per capita ($1,760 compared to $3,912) (U.S. Government Printing Office, 2000a:321, Table 114). Yet Japan has the longest life expectancy of any nation in the world, both at birth and at age sixty-five, for both males and females (U.S. Government Printing Office, 2000a:158, Table 27). Table 8.1 illustrates some of these comparative data.

What is wrong with the U.S. health care system? In short, it is inefficient. We spend more on health care than any other country in the world, yet indicators of population health, such as infant mortality rate and life expectancy, show that we are well below many other nations in terms of the health status of our citizens. Perhaps it is time to consider the following proposal by Woolhandler and Himmelstein (1997):

> Since the gap between health care costs in the United States and those in the rest of the world is widening and the ranks of the uninsured and underinsured are swelling, perhaps it is time to ask whether our experiment with market medicine has failed. (774) (Woolhandler, Steffie and Himmelstein, David U. [1997]. Costs of care and administration at for-profit and other hospitals in the United States. *New England Journal of Medicine,* 336[11]: 769-799. Copyright 1997 Massachusetts Medical Society. All rights reserved.)

Distribution of U.S. health care expenditures. Table 8.2 shows that, in 1998, a total of $1 trillion, 149.1 billion was expended for health care. Over one-half (53.3 percent) of all U.S. health care expenditures went for only two categories: inpatient hospital services (33.3 percent) and physicians' services (20.0 percent). In contrast, only 3.2 percent of all health care expenditures went for government public health services. Presumably, most public health expenditures are for primary prevention, that is, efforts to pre-

TABLE 8.2. Distribution of U.S. National Health Expenditures, 1998, by Object, Percent, Billions of Dollars, and Rank Order

Ranking	Object	Percent	Billions of Dollars	Cumulative Percent
1	Hospital	33.3	382.8	33.3
2	Physician	20.0	229.5	53.3
3	Drugs and other medical nondurables	10.6	121.9	63.9
4	Nursing home	7.6	87.8	71.5
5	Other professional service	6.0	66.6	77.5
6	Insurance and administration	5.0	57.7	82.5
7	Dental	4.7	53.8	87.2
8	Government public health	3.2	36.6	90.4
9	Other health services	3.0	32.1	96.0
10	Home health care	2.6	29.3	93.0
11	Medical research	2.0	19.9	98.0
12	Medical facility construction	1.0	15.5	99.0
13	Vision products and other medical durables	1.0	15.5	100.0
Total		100.0	1,149.1	100.0

Source: U.S. Government Printing Office (2000b). *Statistical Abstracts of the United States.* Washington, DC: Author, 108, Table 152.

vent health problems from occurring, and early intervention, i.e., efforts to prevent early problems from developing further.

Distribution of Medicare expenditures. Table 8.3 provides the distribution of health care expenditures through the Medicare program in 1998. The data show that $134.321 billion was spent through Part A of Medicare and an additional $75.814 billion through Part B of Medicare, for a total of $210.135 billion combined, which was 18.3 percent of total national health care expenditures in 1995 in the United States.

Table 8.3 also illustrates that 65 percent (64.8 percent) of Medicare Part A expenditures in 1998 were for acute inpatient hospital care—the most expensive level of care—while the largest share (42.7 percent) of Medicare Part B expenditures was for outpatient physicians' services. *Long-term*

TABLE 8.3. Distribution of Medicare Expenditures, Part A and Part B, 1998, by Object, Amount, and Percent

Expenditure Category	Amount (Billions of Dollars)	Percent
Part A: Hospital Insurance		
Inpatient hospital	86.998	64.8
Skilled nursing facility	13.630	10.1
Home health agency	13.806	10.3
Hospice	2.080	1.5
Managed care	17.807	13.3
Total Part A	134.321	100.0
Part B: Supplementary Medical Insurance		
Physician	32.341	42.7
Outpatient hospital	9.056	11.9
Home health agency	0.202	0.3
Managed care*	14.132	18.6
Intermediary laboratory	1.470	1.9
Durable medical equipment	4.108	5.4
Physician office lab or independent lab	2.168	2.9
Renal dialysis payments	6.492	8.6
Freestanding surgical centers, ambulance services, and supplies	5.845	7.7
Total Part B	75.814	100.0
Grand Total (Parts A and B combined)	$210.135**	

Source: U.S. Government Printing Office (2000b). *Statistical Abstracts of the United States.* Washington, DC: Author, 114, Table 168.
*Includes costs of experiments, demonstration projects, and peer review activity.
**Grand total 1998 Medicare expenditure source was U.S. Government Printing Office (2000a). *Health, United States.* Washington, DC: Author, 348, Table 133.

care, or the combination of nursing home, home health, and hospice care, constituted only 23.2 percent of total Medicare expenditures.

Distribution of Medicaid expenditures. Table 8.4 indicates that almost one-half (46.2 percent) of Medicaid expenditures in 1998 were for inpatient hospital or nursing home care, that is, institutional services, which are the first three categories listed. The total expended under the Medicaid program in 1998 was $142.318 billion which was about 12.4 percent of total expenditures of $1 trillion, 149.1 billion for national health services that year.

TABLE 8.4. Distribution of Medicaid Expenditures, 1998 by Object, Amount, and Percent

Object	Amount (Billions of Dollars)	Percent
Inpatient hospital		
General hospital	21.499	15.1
Mental hospital	2.801	2.0
Intermediate care facilities (mentally retarded)	9.482	6.7
Nursing facility services	31.892	22.4
Physicians	6.070	4.3
Dental	0.901	0.6
Other practitioner	0.587	0.4
Outpatient hospital	5.759	4.1
Clinic	3.921	2.8
Laboratory	0.939	0.7
Home health	2.702	2.0
Prescribed drugs	13.522	9.5
Family planning	0.449	0.3
Prepaid health care	19.296	16.6
Total	142.318	does not add to 100

Source: U.S. Government Printing Office (2000b). *Statistical Abstracts of the United States,* Washington, DC: Author, 116, Table 172.

Note, too, that less than one-half of 1 percent of Medicaid expenditures was used for family planning, an important aspect of preventive health care.

MANAGED CARE

The Background of Managed Care

Managed care has emerged in the United States as one method to control health care costs, which continued to rise at an increasing rate until the annual rate of increase diminished from 13.6 percent in 1980 to 11.6 percent in 1985. The decreasing rate of increase apparently reflected the introduction in 1983 of the diagnosis-related group (DRG) system under Medicare. In addition, the decrease in the rate of health care cost increases may have reflected the fact that health maintenance organizations more than doubled in number during that same period, 1980 to 1985 (U.S. Government Printing Office, 1997a:271). Amazingly, since 1985, the annual rate of increase in national health care expenditures continued to decrease across subsequent periods until 1996 when it reached an all-time low of only 4.6 percent for the one-year period of 1995 to 1996. However, by 1998, it had begun to rise again, when it was then 5.6 percent (U.S. Government Printing Office, 2000a:325, Table 118).

Still, the actual cost of national health care expenditures in the United States continued to increase, in spite of the reduction in the rate of increase. In 1985, national health care expenditures totaled $428.7 billion, but by 1998, they had more than doubled, reaching $1,149.0 billion (U.S. Government Printing Office, 2000a:325, Table 118).

The Growth and Development of Managed Care

Health maintenance organizations (HMOs) first emerged in the 1930s and 1940s, but since the 1970s a new form of managed care has emerged, called "utilization review firms" or "managed care organizations." The idea behind this new form is that a third party other than the service provider or patient influences which kinds and amounts of service interventions will be approved for reimbursement. The motive is entirely cost control (Freeman and Trabin, 1994, cited in Manderscheid and Henderson, 1998:114). In fact, Munson (1998) has somewhat facetiously referred to managed care organizations as "managed cost organizations" (480).

HMOs had their roots in the nineteenth century in plantation owners, mining companies, and lumber firms providing health care services (not health insurance) as a fringe benefit to attract and retain workers (Friedman, 1996, cited in Kovner, 1999:283). Similarly, the first true HMO was started in the 1930s when what has since become known as the Kaiser Permanente Health Plan was offered to recruit and retain workers to help build the Grand Coulee Dam in Washington and then to attract shipbuilding workers in Oakland, California, during World War II (Kovner, 1999:283).

During the Nixon administration (1969-1974), "The Health Maintenance Organization Act of 1973 (Public Law 93-222) stimulated a sluggish health maintenance industry that has since grown at an explosive rate" (Karger and Stoesz, 1998:187). The HMO Act of 1973 authorized federal aid to establish HMO facilities in many favorable marketing areas that, combined with the coexisting growth in the nursing home and hospital management industries, piqued investor interest. Within ten years of the HMO Act of 1973, sixty proprietary HMOs were operating (Karger and Stoesz, 1998:190).

Managed care organizations in the United States have grown from only 174 in 1976 to 643 organizations in 1999, including 309 (48 percent) independent practice associations (IPAs), 123 (19 percent) group practice associations, and 208 (32 percent) mixed-model organizations (U.S. Government Printing Office, 2000a:345, Table 131). The period of greatest increase in HMOs was between 1980 and 1985, when the number more than doubled from 235 to 478, perhaps related to the introduction of the DRG system to control hospital costs. Since 1997 the number of HMOs has decreased somewhat.

As of 1997, nearly 29 percent (28.7 percent) of insured Americans were enrolled in managed care organizations (U.S. Government Printing Office, 2000a:344, Table 130), with the highest percentage, 41.4 percent, in the West, 36.7 percent in the Northeast, 23.9 percent in the South, and the lowest percentage, 23.3 percent, in the Midwest. This included 12.7 percent of Medicaid recipients and 8 percent of Medicare recipients (U.S. Government Printing Office, 2000a:345, Table 131).

What Is "Managed Care"?

Managed care refers to a cluster of health service systems, including health maintenance organizations (HMOs), with the three main models of (1) group, (2) staff, (3) IPAs, and (4) the newest form of HMO, provider service organizations (PSOs). Managed care includes also other forms that are not HMOs, such as preferred provider organizations (PPOs) and point-of-service (POS) plans.

I will try to clarify the distinguishing features of each variety of managed care model; however, the literature is somewhat confusing because of the lack of consistent use of terms (especially the terms *group model, staff model,* and *network model*), as well as the variance in features not only between models but within models.

The Group Model (e.g., Kaiser Permanente)

According to Mechanic (1999):

> The traditional and most studied HMO type is the group model in which the insurance plan contracts with one or many large multispecialty groups on a capitated basis to provide services exclusively to its insured population. The professional group is responsible for its internal organization and processes and for distributing income within the group, but the insurance plan provides for hospitals or other needed physical facilities. These facilities may be directly owned by the plan, be available through contracts, or both. (154)

In the group model, the provider organization, that is, the professional group, assumes the financial risk of providing services that cost more than the prepaid capitated sum.

The Staff Model (e.g., Group Health Cooperative of Puget Sound)

> Staff model HMOs are similar to group models in many ways, but physicians are typically salaried and not personally at risk, although there may be financial incentives to help shape their behavior. The insurance organization, however, is capitated and is at risk. Physicians tend to dislike staff models, which make physicians employees, and they commonly convert to group models over time. (Mechanic, 1999:154)

Independent Practice Association Model/Network Model

As of 1999, independent practice associations (IPAs) were the predominant model of managed care, with 309 or 48.0 percent of the 643 managed care organizations reported that year (U.S. Government Printing Office, 2000a:345, Table 131). According to Mechanic (1999), the IPA model also is referred to as the network model. The usual pattern is for the insuring organization to develop a network of physicians in solo practice, or group practice of the same specialty, who will serve the insurance enrollees. These are capitated insurance plans and the physicians are also often paid on a capitated basis. The physicians are not required to limit their services only to one HMO, but instead may participate in several and may also see fee-for-service patients. The advantage of the independent practice association, or network model, is that it provides more flexibility and autonomy to the physicians, and greater choice of physicians to patients. However, under the IPA model, the physicians are less likely to attend to preventive and other innovative efforts or to involve other health care professionals in team efforts (Mechanic, 1999:154-155).

Provider Service Organizations

One of the newest HMO types is the provider service organization. According to Rovner (1998):

> PSOs resemble HMOs in that they require patients to receive care from the plan's own doctors and hospitals, and patients must agree to have their care "managed" by the plan. The difference between a PSO and other plans is that a PSO offers its services through the doctors and hospitals who are owners of the PSO. (2)

Dick Davidson, president of the American Hospital Association, refers to PSOs as "community care networks" and apparently views them as a potential solution to the reduction in hospital inpatient usage in recent years and the reduction in hospital income resulting from managed care organization efforts to reduce health care costs by reducing hospital rates. Davidson advocates for PSOs partly because he sees them as having the advantage of local control over vertically integrated health care systems rather than control by huge HMO corporations often located in some other state (Grayson, 1998).

Preferred Provider Organizations

A related type of health care organization is the preferred provider organization, which is not really a form of HMO, but instead simply means that the insuring organization, such as Blue Shield, contracts with a network of physicians and other health service providers to provide services at a discounted price. Presumably, it is not considered a form of HMO because it remains a fee-for-service system, but it is one in which the fees are contracted at reduced amounts.

Point of Service

"Point of service" is a provision that may be associated with any of the HMO models and simply means that the model provides for patients having the choice to utilize health care providers outside the HMO, with the understanding that they must pay more out of pocket for such outside services.
As Kovner (1999) noted:

> Managed care organizations are health care systems under which a broad scope of medical services is provided for a fixed amount of money, negotiated in advance . . . and health maintenance organizations are [but] one model of managed care. (280)

> What differentiates HMOs [not all managed care organizations] from traditional healthcare delivery are the following factors: (1) the combining of the financing and delivery systems under a single organizational entity; (2) a broad scope of benefits; (3) a voluntarily enrolled population (unless the employer offers no alternative plan to the employees); (4) prepayment; (5) an organized provider system; and (6) the assumption of financial risk by the HMO. (282)

Kovner (1999:285-286) identifies "five main elements of HMOs: purchasers, plans, hospital providers, medical providers, and members":

1. The purchaser is an employer seeking a health care coverage plan for his or her employees, who prepays the plan for coverage of the enrolled employees.
2. The members are the employees enrolled in the plan.
3. The plan is both the contract itself and the organization that contracts with the purchaser, which may or may not be the same as the provider.
4. The hospital provider is either owned by the plan organization or contracts with it to provide needed hospital services to members referred by their HMO physician.
5. The physician providers are related to the plan under either the IPA model, the group model, or the staff model.

Many HMO plans are owned by insurance companies, but they are also owned by cooperatives, nonprofit organizations, hospitals, and doctor groups (Kovner, 1999:284).

Trends and Impacts of Managed Care

Since the 1970s, managed care organizations have tended to shift from predominately nonprofit to predominately for-profit organizations with stockholder ownership. Furthermore, the theory behind the original health maintenance organization was that by focusing on primary and preventive care, health care costs could be controlled by reducing the need for more costly repair services from specialists (Mechanic, 1999:155). By shifting from a fee-for-service system to a prepaid service system, a mechanism of financial incentive was provided to physicians and other providers to focus on health maintenance (Mizrahi, 1993).

The Main Features of Health Maintenance Organizations

1. The purchaser is an employer seeking a health care coverage plan for his or her employees, who prepays the plan for coverage of the enrolled employees.
2. The members are the employees enrolled in the plan.
3. The plan is both the contract itself and the organization that contracts with the purchaser, which may or may not be the same as the provider.
4. The hospital provider is either owned by the plan organization or contracts with it to provide needed hospital services to members referred by their HMO physician.
5. The physician providers are related to the plan under either the IPA model, the group model, or the staff model. (Kovner, 1999:285-286)

Today, however, managed care seems little involved in preventive care (Munson, 1997) and more involved in preventing physicians and other health service providers from using interventions that are not established by outcomes research as cost effective. This change in the direction of HMOs has important implications for the concept of "professional" and tends to shift the focus of professional services from the provider-patient relationship and its alleged healing power as a medium of intervention (Munson, 1997; Schuster et al., 1994) to a focus on the independent efficacy of a particular technological intervention, such as a drug, surgical procedure, or form of psychotherapy.

The introduction of managed care also impacts on the meaning of a "professional" because a key ingredient in this concept has long been that a professional must be able to practice with relative autonomy. If, instead, third-party bureaucrats with little or no education or training in the field of practice in question are empowered to refer to computer-recorded protocols for the preferred procedure for treating a particular health problem—and to approve or deny a professional health care provider's intervention plan— professional autonomy, as traditionally conceptualized, is evidently lost (Munson, 1997).

As Cornelius (1994) noted, "In essence, the social worker becomes an agent of managed care and agrees to serve the public within the corporate guidelines and not necessarily according to the assessed needs of the client" (52). Strom-Gottfried (1998b) has expressed concern about the potential barriers imposed by managed care on the obligation of the professional provider to assure clients of the confidentiality of information concerning them, as well as to ensure that all interventions with clients and releases of information are preceded by obtaining their informed consent.

A recent study by Chambliss, Pinto, and McGuigan (1997) found that among 139 mental health care professionals responding to a questionnaire sent to a randomly selected sample of 200 such professionals, considerable concern was expressed about perceived diminished client confidentiality and harmful effects on clients as a result of utilization reviews (149). Davidson and Davidson (1996) noted that "A document containing highly confidential material, in the hands of a managed care administrator, will be used whatever way is most profitable from a business perspective" (209). Concerning the issue of informed consent, reportedly, social work providers often feel compelled to get their clients to sign release of information forms in order to be reimbursed, while knowing that the clients' clinical information may be misused (Davidson and Davidson, 1996).

Strom-Gottfried (1998a) has proposed that it may be possible to resolve many of the current conflicts between providers and case managers in utilization review organizations through applying mediation techniques. Citing

Moore (1986), Strom-Gottfried (1998a) lists the common sources of disputes as including: "inconsistencies in data; relationship issues; value conflicts; structural problems such as unequal power or resources or geographic or physical barriers; and conflicts about interests" and makes the interesting observation that "a primary principle in conflict resolution is to focus on interests, broadly defined, rather than positions" (395).

In a sense, proprietary managed care organizations are the current answer of the free-market health insurance industry to the perceived threat of a single-payer plan, such as national health insurance, a national health service, or other government intervention as a mechanism of controlling health care costs.

"The HMO's response to traditional indemnity financing is offer a price to the purchaser of only 80 percent of the traditional price and at the same time achieve a bottom line profit that is 50 percent greater than that of the traditional indemnity insurer" (Hodge, 1996, cited in Kovner, 1999:297). This private reduction typically comes from three sources—reductions of about one-third each in payments to specialists, drug suppliers, and hospitals (Kovner, 1999:297).

Some HMO executives have made as much as $10 million a year in salary and bonuses and much more than that as a result of increases in the stock prices of the HMO (Kovner, 1999:299). The for-profits have been growing rapidly, in large part because of their advantages over nonprofits in securing large amounts of capital (Kovner, 1999:284). "In 1997, on average, CEO's at for-profit HMO's made annual salaries equaling $2 million" (Shindul-Rothschild, 2001:25). According to Shindul-Rothschild (2001), in 1997, the CEO of Oxford Health Plans, a for-profit HMO, was the highest paid executive, with $30.7 million in salary and $8.7 million in stock options. Curiously, this represented a salary increase of $10 million, even though the HMO had lost more than $80 million that year.

Underscoring the evidence that our profit-oriented health care system is not primarily driven by a public-good motive, Shindul-Rothschild (2001: 25, citing Limbacher, 1998) noted that "Columbia-HCA, the nation's largest hospital chain, reported its net earnings were up 51 percent even as it was subject of the largest Medicare fraud case in history."

Commenting on the current market-driven takeover of the U.S. health care system, Robert B. Friedland (1996), director of the National Academy on Aging, predicted:

> in about twenty years, what was once a market-based evolution will become a state-based public enterprise. Managed care will still be with us, but so too will managed financing, as state utility commis-

sions set the rates and the policies concerning the care provided by the publicly regulated health plans. (41)

SUMMARY

The strengths of the U.S. health care system include a generally high quality of medical care and highly advanced technological interventions to repair and manage health problems. In addition, generally high standards, both legal and professional, exist for the training and practice of physicians and other health and allied health professionals in the United States. Although often critical of the nation's health care system, most Americans are quite satisfied with their own health care services.

On the other hand, the U.S. health care system does have significant problems, for example, the health status indicators of the population do not sufficiently reflect the proportion of our economic resources expended for health care. While stubbornly resisting a sincere and careful consideration of the possible advantages of other countries' health care systems, we have instead turned to such approaches as for-profit managed care (or managed cost?) organizations and to prospective payment systems, for hospitals in 1984 and for home care organizations and nursing homes in 1997, in an effort to control costs of health services.

The major value of managed care would be realized if only it reduced waste in the health care system without reducing the quality of care. Unfortunately, however, the effect of our efforts to control costs has been more to ration services, which has helped to reduce the annual rates of increase in the corresponding health care costs.

However, one wonders what has become of the people and health-related problems that are dropped from such services. Have they turned to alternative medicine or to informal family care at home, or what?

That our American health care system is in trouble is suggested by a glance at the table of contents of the March 2001 issue of *Hospitals and Health Networks,* a publication of the American Hospital Association. The topics include a shortage of nursing and other emergency room staff; a shortage of physicians, who are increasingly retiring earlier; the problem of medication errors; and the danger of defective infusion pumps, which the HCFA has warned may suddenly open and allow too much medication to enter the patient.

Although the annual rate of increase in health care costs has generally declined, our total health care costs continue to increase and to exceed those of any other country in the world, both per capita and relative to the gross domestic product. Presumably, our excessive health care costs are the result of our tendency to focus on the acute (repair) level of health care, with comparatively little in the way of supportive interventions to (1) promote health and prevent disease onset; (2) prevent disease development and complication, by providing supportive assistance to supplement cure efforts, once disease onset is evident; or (3) prevent avoidable impairment of comfort and function of persons with chronic or terminal, mental or physical, health conditions and to prevent secondary disabilities. In other words, we are preoccupied with curing to the neglect of caring, at all levels of health service. We also tend to overuse diagnostic and repair technology in the sense that health care providers often use it even when its cost effectiveness is not well established.

We have come to equate "doing something" with the diagnosis and treatment of already existing mental and physical health problems in individuals and have sometimes lost sight of the things we *could* do in the way of social interventions with the larger community to promote health, to prevent injury and disease, and to reduce the avoidable effects of injury and disease that impair comfort and function and thus reduce the quality of life. We also need to reexamine our tendency in America to think of private specialized practice and high technology as exciting and to think of public health, generalist practice, primary care, and long-term care as dull and unchallenging. In short, we need to review the current literature on the role of social inequality in the production of health problems and return to a greater public health perspective, and less of a medical model perspective.

Some trends in our health care system hold promise, I think, such as the move toward greater continuity of health care via vertically integrated health care systems, greater concentration of resources on primary care, more attention to outcomes research as criteria for intervention planning, and setting limits on available resources to pay for health care and forcing providers to think more about the cost effectiveness of intervention options.

On the other hand, some of us question the morality of CEOs of profit-making managed care organizations being rewarded with multimillion dollar annual salaries and benefits packages in a nation where about 44 million citizens have no health insurance, and millions more must regularly choose between groceries or uncovered health care needs. Here the issue is equity, that is, what is fair and just.

Furthermore, it does seem to make sense that a single-payer system like Canada's would likely reduce the current administrative costs in the United States caused by having multiple insurance organizations. Shindul-Rothschild (2001) cited some Organization for Economic Cooperation and Development (OECD) (1997) findings explaining that because the United States has some 1,500 different private health insurers, the United States in 1994 spent $194 per capita on administrative costs, compared to Canada's administrative costs of only $42 per capita. In addition, a single-payer system under national health insurance eliminates "bad debts" and so reduces provider overhead costs, which in the United States currently get shifted to the fees of those who do pay (Belcher, 1993). That is, Canadian hospitals receive an annual global budget at the beginning of each year and must operate within it; they also do not have the expense of filing claims for reimbursement, as they have already been funded for the year, adding to administrative cost savings.

In addition, I think we need more HMOs of the Kaiser Permanente type, that is, nonprofit, health care providers who make their own decisions about choice of interventions and assume the financial risk of exceeding the capitated prepayment, and within which considerable interprofessional teamwork is the norm, including efforts at disease prevention and early intervention. Recall that a "true HMO" knows that if it fails to keep the patients healthy and functional and prevent serious health problems, more extensive and more expensive procedures will be required, which will reduce the HMO's profits.

Chapter 9

A Vision of Future Social Work Practice in Health Care

INTRODUCTION

This final chapter deals with reflections on the past and future of social work in the health field, in light of changes that are occurring in the health field and in the knowledge about the determinants of health and disease, in the context of current and needed knowledge, skills, values, and ethics of professional social workers.

EMERGING TRENDS IN HEALTH CARE DELIVERY

Among the changes occurring in health care in the United States are the following:

1. Shift from the hospital to the community as the center of health care delivery
2. Increase in health problems with social and environmental etiology
3. Public demand for more input into personal health care decisions, in the context of increasing complex medical and surgical intervention options
4. Growing expectation that families will have to do more of the care-giving of their own members, at all levels of caring
5. Gradual transformation of once-terminal health problems into more chronic long-term care ones
6. Interaction of profit-oriented managed care and its principles with these changes (Vaghy, 1998:8)

Worded slightly differently, the major trends in health care delivery are as follows:

1. Move from acute care to chronic illness and diseases of aging
2. Increased emphasis on market forces and cost control

3. Emphasis on measuring outcomes of health care interventions
4. Increased recognition of social and environmental determinants of diseases
5. Increasing role of families, broadly defined, in provision of home care
6. Increased patient participation in health care decisions (Volland et al., 2000:1)

These trends in health care have the following implications for all health professionals:

- Long-term management of chronic illnesses as a primary focus within health care delivery systems
- Shift from acute care settings to ambulatory settings
- Use of population-focused interventions to improve health status
- Increased focus on disease prevention and health promotion (Volland et al., 2000:1)

Changes in U.S. Health Care

1. Shift from the hospital to the community as the center of health care delivery
2. Increase in health problems with social and environmental etiology
3. Public demand for more input into personal health care decisions, in the context of increasing complex medical and surgical intervention options
4. Growing expectation that families will have to do more of the caregiving of their own members, at all levels of caring
5. Gradual transformation of once-terminal health problems into more chronic long-term care ones;
6. Interaction of profit-oriented managed care and its principles with these changes (Vaghy, 1998:8)

Among the trends in health care with clear implications for social work are these:

- A move away from hierarchical practice and toward a team-based approach
- New attention to brief interventions, critical path models, and solution-focused therapy
- Increased need for and importance of case management
- Greater emphasis on patient outcomes research and evaluation of social work services
- Increased need for patient education about health care coverage and financing

- Increased emphasis on health promotion and preventive interventions
- Population-specific social work practice, such as older patients, HIV/AIDS patients, patients with chronic physical illness, patients with chronic mental illness. Other examples include such special populations as persons with addictions, nephrology patients, and oncology patients. (Volland et al., 2000:2)

The Background of These and Other Trends in Health Care

The Shift in the Nature of Prominent Health Problems: From Acute to Chronic Care Management

The general shift in major health problems has moved away from acute diseases due to bacterial and viral infection being controlled largely through public health measures. Also, improved medical management has reduced the number of acute episodes of many chronic diseases, such as diabetes, epilepsy, heart disease, and hypertension. Thus, the health conditions that have now assumed a more prominent position are largely chronic ones that can more easily be managed outside of institutional settings, which is especially important as the aging population increases.

A Trend Toward a More Team-Based Approach

Probably as a result of both increased knowledge about the biopsychosocial interaction in both mental and physical health disorders and the trend toward chronic disease case management, the need for greater coordination and cooperation across both professional services and informal social supports is suggested.

Major Trends in Health Care Delivery

1. Move from acute care to chronic illness and diseases of aging
2. Increased emphasis on market forces and cost control
3. Emphasis on measuring outcomes of health care interventions
4. Increased recognition of social and environmental determinants of diseases
5. Increasing role of families, broadly defined, in provision of home care
6. Increased patient participation in health care decisions (Volland et al., 2000:1)

The Implications of Health Care Trends

For All Health Professionals:
- Long-term management of chronic illnesses as a primary focus within health care delivery systems
- Shift from acute care settings to ambulatory settings
- Use of population-focused interventions to improve health status
- Increased focus on disease prevention and health promotion

For Social Work Professionals:
- A move away from hierarchical practice and toward a team-based approach
- New attention to brief interventions, critical path models, and solution-focused therapy
- Increased need for and importance of case management
- Greater emphasis on patient outcomes research and evaluation of social work services
- Increased need for patient education about health care coverage and financing
- Increased emphasis on health promotion and preventive interventions
- Population-specific social work practice, such as older patients, HIV/AIDS patients, patients with chronic physical illness, patients with chronic mental illness. Other examples include such special populations as persons with addictions, nephrology patients, and oncology patients (Volland et al., 2000:1-2)

The Trend Toward More Case Management/Care Management

Chronic disease management requires doing all that is necessary to obtain and sustain a stable status with the chronic disease, via proper diet, exercises, medication regimen, and appropriate social, emotional, and physical environments, with available assistance for whatever services are required. This implies a focus on linkage with and coordination of multiple service providers and informal helpers, as well as sustained contact with the patients and providers to monitor their status and demonstrate interpersonal support; that is, case management/care management is clearly indicated.

Increased Population-Specific Social Work Practice

Presumably, expectation of more population-specific social work practice is a reflection of the prominence of certain health-related-problem groups, both in numbers and high costs to society, as well as with group-specific problems and needs, such as with the older population, those with chronic kidney disease, and people with HIV/AIDS. Such groups require health provider specialization to achieve a level of optimal knowledge and skills to address their various problems effectively. However, unless working in a special unit of a hospital or another setting that focuses on a specific population, health care social workers will encounter patients who represent a broad range of health problems, each of which has a set of problem-specific needs.

Increased Need for Patient Education About Health Care Coverage and Financing

In lieu of a single-payer health care system, as is found in every other industrial country in the world except for South Africa, the United States has a multiple-payer, patchwork nonsystem of financing, with complex variations in coverage. As a result, many people are unable to navigate the path to the services they need and are eligible to access. Thus, ideally, social workers in health care could be helpful to patients and their families by assisting them in understanding their particular health insurance coverage and associated options.

The Increase in Psychosocial Problems Resulting in Physical Health Impairment

At the same time, a number of psychosocial problems have risen to positions of prominence in health care, such as depression, homicide, suicide, domestic violence, child maltreatment, elder abuse, eating disorders, drug abuse, tobacco addiction, alcoholism, personality disorders, and motor vehicle accidents. Emergency rooms increasingly encounter all of these types of problems that affect physical health but have behavioral causes, at least partly in response to social-environmental conditions. Most hospitals utilize emergency room social workers with clinical social work licenses to handle such cases beyond the immediate medical intervention needs. However, there may be a need for more intervention, not only at a personal level, but also at a community and population level.

Increased Role of Market Forces and Cost Control

The increased role of market forces and emphasis on cost control probably initially resulted from the rapidly growing costs of a hospital-centered health services system as medical technology accelerated in the mid-1960s. At the same time, employers were burdened with the associated increasing costs of health insurance, which, they complained, added to the costs of their products and impaired their ability to compete effectively with foreign companies whose governments provided health coverage to their citizens from general revenues.

Concomitantly, a few true nonprofit HMOs (e.g., Kaiser Permanente) began to receive public attention for their focus on "keeping people well" and thereby reducing the costs of health insurance. Richard Nixon and his conservative associates apparently thought that if the HMO approach worked so well as a nonprofit organization, it could well be a boon to reducing costs if they were for-profit organizations, and the HMO Act of 1973 was passed. However, gradually, the terminology shifted from "health maintenance" to "managed care," as the philosophy moved from one of "keeping people well and preventing health problems from developing" to one of "managing the health care providers" to promote more efficient business practices.

With the passage of Title XVIII and XIX in the mid-1960s, Medicare and Medicaid were born and eventually began to help cover costs of services such as home health care and nursing home care, which helped to promote a for-profit industry in those sectors too.

These changes in the nature of our health problems, in addition to America's unexamined adherence to a market-based health insurance system and a general decline in public health funding for disease prevention and health promotion, all combined to produce annual national health care costs that increased at an almost geometric annual rate. A result of this has been extended government cost-control efforts to reduce the use of health care, first, in inpatient settings such as hospitals, with the prospective payment system begun in 1983, and, more recently, a comparable system to reduce the use of both Medicare-funded home health care and Medicare-funded nursing home care.

Increased Public Participation in Personal
Health Care Decisions

With the steady growth in the population with little or no health insurance coverage, and decreasing access to affordable traditional health services, increasing numbers of Americans have turned to alternative medicine, including over-the-counter drugs, herbal remedies, massage therapy, relaxation therapy, self-hypnosis, naturopathic providers, aromatherapy, hot tubs, extremist diets, prayer, meditation, yoga, chanting, drumming, physical exercise equipment, sweat lodges, and so forth.

As people have taken more interest in health and disease, they have become more empowered and increasingly want to know what their options are, and what the implications of each option are. This increased interest in personal health is probably nurtured by health-related Web sites and TV ads promoting both self-help products and pharmaceutical companies, which have started to inform the public about new drugs they have available for various health problems, suggesting the patient might wish to "ask your doctor if this might be right for you."

Reduction in Hospitals As the Seat of Health Service and Increase in Outpatient Settings in the Community

However, the overall trend has been to reduce the use of both mental hospitals and general hospitals and to increase the use of ambulatory care settings such as the following:

- Outpatient clinics
- Outpatient surgery centers
- Outpatient rehabilitation centers
- Patient and family support-group meetings in community settings
- Visiting home care and hospice services
- Family caregiver-provided home care services
- Mental health professional case management team outreach to persons with chronic mental illness (i.e., assertive community treatment [ACT] teams)
- Child and adult day care programs in community settings for persons with special care needs
- Group homes/assisted living facilities for persons with chronic illness or other mental and/or physical impairments (e.g., early stage Alzheimer's disease or HIV/AIDS)
- Programs such as PACE (Program of All-Inclusive Care for the Elderly), an adult day care program with high-quality interprofessional team services that enables older people to remain at home with a higher quality of life and to avoid institutional care (Lee et al., 1998)

From Health Profession-Controlled Health Care to Business Management of Health Professionals

Clearly, the U.S. health care system is at a crossroads, with considerable uncertainty about what path to take from here. For now, however, our for-profit managed care financing system requires that we all become more efficient, that is, get better outcomes for less cost (in terms of compensation to professional health care service providers). The required techniques for controlling costs include such approaches as

- short-term, solution-focused interventions
- critical path models, and
- outcomes research

Short-term solution-focused interventions refers to brief interventions that focus on resolving the immediate problem, whether the need is to

1. discharge the patient back to the community within the Medicare limit on DRG days;
2. reduce the frequency with which the patient keeps returning to the emergency room;
3. enable the family to regulate the child's medication to reduce the cost of doctor visits; or
4. link the young adult with severe mental illness to some community-based case management program to prevent decompensation and resultant need for costly acute crisis care services.

Technically, solution-focused therapy seeks to engage the client's own cognitive framework in constructing behavioral tasks that will lead to a speedy solution, reinforcing the clients' ideas and prompting the client to relate them to the desired outcome (Robbins, Chatterjee, and Canda, 1998: 314-315).

Critical path models are similar to *protocols* (sets of rules governing some procedure or process) or *algorithms* (specific methods of solving a problem) that spell out a preplanned sequence of steps to follow, given *x, y,* or *z* (i.e., "if," "then . . ."). The idea behind critical path models is to avoid reinventing the wheel, so to speak, to avoid approaching every situation as if it were unique, and instead to *use brief and rapid assessment tools* (i.e., scales with established validity and reliability) to quickly identify the patient's status, and then follow the preestablished step or series of steps to try to address it, based on previous outcomes research that suggests which intervention is likely to be effective.

Outcomes research requires specifying one or more measurable objectives of intervention and measuring the client's status on that variable, again using brief and rapid assessment tools, before and after the intervention, so that the social worker has some sort of evidence of whether the desired changes actually were achieved.

Shifts in the Burden Bearers of Health Care

An impact of these trends in the U.S. health care system is that the burden of health care costs is shifting from employers, in the form of employee benefits, to employees and government, and from professional health care providers to family lay providers.

Shifts in the Profit Receivers in the Health Care System

Increasingly, those who benefit economically are not the professional health service providers but the CEOs of profit-oriented managed care organizations, nursing home corporations, and other chains of for-profit, health-related businesses, which tend to compromise service quality by shifting costs from service overhead to executive salaries and benefits and stockholder dividends.

The Call of Science for Increased Focus on Disease Prevention and Community Health Promotion

The *NASW NEWS* has reported a number of recent studies of the National Institutes of Health and National Academies with the common theme of "the need for emphasis, not just on medical interventions, but on the social, cultural, economic, family and community factors in prevention and treatment of health conditions" (O'Neill, 2001:3). Ten *priority areas* for research spending to integrate the behavioral, social, and biomedical sciences at NIH are recommended by the National Research Council. Following is a list of seven of these:

1. *Predisease pathways*—identify the precursors to disease, both brief and long-term biological, social, psychological, and behavioral ones
2. *Positive health*—identify the positive factors, biological, social, psychological, and behavioral, that provide resistance to disease and promote wellness
3. *Personal ties*—detail the mechanisms by which close social interactions influence health and disease outcomes
4. *Healthy communities*—identify the collective properties of social and physical environments that influence health and disease outcomes
5. *Inequality*—clarify the mechanisms through which socioeconomic hierarchies, racism, discrimination, and stigmatization influence health and disease outcomes
6. *Interventions*—expand the scope and effectiveness of strategies for social and behavioral interventions to improve health
7. *Methodology*—develop new measurement techniques and research designs that link information across levels of analysis (molecular, cellular, behavioral, psychosocial, community, and across time) (O'Neill, 2001)

It has been well documented through multiple controlled empirical studies in the social sciences that the health status of populations is very much influenced by social inequality and other sources of stress (some such data were cited in Chapter 3) (see Evans, Barer, and Marmor, 1994; Kawachi, Kennedy, and Wilkinson, 1999; see also Poland, Green, and Rootman, 2000; Bracht, 1999; Raczynski and DiClemente, 1999).

At the same time that the government is desperately attempting to restrain health care costs funded by Medicare and Medicaid, it is constrained by market economy forces that control national politics from taking more effective action to strengthen the health care system and improve the national indicators of the health status of the nation. In short, it is difficult to make changes in a society when powerful sectors have vested interests in avoiding such changes. I am referring to such needed policy changes as these:

- A national health insurance system similar to the Canadian system*
- A considerable increase in the minimum wage to above the poverty level
- A more progressive income tax scale to reduce income inequality
- A shift in funding for public education to more state and federal funding in an effort to elevate all public schools to a high level of quality
- Increased funding from the federal level for more effective child protection services provided by sufficient numbers of MSW-level social workers
- Automatic Medicaid coverage of all persons whose income is near or below the poverty level (pending extension of Medicare to all Americans to provide a national health insurance system)
- Mandatory parenting-education programs to help prepare people for parenthood and to provide refresher courses for those who need it

- Funding for public health nurse and public health social worker teams to visit with every parent with a new baby before leaving the hospital to explore the level of knowledge and skill to assume care responsibilities

Such funding would also provide automatic follow-up home visits to offer support, education, and troubleshooting until the child enters school, whereupon the same sort of team would be available in every public school, with

---

*Readers who wish to know more about the Canadian health care system should read *Universal Healthcare: What the United States Can Learn from the Canadian Experience* (1998), by Pat and Hugh Armstrong with Claudia Fedan and *The Canadian Health Care System: Lessons for the United States* (1995), by Susan Brown Eve, Betty Havens, and Stanley R. Ingman.

federal funding to assist those states that claim they cannot afford such services. (This is a Scandinavian model, where child abuse and neglect reports are negligible, apparently as a result of this prevention-type outreach service.)

- Restoration of a nationwide system of publicly funded comprehensive community mental health centers (CMHCs), with a sliding-fee scale, focused on prevention and early intervention, including drug and alcohol and cigarette smoking prevention and treatment services, as well as treatment for eating disorders and counseling services for parent-child problems, couple relationship issues, and teenagers who feel they need a professional to talk with about something of concern to them

In addition, such CMHCs would have both inpatient and outpatient services, and take major responsibility for lifetime outreach and follow-up support services to persons with chronic mental illness, so that the streets and jails would no longer be their plight. CMHCs would be centers of public education via small groups and public lectures about issues relating to mental health which could help people to know how to avoid and how to recognize and respond to what could be signs and symptoms of mental health problems.

- Extension of Head Start so that all children who need it can access it

In light of the values and ethics of the profession, it seems that health care social workers ought to consider what is really needed to make fundamental improvements in our nation in order to

- elevate the health status of populations;
- reduce social inequality;
- increase funding and programs for health promotion and disease prevention;
- improve the quality and accessibility of publicly supported care services, as an alternative to family caregiving as the only ethical option;
- promote in social work more research of an experimental design nature to develop a solid body of effective social work interventions in health care; and
- further develop a body of knowledge about the social and environmental determinants of disease and about effective interventions to promote health and prevent disease at a population level.

Note: Bloom (2000), a medical sociologist with the Mount Sinai School of Medicine, proposed that social work in the health field and medical sociology join forces again. He discussed their historical background and early close partnership, followed by their unfortunate division as they both sought professional status, when social work became a client-centered clinical enterprise with ethical concerns, and sociology sought to become a value-free, research-oriented field. Bloom calls this "the tension between advocacy and objectivity" (32). Medical sociology emerged after World War II, focused on population-based studies reflecting sociocultural theory.

Now, however, Bloom argues, the time is ripe for a renewed partnership between the fields of medical sociology and social work in health care, because

> [i]n the face of pressures for commodification and dehumanization, the parochialism that is always potential in relations between academic disciplines is no longer a rational choice. The nature of the problems for both inquiry and application have changed, and must, inevitably, influence the choice of methods and practice. (35)

Bloom anticipates that such a partnership could "meet the challenges of educating doctors to be more effective in meeting the needs of patients in the health care system that they face today" (35).

Bloom's proposal is appealing, I think, because it could be mutually beneficial, with social work acquiring the research knowledge and skills and population-focused perspective of sociology, and medical sociology heightening its sensitivity to the complex biopsychosociocultural interaction between a unique individual and the multilayered external social system.

IMPLICATIONS

In any case, Volland and colleagues (2000) identified three groups of social work skills especially needed in light of the trends in health care affecting social work in the field:

1. Basic skills: interviewing and assessment techniques that retain biopsychosocial emphasis but incorporate standardized screening measures, data management, setting of goal-based outcomes, and application of analytic skills to evaluate data and outcomes
2. Population-specific skills: knowledge of racial, ethnic, and cultural characteristics of populations; knowledge of treatment modalities appropriate to the patient's social situation; and knowledge of terminology, policies, regulations, and ways to access systems of care specific to the disease or population in question

3. Autonomy-building skills: ability to assist in securing grants and other financial resources; enhanced training in making ethical decisions; knowledge of program and finance management; ability to help patients and families negotiate health care systems; and training in interdisciplinary collaboration, conflict mediation, and advocacy within the health care setting and in the larger arena of health care legislation and regulation

---

Social Work Skills Needed to Navigate the Health Care System

Basic skills: interviewing and assessment techniques that retain biopsychosocial emphasis but incorporate standardized screening measures, data management, setting of goal-based outcomes, and application of analytic skills to evaluate data and outcomes

Population-specific skills: knowledge of racial, ethnic, and cultural characteristics of populations; knowledge of treatment modalities appropriate to the patient's social situation; and knowledge of terminology, policies, regulations, and ways to access systems of care specific to the disease or population in question

Autonomy-building skills: ability to assist in securing grants and other financial resources; enhanced training in making ethical decisions; knowledge of program and finance management; ability to help patients and families negotiate health care systems; and training in interdisciplinary collaboration, conflict mediation, and advocacy within the health care setting and in the larger arena of health care legislation and regulation (Volland et al., 2000)

Given these needs, Volland and colleagues (2000) recommended the following:

1. Health care education at the graduate social work level should be offered in more schools of social work and be more extensive in terms of the number and range of courses offered.
2. The education materials used should be more current and relevant to the reality of the health care system in which social workers will be employed, such as
   - more education about what managed care is, how it works, and what it requires of social work;*
   - more training in research methodology and statistics, especially in the use of appropriate rapid assessment tools and outcomes research;

---

*For a thorough understanding of managed care in the current U.S. health care system and the implications for social work, the following texts are highly recommended: *Humane Managed Care* (1998), edited by Gerald Schamess and Anita Lightburn, and *Managed Care in Human Services* (1999), edited by Stephen Wernet.

- increased coordination between classroom and practicum experiences;
- more education in case management requirements;
- more training in data management systems, to have systematic computerized records of case-related information that can be used to do research and evaluation on the social work program; and
- more training in ethical decision making.

3. Graduate schools should provide more specialized knowledge pertinent to special populations, such as older persons; persons with traumatic brain injury; sexually abused children; persons with chronic fatigue syndrome, fibromyalgia, Alzheimer's disease, and so forth, in terms of available insurance and managed care coverage, available medical treatments, relevant terminology, and so on.

4. Health care social workers need to be prepared to work with little or no supervision; this includes having knowledge and skills in such areas as
   - community resources networking;
   - grant writing for funds to, for example, enable the social workers to conduct research or develop some experimental program;
   - program and fiscal management requirements, so as to be sufficiently informed to be able to advise the patient and family about their options;
   - teamwork, such as conflict resolution, to enable the social workers to assume leadership roles on these teams; and
   - policy advocacy, to enable them to be vocal and impressive advocates, capable of rallying community support for needed policy changes.

In addition, I would add that health care social workers need to learn to do the following:

- Perform experimental design research

Often misunderstood in social work, this is needed because it is the only research approach that can be said to measure the effect of an intervention through the use of random selection and random assignment to two or more groups to be studied. Outcomes research, on the other hand, does not provide for internal validity, that is, any means to establish that the outcome was the result of the intervention, rather than some other variable, since random selection and random assignment to experimental and control groups are not utilized. As Ell (1996) noted:

Interventions that have been studied with controlled clinical trial designs and that have demonstrated efficacy are among those most widely accepted in health care. . . . Given that social work is a practice-based profession, it is both surprising and cause for concern that there have been few controlled studies of social work interventions. (585)

A recent example of experimental design employed by social workers (McKay et al., 1998) compared the effectiveness of two varied telephone interventions to encourage urban parents to use available mental health services for themselves and their children.

- Gain practicum experience in health care settings other than hospitals

Such settings include public health agencies, nursing homes, home care agencies and hospice programs, support groups for patients with specific types of health problems, ACT teams, day care programs for children or adults with special needs, group homes/assisted-living facilities, and PACE programs. Perhaps a rotational experience across a range of settings would be useful, followed by a longer experience in the setting of special interest.

- Work with clients who are elderly and/or have disabilities due to chronic health conditions, whether mental or physical, directed to maximizing their function, integration with the community, and overall sense of well-being
- Work collaboratively with other professional groups linked with client network systems (open teamwork with networking, as Payne [2000] calls it)
- Develop and utilize a variety of community-based supportive resources, such as caregiver support resources
- Think outside the box about technologies for problem-solving, whether the need is for tools and equipment, services, income supports, environmental adaptations, interpersonal supports, or other resources
- Engage in more community-organization/community-development work to enhance health promotion objectives in the community, increased training in public health theory and methods
- Focus on social group work as a medium of mutual social support, health-related education, empowerment, consciousness raising, advocacy skill development, and mutual problem solving

- Document data on community needs and participate in professional advocacy to correct conditions that worsen rather than support community health conditions
- Conduct outcomes research on intervention efforts as part of an ongoing process of building a solid body of practice research and evidence of effectiveness

The Need for Social Work to Develop a Body of Practice Research

Auslander (2000) indicated four types of outcomes: (1) mission-oriented, (2) enabling (ones that are instrumental in enabling another profession to achieve its objective with the patient), (3) maintenance (ones that enable the host organization to achieve its goals), and (4) departmental or psychosocial (reducing, resolving, or preventing a negative impact on a patient or family member of a medical intervention or event). Auslander (2000) found that most of the journal articles including any report of service outcome fell into the fourth category and generally lacked evidence of the intervention being either useful or cost effective to the organization, although many dealt with client satisfaction with social work service—albeit a weak indicator of service quality.

For years, the call has been going out in the social work in health care literature for social workers to demonstrate their effectiveness if they hope to retain their positions in the field. Unfortunately, this call has not been sufficiently heeded. Growing evidence suggests that social work is not widely recognized as a key health care profession (Rosenberg, 1998:9-10).

Volland (1996) warned that "[t]he results of outcome management studies will play an increasingly important role in determining the level and type of financial support a specific health care service [such as social work] will receive" (49).

Managed care itself is such a dilemma for social workers that, as Veeder and Peebles-Wilkins (1998) admonished:

> A commitment must be made to evaluate every aspect of managed care, from services delivered and *their outcomes,* to administrative issues, to ethical concerns, to policies generated and implemented, to protocol proprietorship and other legal and statutory issues, and to the comparative viability of managed care approaches to behavioral health care. (489) (emphasis added)

A basic text concerning outcomes measurement for social workers is the recent publication of the NASW Press: *Outcomes Measurement in the Human Services: Cross-Cutting Issues and Methods* (Mullen and Magnabosco, 1997). This compilation of thirty brief chapters addresses a wide variety of practical and crucial issues in outcomes research. For example, one chapter (Berman and Hurt, 1997) from this text discusses the four basic types of outcomes one may choose to research—services, costs, satisfaction, and clinical outcomes—and cites examples of each, noting that clinical outcomes (measures of clinical change or effect of intervention) is least developed, although most important from the perspective of the issue of service effectiveness. Curiously, managed care tends to attend more to client satisfaction and compliance with management standards for service delivery—again reflecting a priority of business concerns over service effectiveness. Presumably, some examples of clinical outcomes would include:

1. improved or maintained function;
2. improved or maintained client sense of well-being;
3. reduction in relapses;
4. reduction in ER use;
5. reduction in rehospitalization;
6. improvement in symptoms (e.g., blood pressure, frequency of falls, conflicts with police, or acute episodes of congestive heart failure); or
7. improvement in proper medication intake.

Some Tools for Outcomes Research

In response to the increased demand for outcomes research and documentation of diagnostic accuracy and intervention effectiveness at the primary care level, Van Hook, Berkman, and Dunkle (1996) have proposed that social workers in primary care settings make increased use of some of the existing instruments appropriate to (1) mental health problem assessment, such as PRIME-MD; (2) the functional assessment of older persons, such as OARS; and (3) assessment of the health-related quality of life, such as the HRQL instrument (SF-36).

PRIME-MD (Primary Care Evaluation of Mental Health Disorders) targets (1) mood, (2) anxiety, (3) somataform disorders, (4) eating disorders, and (5) alcohol abuse and facilitates identification of any of eighteen common diagnostic categories of the DSM-IV (Van Hook, Berkman, and Dunkle, 1996).

The OARS questionnaire (Older Americans Resources Survey) is instrumental in assessing older persons' level of ability to perform ADLs and IADLs in addition to their social resources, economic resources, mental health and physical health. It also "can be used for screening, evaluating outcomes, and modeling the cost-effectiveness of alternative approaches of care" (McDowell and Newell, 1987, cited in Van Hook, Berkman, and Dunkle, 1996:231).

Finally, the SF-36 instrument focuses on health-related quality of life (HRQL) indicators, from a patient's perspective. Essentially, it addresses issues of the impact of physical or mental health problems on ability to perform physical activities, usual roles, social activities, mental health and well-being, energy level, and perceptions of overall health. An advantage of the tool is that it can be completed by clients age fourteen or older in ten minutes or less. It is currently believed to be most appropriately used in measuring outcomes at a group level and has yet to be assessed in terms of use at the individual level (Van Hook, Berkman, and Dunkle, 1996; Berkman, 1998).

Davis (1998:417) wrote, "Clinical practice in managed care emphasizes a short-term, problem-focused acute care model based in part on measurement scales designed to aid in diagnosis and outcome assessment."

Two volumes of outcomes research tools are useful to social workers:

1. *Measures for Clinical Practice: A Sourcebook* (Concoran and Fischer, 2000). Although the instruments included are not all addressed to health-related issues, many of them are. Examples include scales for pain appraisal, client satisfaction, cognitive processes, self-esteem, cultural congruity, acculturation rating for Mexican Americans, geriatric depression, General Health Status, illness behavior scale, perceived social support, life satisfaction, self-efficacy, severity of compulsive behavior, trust in physicians, willingness to care scale (a caregiver potential scale), as well as a caregiver strain scale, a caregiver burden scale, and a depression screening instrument.

2. *Measuring Health: A Guide to Rating Scales and Questionnaires* (McDowell and Newell, 1996). Over 100 measurement instruments are included, such as the Sickness Impact Profile, Short-Form 20 (SF-20) and Short-Form 36 (SF-36), various functional assessment scales, the Illness Behavior Questionnaire, several quality of well-being scales, the Social Dysfunction Rating Scale, social support scales, the Alzheimer's Disease Assessment Scale, OARS (Older Americans Resources and Services), and other activities of daily living assessment scales, in addition to many others.

The Need for a Technology of Caring

As was stated in the preface, professionals in health care need to *expand* the focus of their attention from preoccupation with repairing human health problems (curing) to achieve a more supportive intervention approach (caring) at each level of health services. In a sense, *caring is prevention,* at all three levels of health service: (1) promotion of health and prevention of disease onset, (2) prevention of compounding already existing health problems, and (3) prevention of avoidable suffering and impairment of function, i.e., prevention of secondary disabilities.

> Interventions are needed to address [health] behavior and to promote the creation and maintenance of social support. . . . The need is growing for social work to step back from health care, aging, disability, mental health, and managed care and to reconceptualize its roles in the entire dynamic holistic continuum of care and services: prevention, health promotion, service delivery design, acute and chronic care, treatment, rehabilitation, and long-term care. (Keigher, 1997:151)

As David Mechanic advised over twenty years ago, we need to develop a technology of caring to more effectively address the chronic and psychosocial health problems that predominate today. According to Mechanic (1978), caring consists of techniques based on scientific knowledge of how to provide human support.

Davidson (1998), citing Monkman (1991) and Ell (1996), wrote:

> the psychosocial arena is too often perceived as everyone's area of expertise. It remains imperative for social workers to demonstrate through research studies that the professional expertise that allows us to provide *supportive services* to families provides positive and welcome results, such as reduction of lost work or school days; decreased stress-induced illness; and fewer of the medical crises that are often related to lack of knowledge, non-compliance with treatment, and overburdened caretakers. Research can then be used to advocate for provision of psychosocial services throughout health care programs. (426) (emphasis added)

The Etiological Role of Psychosocial Factors

Most of the health problems we face today are significantly caused by destructive human behavior or by ignorance, unrelieved environmental stress, social injustice, and other social or emotional conditions that are the arena of social workers more than physicians. Caring at the primary level seems to point to needed changes in communities, and in the entire social system, which will empower its members through building a greater sense of community. This sense of belonging, of being valued members of their community, and being respected, is enhanced through equitable educational opportunities, satisfying work with good wages, encouragement to be active participants in community decision making, and having accessible community resources for personal and family needs.

As the Ottowa Charter for Health Promotion states, "the fundamental conditions and resources for health are peace, shelter, education, food, income, a stable ecosystem, sustainable resources, social justice, and equity. Improvement in health requires a secure foundation in these basic requirements" (WHO, 1986:1).

"[T]he fundamental conditions and resources for health are peace, shelter, education, food, income, a stable ecosystem, sustainable resources, social justice, and equity. Improvement in health requires a secure foundation in these basic requirements." (WHO, 1986:1)

All that is necessary to get a sense of what needs to be improved in our communities and nation is to examine the book *The Social Health of the Nation: How America is Really Doing* (Miringoff and Miringoff, 1999), cited in Chapter 3.

Some common biopsychosocial problems that social workers can help to address include drug and alcohol abuse, child abuse and neglect, domestic violence, elder abuse, teenage pregnancy, sexually transmitted diseases, suicide, depression, homicide, motor vehicle accidents, tobacco addiction, eating disorders, obsessive-compulsive behaviors, panic disorders, agoraphobia, social isolation, emotional withdrawal, and self-mutilation behavior.

The Mediating Role of Social Support

Perhaps the strongest argument for professional social workers playing a major role in health care in the future is the evidence that some *mediating structures,* such as social support, *are the most powerful determinant of health.* The key role of such community support in promoting a healthy society cannot be overemphasized (Kelner, 1985). Social support is not just an emotional experience, however, but often involves concrete material forms. Examples of the lack of caring in the United States include the following:

- The high rate of child poverty
- The low minimum wage
- The thousands of homeless people
- The majority of correctional institutions being filled with victims of child abuse, poverty, and lack of education, drug addiction, mental illness, and functional illiteracy, and the excessive use of incarceration as an alternative to a responsible and caring society (We have a higher percentage of our own population in prison than any other country in the world.)
- About 15 percent of the U.S. population going without health insurance
- Insufficient U.S. national health expenditures allocated for health promotion
- Many elderly people unable to afford or obtain prescribed medications, many of which are not covered by Medicare
- A public child welfare system that is in shambles in terms of the quality of its services, due to a general lack of adequate funding and inferior standards for staff qualifications

Finally, it is thought provoking that the U.S. government is reported to have a defense budget that exceeds the combined defense budgets of all other countries in the world.

CONCLUSION

Essentially, we need to develop a repertoire of effective supportive interventions to address the needs of the aged and others with chronic impairments, as well as those who are temporarily impaired, terminally ill, or need supportive assistance to prevent impairment—such as those whose lifestyle is reckless, as well as those who simply need care to grow and develop. The key to effective caring is to relieve helplessness, assessed objectively and subjectively, by both the helper and the one who needs caring.

As quoted in Chapter 2, David Mechanic (1978), medical sociologist observed:

> It is unfortunately common for many physicians to conceive of the caring functions of medical care as simply the expression of kindness and acceptance of the patient. While this is no trivial aspect, *caring constitutes* a much wider *range of techniques based* not only on human feeling, or even on the techniques usually associated with psychotherapy, but *on scientific knowledge of how to provide human*

support. . . . In short, caring is a technology, the dimensions of which can be concretely identified, studied, manipulated and transmitted to practitioners who apply the technology in concrete situations. Caring is thus much more than a communication of feeling. (309) (emphasis added)

These needs may relate to prevention of such problems, to support of function or comfort during a problem episode, or to adjustment, adaption, or compensation for an incurable problem. Caring refers to interventions aimed at strengthening the ability of another person to deal with the impairing effect of any circumstance—whether childhood, old age, illness or injury, loss of a loved one, loss of employment, a natural disaster, or other stressful life situation.

In summary, whether the supports are interpersonal or concrete, the essence of care or caring is to strengthen the ability of people to cope with the challenges they face, so they can have an improved quality of life.

Perhaps social work should take the lead in drawing representatives of other relevant groups into a proposal for foundation funding to establish an Interdisciplinary Institute for Research and Development of Care Technology. This center would include, for example, architects, engineers, nurses, occupational therapists, patients, physicians, physical therapists, social workers, speech therapists, sociologists, economists, and medical anthropologists, who would together identify current dilemmas in the health care field, prioritize them, and form interdisciplinary work groups to jointly develop efficacious interventions to address them. Such work and products would constitute a new "science of caring."

References

Chapter 1

American Hospital Association (2002). *Hospital statistics.* Chicago: Health Forum, an affiliate of the American Hospital Association.

Bope, Edward T., and Jost, Timothy S. (1994). Interprofessional collaboration: Factors that affect form, function, and structure. In Casto, R. Michael, Julia, Maria C., Platt, Larry J., Harbaugh, Gary L., Waugaman, Wynne R., Thompson, Arlene, Jost, Timothy S., Bope, Edward T., Williams, Tennyson, and Lee, Daniel B. *Interprofessional care and collaborative practice.* Pacific Grove, CA: Brooks-Cole, 61-69.

Bracht, Neil F. (1978). *Social work in health care: A guide to professional practice.* Binghamton, NY: The Haworth Press, Inc.

Briggs, Margaret H. (1997). *Building early intervention teams.* Gaithersburg, MD: Aspen Publications.

Bucher, Rue, and Stelling, Joan (1978). Characteristics of professional organizations. In Schwartz, Howard D. and Kart, Cary S. (Eds.), *Dominant issues in medical sociology.* Reading, MA: Addison-Wesley, 340-351.

Cabot, Richard C. (1928). Hospital and dispensary social work. In Goldstine, Dora (Ed.) (1955), *Expanding horizons in medical social work.* Chicago: University of Chicago Press, 255-270.

Cannon, Ida M. (1923). *Social work in hospitals.* New York: Russell Sage.

Caputi, Marie A. (1978). Social work in health care: Past and future. *Health and Social Work,* 3 (1): 9-29.

Casto, R. Michael (1994). Education for interprofessional practice. In Casto, R. Michael, Julia, Maria C., Platt, Larry J., Harbaugh, Gary L., Waugaman, Wynne R., Thompson, Arlene, Jost, Timothy S., Bope, Edward T., Williams, Tennyson, and Lee, Daniel B. *Interprofessional care and collaborative practice.* Pacific Grove, CA: Brooks-Cole, 95-110.

Coe, R. (1978). *Sociology of medicine.* New York: McGraw-Hill.

Cowles, Lois A. (1990). Medical social work in hospitals: Interdisciplinary expectations of the role. Unpublished doctoral dissertation, University of Wisconsin Library, Madison. University Microfilms No. 9020434.

Cowles, Lois A., and Lefcowitz, Myron J. (1995). Interdisciplinary expectations of the medical social worker in the hospital setting: Part 2. *Health and Social Work,* 20 (4): 279-286.

Engel, George (1977). The need for a new medical model: A challenge for biomedicine. *Science,* 196: 129-136.

French, Ruth (1979). *Dynamics of health care.* New York: McGraw-Hill.

Friedson, Elliot (1978). The prospects for health services in the U.S. *Medical Care,* 16 (12): 971-983.

Gibelman, Margaret, and Schervish, Phillip H. (1996). *Who we are.* Washington, DC: NASW Press.

Ginsberg, Leon (1995). *The social work almanac* (Second edition). Washington, DC: NASW Press.

Given, Barbara, and Simmons, Sandra (1977). The interdisciplinary health care team: Fact or fiction. *Nursing Forum,* 16 (2): 165-177.

Goffman, Erving (1961). *Asylums: Essays on the social situation of mental patients and other inmates.* Garden City, NJ: Doubleday.

Grob, Gerald N. (1983). *Mental illness and American society: 1875-1940.* Princeton, NJ: Princeton University Press.

Harris, J.W., Saunders, D.N., and Zasorin-Conners, J. (1978). A training program for interprofessional health care teams. *Health and Social Work,* 3 (2): 35-53.

Jonas, Steve (1981). *Health care delivery in the United States.* New York: Springer.

Julia, Maria C., and Thompson, Arlene (1994a). Essential elements of interprofessional teamwork. In Casto, R. Michael, Julia, Maria C., Platt, Larry J., Harbaugh, Gary L., Waugaman, Wynne R., Thompson, Arlene, Jost, Timothy S., Bope, Edward T., Williams, Tennyson, and Lee, Daniel B. *Interprofessional care and collaborative practice.* Pacific Grove, CA: Brooks-Cole, 43-58.

Julia, Maria C., and Thompson, Arlene (1994b). Group process and interprofessional teamwork. In Casto, R. Michael, Julia, Maria C., Platt, Larry J., Harbaugh, Gary L., Waugaman, Wynne R., Thompson, Arlene, Jost, Timothy S., Bope, Edward T., Williams, Tennyson, and Lee, Daniel B. *Interprofessional care and collaborative practice.* Pacific Grove, CA: Brooks-Cole, 35-42.

Kane, Rosalie (1976-1977). Interprofessional education and social work: A survey. *Social Work in Health Care,* 2 (2): 229-238.

Kane, Rosalie (1978). The interprofessional team as a small group. In Bracht, Neil (Ed.), *Social work in health care: A guide to professional practice.* Binghamton, NY: The Haworth Press, Inc., 85-97.

Kane, Rosalie (1980). Multidisciplinary teamwork in the U.S.: Trends, issues, and implications for the social worker. In Lonsdale, Susan, Webb, Adrian, and Briggs, Thomas L. (Eds.), *Teamwork in the personal social services and health care.* Syracuse, NY: Syracuse University School of Social Work, 138-151.

Karger, Howard Jacob, and Stoesz, David (1994). *American social welfare policy: A pluralist approach* (Second edition). New York: Longman.

Karger, Howard Jacob, and Stoesz, David (1998). *American social welfare policy: A pluralist approach* (Third edition). New York: Longman.

Levy, Norman B. (1974). The giving-up-given-up complex. In Simons, Richard C. and Pardes, Herbert (Eds.), *Understanding human behavior in health and illness.* Baltimore, MD: Williams and Wilkins, 430-435.

Lodge, Richard (1974). University education in interprofessional perspectives. In Rehr, Helen (Ed.), *Medicine and social work: An exploration of interprofessionalism.* New York: Prodist, 26-32.

Lonsdale, Susan, Webb, Adrian, and Briggs, Thomas L. (Eds.) (1980). *Teamwork in the personal social services and health care.* Syracuse, NY: Syracuse University School of Social Work.

Lubove, Roy (1965). *The professional altruist: The emergence of social work as a career.* Cambridge, MA: Harvard University Press.

Mailick, Mildred D., and Jordon, Pearl (1977). A multimodal approach to collaborative practice in health settings. *Social Work in Health Care,* 2 (4): 445-455.

McLachlan, Gordon, and McKeown, Thomas (Eds.) (1971). *Medical history and medical care.* London: Oxford University Press.

Nagi, Saad Z. (1978). Teamwork in health care in the U.S.: A sociological perspective. In Schwartz, Howard D. and Kart, Cary S. (Eds.), *Dominant issues in medical sociology.* Reading, MA: Addison-Wesley, 490-498.

National Association of Social Workers (1983). Membership survey data obtained through phone conversation with an NASW research associate during Summer 1992.

National Association of Social Workers (1987). *NASW standards for social work in health care settings.* Washington, DC: NASW Press.

National Association of Social Workers (2000). Practice research survey. Washington, DC: Practice Research Network; NASW. April.

Payne, Malcolm (2000). *Teamwork in multiprofessional care.* Chicago: Lyceum Books, Inc.

Platt, Larry J. (1994). Why bother with teams: An overview. In Casto, R. Michael, Julia, Maria C., Platt, Larry J., Harbaugh, Gary L., Waugaman, Wynne R., Thompson, Arlene, Jost, Timothy S., Bope, Edward T., Williams, Tennyson, and Lee, Daniel B. *Interprofessional care and collaborative practice.* Pacific Grove, CA: Brooks-Cole, 3-10.

Popple, Philip R., and Leighninger, Leslie (1993). *Social work, social welfare, and American society* (Second edition). Boston, MA: Allyn and Bacon.

Rubin, Irwin M., and Beckhard, Richard (1972). Factors influencing the effectiveness of health teams. *Milbank Memorial Fund Quarterly,* 50 (Part 1): 317-335.

Schmale, Arthur H. (1972). Giving up as a final common pathway to changes in health. *Advances in Psychosomatic Medicine,* 8: 20-40.

Sheps, Cecil G. (1974). Developmental perspectives on interprofessional education. In Rehr, Helen (Ed.), *Medicine and social work: An exploration of interprofessionalism.* New York: Prodist, 3-13.

Smith, Harvey L. (1978). Two lines of authority: The hospitals' dilemma. In Swartz, Howard D. and Kart, Cary S. (Eds.), *Dominant issues in medical sociology.* Reading, MA: Addison-Wesley, 315-322.

Stuart, Paul H. (1997). Community care and the origins of psychiatric social work. *Social Work in Health Care,* 25 (3): 25-36.

Trattner, Walter I. (1989). *From poor law to welfare state: A history of social welfare in America* (Fourth edition). New York: The Free Press.

U.S. Department of Labor, Bureau of Labor Statistics (2000). National occupational employment and wage estimates. <http://www.bls.gov/oes/2000/oes 211022>.

Waugaman, Wynne R. (1994). Professionalization and socialization in interprofessional collaboration. In Casto, R. Michael, Julia, Maria C., Platt, Larry J., Harbaugh, Gary L., Waugaman, Wynne R., Thompson, Arlene, Jost, Timothy S., Bope, Edward T., Williams, Tennyson, and Lee, Daniel B. *Interprofessional care and collaborative practice.* Pacific Grove, CA: Brooks-Cole, 23-32.

Wenger, G.C. (1994). *Understanding support networks and community care: Network assessment for elderly people.* Aldershot: Avebury.

World Health Organization (1978). *Alma-Ata 1978: Primary health care: Report of the international conference on primary health care.* Alma-Ata, Union of Soviet Socialist Republics, September 6-12. Geneva: WHO.

Chapter 2

Blazyk, Stan, and Canavan, Margaret (1985). Therapeutic aspects of discharge planning. *Social Work,* 30 (6): 489-496.

DeCoster, Vaughn (2000). Health care treatment of patient and family emotion: A synthesis and comparison across patient populations and practice settings. *Social Work in Health Care,* 30 (4): 7-24.

DiNitto, Diana M., and McNeece, C. Aaron (1997). *Social work: Issues and opportunities in a challenging profession* (Second edition). Boston, MA: Allyn and Bacon.

Germain, Carel B., and Gitterman, Alex (1980). *The life model of social work practice.* New York: Columbia University Press.

Goffman, Erving (1961). *Asylums: Essays on the social situation of mental patients and other inmates.* Garden City, NJ: Doubleday.

Greenwood, Ernest (1957). Attributes of a profession. *Social Work,* 2 (3): 45-55.

Kerson, Toba Schwaber (Ed.) (1989). *Social work in health settings: Practice in context.* Binghamton, NY: The Haworth Press, Inc.

Kerson, Toba Schwaber (1997). *Social Work in health settings: Practice in context* (Second edition). Binghamton, NY: The Haworth Press, Inc.

Levy, Norman B. (1974). The giving-up-given-up complex. In Simons, Richard C. and Pardes, Herbert (Eds.), *Understanding human behavior in health and illness.* Baltimore, MD: Williams and Wilkins, 430-435.

Maslow, A.H. (1968). *Toward a psychology of being* (Second edition). Princeton, NJ: Van Nostrand.

McLachlan, Gordon, and McKeown, Thomas (Eds.) (1971). *Medical history and medical care.* London: Oxford University Press.

Mechanic, David (1978). *Medical sociology.* New York: The Free Press.

Morales, Armando, and Sheafor, Bradford (1989). *Social work: A profession of many faces.* Boston, MA: Allyn and Bacon.

Morris, Robert, and Anderson, Delwin (1975). Personal care services: An identity for social work. *Social Service Review,* 41 (2): 157-174.

National Association of Social Workers (1987). *NASW standards for social work in health care settings.* Washington, DC: NASW Press.

National Association of Social Workers (1991). *The social work dictionary.* Washington, DC: NASW Press.

National Association of Social Workers (1996). *NASW code of ethics.* Washington, DC: NASW Press.

Neuman, W. Lawrence (1994). *Social research methods: Qualitative and quantitative approaches.* Boston, MA: Allyn and Bacon.

Schmale, Arthur H. (1972). Giving up as a final common pathway to changes in health. *Advances in Psychosomatic Medicine,* 8: 20-40.

Seligman, Martin E. (1975). *Helplessness.* San Francisco, CA: W.H. Freeman and Co.

Wing, John W. (1978). *Reasoning about madness.* Oxford, England: Oxford Press.

World Health Organization (1978). *Alma-Ata 1978: Primary health care: Report of the international conference on primary health care.* Alma-Ata, Union of Soviet Socialist Republics, September 6-12. Geneva: WHO.

Chapter 3

Ajzen, I., and Fishbein, M. (1980). *Understanding attitudes and predicting social behavior.* Englewood Cliffs, NJ: Prentice-Hall.

American Psychiatric Association (1995). *Diagnostic and statistical manual of mental disorders: Primary care version* (Fourth edition). Washington, DC: APA.

American Public Health Association (2001a). Overweight, not just obesity, leads to chronic health risks. *The Nation's Health* (October): 32.

American Public Health Association (2001b). School-based health centers growing in numbers. *The Nation's Health* (May): 7.

Amick, Terrence L., and Ockene, Judith K. (1994). The role of social support in the modification of risk factors for cardiovascular disease. In Shumaker, Sally A. and Czajkowski, Susan M. (Eds.), *Social support and cardiovascular disease.* New York: Plenum Press, 260-264.

Angel, Ronald J., and Williams, Kristi (2000). Cultural models of health and illness. In Cuellar, Israel and Paniagua, Freddy A. (Eds.), *Handbook of multicultural mental health.* San Diego, CA: Academic Press, 25-44. Copyright© 2000. Reprinted with permission from Elsevier Science.

Ashton, J. (Ed.) (1992). *Healthy cities.* Philadelphia, PA: Open University Press.

Badger, Lee W., Ackerson, Barry, Buttell, Frederick, and Rand, Elizabeth H. (1997). The case for integration of social work psychosocial services into rural primary care practice. *Health and Social Work,* 22 (1): 20-29.

Bandura, A. (1986). *Social foundations of thought and action: A social cognitive theory.* Englewood Cliffs, NJ: Prentice-Hall.

Bandura, A. (1997). Self-efficacy: The exercise of control. New York: W. H. Freeman Co.

Beer, John S., Kivlahan, Daniel R., Blume, Arthur W., McKnight, Patrick, and Marlatt, G. Alan (2001). Brief intervention for heavy drinking college students: 4-year followup and natural history. *American Journal of Public Health,* 91 (8): 1310-1316.

Berkman, Lisa (2000). Social support, social networks, and social cohesion and health. *Social Work in Health Care,* 31 (2): 3-14.

Bird, Michael (2001). Community is power. *The Nation's Health* (August): 3.

Blair, Robert G. (2000). Risk factors associated with PTSD and major depression among Cambodian refugees in Utah. *Health and Social Work,* 25 (1): 23-30.

Bloom, Martin (1987). Prevention. In Minahan, Anne (Ed.), *Encyclopedia of social work* (Eighteenth edition). Washington, DC: NASW Press, 303-311.

Bloom, Martin (1995). Primary prevention overview. In Edwards, Richard L. (Ed.), *The encyclopedia of social work* (Nineteenth edition). Washington, DC: NASW Press, 1895-1904.

Bracht, Neil (Ed.) (1990). *Health promotion at the community level.* Thousand Oaks, CA: Sage Publications.

Bracht, Neil (Ed.) (1999). *Health promotion at the community level: New advances* (Second edition). Thousand Oaks, CA: Sage Publications.

Cabot, Richard C. (1928). Hospital and dispensary social work. In Goldstine, D. (Ed.) (1955), *Expanding horizons in medical social work.* Chicago: University of Chicago Press, 255-270.

Cannon, Ida M. (1923). *Social work in hospitals.* New York: Russell Sage.

Cassell, Eric (1995). Teaching the fundamentals of primary care: A point of view. *The Milbank Quarterly,* 75 (3): 373-405.

Clare, Anthony W. (1982). Social aspects of ill-health in general practice. In Clare, Anthony W. and Corney, Roslyn H. (Eds.), *Social work and primary health care.* London: Academic Press, 9-22.

Cleveland, Tessie (1981). Where are we going with specialty interest groups? *Health and Social Work,* 6 (4): 95-125.

Cochrane, Glynn (1979). *The cultural appraisal of development projects.* New York: Praeger.

Cockerham, William C. (1992). *Medical sociology.* Englewood Cliffs, NJ: Prentice-Hall.

Cook, Cynthia Loveland, Becvar, Dorothy S., and Pontious, Sharon L. (2000). Complementary alternative medicine in health and mental health: Implications for social work practice. *Social Work in Health Care,* 31 (3): 39-57.

Corin, Ellen E. (1994). The social and cultural matrix of health and disease. In Evans, Robert G., Barer, Morris L., and Marmor, Theodore R. (Eds.), *Why are some people healthy and others not? The determinants of health of populations.* New York: Aldine De Gruyter, 93-132.

Cowles, Lois A., and Lefcowitz, Myron J. (1995). Interdisciplinary expectations of the medical social worker in the hospital setting: Part 2. *Health and Social Work,* 20 (4): 279-286.

Currie, E. (1998). *Crime and punishment in America.* New York: Metropolitan Books.

Davis, King E. (1996). Primary health care and severe mental illness: The need for national and state policy. *Health and Social Work,* 21 (2): 83-87.

Dobrof, Judith, Umpierre, Mari, Rocha, Loraine, and Silverton, Marsha (1990). Group work in a primary care medical setting. *Health and Social Work,* 15 (1): 32-37.

Donaldson, Molla S., Yordy, Karl D., Lohr, Kathleen N., and Vanselow, Neal A. (Eds.) (1996). *Primary care: America's health in a new era.* Washington, DC: National Academy Press.

Dunlop, Judith, and Holosko, Michael (1992). Community social work practice: Health promotion in action. In Holosko, Michael J. and Taylor, Patricia A. (Eds.), *Social work practice in health settings.* Toronto, Canada: Canadian Scholar's Press, 643-656.

Ell, Kathleen, and Morrison, Diane R. (1981). Primary care. *Health and Social Work,* 6 (4) (supplement): 35s-43s.

Engel, George (1977). The need for a new medical model: A challenge for bio-medicine. *Science,* 196: 129-136.

Evans, Robert G., Barer, Morris L., and Marmor, Theodore R. (Eds.) (1994). *Why are some people healthy and others not? The determinants of health of populations.* New York: Aldine De Gruyter.

Fitzpatrick, Tanya R., and Bosse, Raymond (2000). Employment and health among older bereaved men in the normative aging study: One year and three years following a bereavement event. *Social Work in Health Care,* 32 (2): 41-60.

Freund, Peter E.S., and McGuire, Meridith B. (1991). *Health, illness, and the social body: A critical sociology.* Englewood Cliffs, NJ: Prentice-Hall.

Friis, Robert H., and Sellers, Thomas A. (1996). *Epidemiology for public health practice.* Gaithersburg, MD: Aspen Publishers.

Garrett, Laurie (2000). *Betrayal of trust: The collapse of global public health.* New York: Hyperion Publishers.

Gaston, Marilyn H., Barrett, Sharon E., Johnson, Tamara Lewis, and Epstein, Leonard G. (1998). Health care needs of medically underserved women of color: The role of the Bureau of Primary Health Care. *Health and Social Work,* 23 (2): 86-95.

Gilliland, M. Janice, and Taylor, Judith E. (1999). Planning community heath interventions. In Raczynski, James M. and DiClemente, Ralph J. (Eds.), *Handbook of health promotion and disease prevention.* New York: Kluwer Academic/Plenum Publishers, 427-441.

Girois, Susan B., Kumanyika, Shiriki K., Morabia, Alfredo, and Mauger, Elizabeth (2001). A comparison of knowledge and attitudes about diet and health among 35-75 year old adults in the United States and Geneva, Switzerland. *American Journal of Public Health,* 91 (3): 418-424.

Goel,Vivek, and McIsaac, Warren (2000). Health promotion in clinical practice. In Poland, Blake D., Green, Lawrence W., and Rootman, Irving (Eds.), *Settings for health promotion: Linking theory and practice.* Thousand Oaks, CA: Sage Publications, 217-249.

Gorin, Stephen H. (2001). The crisis for public health: Implications for social workers. *Health and Social Work,* 26 (1): 49-53.

Gorin, Stephen K. (2000). Inequality and health: Implications for social work. *Health and Social Work,* 25 (4): 270-275.

Green, Gilbert J. and Kulper, Teresa (1990). Autonomy and professional activities of social workers in hospital and primary health care settings. *Health and Social Work,* 15 (1): 38-44.

Green, James W. (1995). *Cultural awareness in the human services: A multi-ethnic approach* (Second edition). Boston, MA: Allyn and Bacon.

Gross, Revital, Rabinowitz, Johnothan, Feldman, Dina, and Boerma, Wienke (1996). Primary health care physician's treatment of psychosocial problems. *Health and Social Work*, 21 (2): 89-95.

Gullotta, T.P. (1987). Prevention's technology. *Journal of Primary Prevention*, 8 (1): 4-24.

Hafen, Brent Q., Karren, Keith J., Frandsen, Kathryn J., and Smith, N. Lee (1996). *Mind/body health: The effects of attitudes, emotions, and relationships*. Boston: Allyn and Bacon.

Henk, Mat L. (1989). *Social work in primary care*. Thousand Oaks, CA: Sage.

Hess, Howard (1985). Social work clinical practice in family medicine centers: The need for a practice model. *Journal of Social Work Education*, 21 (1): 56-65. (Quoted material reprinted with permission of the Council on Social Work Education, Department of Sociology, Social Work, and Criminal Justice, 1600 Duke Street, Alexandria, VA.)

Hill, Dana Robin, Kelleher, K., and Shumaker, Sally A. (1992). Psychosocial interventions in adult patients with coronary heart disease and cancer: A literature review. *General Hospital Psychiatry*, 145 (65): 28s-42s.

Katon, Wayne (1987). The epidemiology of depression in medical care. *International Journal of Psychiatry in Medicine*, 17 (1): 93-112.

Katon, Wayne and Schulberg, Herbert (1992). Epidemiology of depression in primary care. *General Hospital Psychiatry*, 14 (4) (Supplement 6): 237-247.

Kawachi, Ichiro, Kennedy, Bruce, and Wilkinson, Richard (1999). *The society and population health reader: Income Inequality and Health*. New York: The New Press.

Keigher, Sharon (1999). Editorial: Including "mental" in health and social work. *Health and Social Work*, 24 (2).

Kelner, M. (1985). Community support networks: Current issues. *Canadian Journal of Public Health*, 76 (Supplement 1): 69-70.

Kerson, Toba Schwaber and Peachey, Helen (1989). Family planning agency: An unsuccessful contraceptor. In Kerson, Toba Schwaber (Ed.), *Social work in health settings: Practice in context*. Binghamton, NY: The Haworth Press, Inc., 231-245.

Kohler, Connie L., Grimley, Diane M., and Reynolds, Kim D. (1999). Theoretical models and evaluation methods in health promotion and disease prevention. In Raczynski, James M. and DiClemente, Ralph J. (Eds.), *Handbook of health promotion and disease prevention*. New York: Kluwer Academic/Plenum Press, 23-51.

Kozol, Jonathan (1991). *Savage inequalities: Children in America's schools*. New York: HarperCollins.

Kozol, Jonathan (1995). *Amazing grace: The lives of children and the conscience of a nation*. New York: Crown Publishing Group.

Lesser, Joan Granucci (2000). Clinical social work and family medicine: A partnership in community service. *Health and Social Work*, 25 (2): 119-126.

Levy, Jerrold E., and Kunitz, Stephen (1987). A suicide prevention program for Hopi youth. *Science and Medicine*, 25: 931-940.

Macrina, David M. (1999). Historical and conceptual perspectives. In Raczynski, James M. and DiClemente, Ralph J. (Eds.), *Handbook of health promotion and disease prevention.* New York: Kluwer Academic/Plenum Publishers, 11-20.

Marsella, Anthony J., and Yamada, Ann Marie (2000). Culture and mental health: An introduction and overview of foundations, concepts and issues. In Cuellar, Israel and Paniagua, Freddy A. (Eds.), *Handbook of multicultural mental health.* San Diego, CA: Academic Press, 3-24. Copyright© 2000. Reprinted with permission from Elsevier Science.

Marshack, Elaine, Davidson, Kay, and Mizrahi, Terry (1988). Preparation of social workers for a changing health care environment. *Health and Social Work,* 13 (3): 226-233.

McLeroy, K.R., Bibeau, D., Steckler, A., and Glanz, K. (1988). An ecological perspective on health promotion programs. *Health Education Quarterly,* 15 (4): 351-377.

Mechanic, David (1994). Integrating mental health into a general health care system. *Hospital and Community Psychiatry,* 45 (9): 893-897.

Miller, Rosalind (1987). Primary health care. In Minahan, Anne (Ed.), *Encyclopedia of social work* (Eighteenth edition). Washington, DC: NASW Press.

Miringoff, Marc, and Miringoff, Marque-Luisa (1999). *The social health of the nation: How America is really doing.* New York/Oxford: Oxford University Press.

Mittelmark, Maurice (1999). Health promotion at the communitywide level: Lessons from diverse perspectives. In Bracht, Neil (Ed.), *Health promotion at the community level: New advances* (Second edition). Thousand Oaks, CA: Sage Publications, 3-26.

Monahan, Kathleen, and O'Leary, Dan (1999). Head injury and battered women: An initial inquiry. *Health and Social Work,* 24 (4): 269-278.

National Association of Community Health Centers (1993). *National directory of community health centers, migrant health centers, health care for the homeless projects and primary care associations.* Washington, DC: Author.

National Association of Social Workers (1987). *NASW standards for social work in health care settings.* Washington, DC: NASW Press.

National Association of Social Workers (1996). *NASW code of ethics.* Washington, DC: NASW Press.

Netting, F. Ellen, and Williams, Frank G. (2000). Expanding the boundaries of primary care for elderly people. *Health and Social Work,* 25 (4): 233-241.

Neugebauer, R. (2001). Editorial: Minding the world's health day, World Health Day 2001. *American Journal of Public Health,* 91 (4): 551-552.

Oktay, Julianne S. (1984). Social workers in primary health care: A national study of tasks and functions. Presented at the CSWE Annual Program Meeting, Detroit, MI, March.

Oktay, Julianne S. (1995). Primary health care. In Edwards, Richard L. (Ed.), *The encyclopedia of social work* (Nineteenth edition). Washington, DC: NASW Press, 1887-1894.

Oliver, M.T., and Shapiro, T.M. (1995). *The black wealth/white wealth.* New York: Routledge.

Paniagua, Freddy A. (2000). Culture-bound syndromes, cultural variations, and psychopathology. In Cuellar, Israel and Paniagua, Freddy A. (Eds.), *Handbook of multicultural mental heatlh.* San Diego: Academic Press, 140-167.

Paster, Zorba (2001). Rx for a long life. *On Wisconsin* (the alumni magazine of the University of Wisconsin) 102 (1): 33-35.

Pert, Candace, Ruff, Michael, Weber, Richard, and Herkenham, Miles (1985). Neuropeptides and their receptors: A psychosomatic network. *Journal of Immunology,* 135 (Supplement 2): 820s-826s.

Poland, Blake (1992). Learning to "walk our talk": The implications of sociological theory for research methodologies in health promotion. *Canadian Journal of Public Health,* 83 (Supplement 1): S31-S46.

Poland, Blake, D., Green, Lawrence, and Rootman, Irving (Eds.) (2000). *Settings for health promotion: Linking theory and practice.* Thousand Oaks, CA: Sage Publications.

Poole, Dennis L. (1995). Editorial: Public health social work: Pro bono publico. *Health and Social Work,* 20 (4): 243-245.

Pray, Kenneth (1995). Prevention and wellness. In Edwards, Richard L. (Ed.), *The encyclopedia of social work* (Nineteenth edition). Washington, DC: NASW Press, 1879-1886.

Prochaska, J.O., and DiClemente, Ralph J. (1983). Stages and processes of self-change in smoking cessation: Toward an integrated model of change. *Journal of Counseling and Clinical Psychology,* 51: 390-395.

Prochaska, J.O., and DiClemente, Ralph J. (1984). *The transtheoretical approach: Crossing the traditional boundaries of therapy.* Homewood, IL: Dow Jones/Irwin.

Prochaska, J.O., and DiClemente, Ralph J. (1986). Toward a comprehensive model of change. In Miller, W.R. and Healther, N. (Eds.), *Treating addictive behaviors: Processes of change.* New York: Plenum Press, 3-28.

Raczynski, James M., and DiClemente, Ralph J. (1999). Future directions in research and practice. In Raczynski, James M. and DiClemente, Ralph J. (Eds.), *Handbook of health promotion and disease prevention.* New York. Kluwer Academic/Plenum Publishers, 661.

Richardson, Jean, Barkan, Susan, Cohen, Mardge, Back, Sara, Fitzgerald, Gordon, Feldman, Joseph, Young, Mary, and Palacio, Herminia (2001). Experience and covariates of depressive symptoms among a cohort of HIV infected women. *Social Work in Health Care,* 32 (4): 93-111.

Rock, Barry D., and Cooper, Marlene (2000). Social work in primary care: A demonstration student unit utilizing practice research. *Social Work in Health Care,* 31 (1): 1-17.

Rockhill, Beverly (2001). The privatization of risk. *American Journal of Public Health,* 91 (3): 365-368.

Rodriguez, Eunice (2001). Keeping the unemployed healthy: The effect of means-tested and entitlement benefits in Britain, Germany, and the United States. *American Journal of Public Health,* 91 (9): 1403-1411.

Rosenstock, I.M. (1974). Historical origins of the health belief model. *Health Education Monographs,* 2: 328-335.

Satcher, David (2001). Editorial: Why we need an international agreement on tobacco control. *American Journal of Public Health,* 91 (2): 191-193.

Seligman, M.E.P. (1975). Helplessness: On depression, development, and death. San Francisco: W.H. Freeman and Co.

Shannon, Mary T. (1989). Health promotion and illness prevention: A biopsychosocial perspective. *Health and Social Work,* 14 (1): 32-40.

Sidel, Victor W., Cohen, Hillel W., and Gould, Robert M. (2001). Good intentions and the road to bioterrorism preparedness. *American Journal of Public Health,* 91 (5): 716-726.

Siefert, Kristine (1995). Future directions for social work practice in maternal and child health. Paper presented at a meeting of the Ad Hoc Committee on Education for Maternal and Child Health Social Work Practice in the year 2010, Baltimore.

Siefert, Kristine, Jayaratne, Srinika, and Martin, Louise Doss (1992). Implementing the public health social work forward plan: A research-based prevention curriculum for schools of social work. *Health and Social Work,* 17 (1): 17-27.

Smith, George D. (2000). Learning to live with complexity: Ethnicity, socioeconomic position, and health in Britain and the United States. *American Journal of Public Health,* 90 (1): 1694-1697.

Smyre, Patricia (1993). *Women and health.* London and Atlantic Highlands, NJ: Zed Books.

Telfair, Joseph, and Gardner, Marilyn M. (1997). Adolescents with sickle cell disease: Determinants of support group attendance and satisfaction. *Health and Social Work,* 25 (1): 43-50.

Thompson, Beti, and Kinne, Susan (1999). Social change theory: Applications to community health. In Bracht, Neil (Ed.), *Health promotion at the community level: New advances* (Second edition). Thousand Oaks, CA: Sage Publications, 29-46.

Trattner, Walter I. (1989). *From poor law to welfare state: A history of social welfare in America* (Fourth edition). New York: The Free Press.

U.S. Census Bureau (2000). Poverty in the United States. September. <http://www.census.gov/hhes/www.poverty.html>.

U.S. Department of Health and Human Services (DHHS) (1999). Mental health: A report of the surgeon general. <http://www.surgeongeneral.gov/library/mental health/>.

U.S. Government Printing Office (2000a). *Health, United States.* Washington, DC: Author.

U.S. Government Printing Office (2000b). *Statistical Abstracts of the United States.* Washington, DC: Author.

Weiss, Gregory L., and Lonnquist, Lynne E. (1994). *The sociology of health, healing, and illness.* Englewood Cliffs, NJ: Prentice-Hall.

Wheaton, Blair (1980). The sociogenesis of psychological disorder: An attributional theory. *Journal of Health and Social Behavior,* 21 (2): 100-124.

Winslow, Charles-Edward Amory (1920). The untilled field of public health. *Modern Medicine,* 2 (March): 183-191.

World Health Organization (1978). *Alma-Ata 1978: Primary health care: Report of the international conference on primary health care.* Alma-Ata, Union of Soviet Socialist Republics, September 6-12. Geneva: WHO.

World Health Organization (1986). *Ottawa Charter for Health Promotion.* <http://www.who.dk/policy/ottawa.html>.

Young, Christine L., and Martin, Louise Doss (1989). Social services in rural and urban primary care projects. *Human Services in the Rural Environment,* 13 (2): 30-35.

Zayas, Luis H., and Dyche, Larry A. (1992). Social workers training primary care physicians: Essential psychosocial principles. *Social Work,* 37 (3): 247-252.

Zayas, Luis H., Kaplan, Carol, Turner, Sandra, Romano, Kathleen, and Gonzalez-Ramos, Gladys (2000). Understanding suicide attempts by adolescent hispanic females. *Health and Social Work,* 45 (1): 53-63.

Chapter 4

Abramson, Julie S. (1990). Enhancing patient participation: Clinical strategies in the discharge planning process. *Social Work in Health Care,* 14 (4): 53-70.

Abramson, Julie, Donnelly, James, King, Michael A., and Mailick, Mildred D. (1993). Disagreements in discharge planning: A normative phenomenon. *Health and Social Work,* 18 (1): 57-64.

Abramson, Marcia (1996). Toward a more holistic understanding of ethics in social work. *Social Work in Health Care,* 23 (2): 1-14.

American Hospital Association (1977). *Development of professional standards review for hospital social work.* Chicago, IL: Author.

American Hospital Association (1985). *Hospital statistics.* Chicago: American Hospital Association.

American Hospital Association (1993/1994). American Hospital Association profile of United States hospitals. *AHA Hospital Statistics.* Chicago, IL: Author.

American Hospital Association (1995). *1994 AHA annual survey.* Chicago: American Hospital Association.

American Hospital Association (2002). *Hospital statistics.* Chicago: Health Forum, an affiliation of the American Hospital Association.

Auerbach, Charles, Rock, Barry D., Goldstein, Marian, Kaminsky, Paula, Heft-Laporte, Heidi (2000). A department of social work uses data to provide its case (88-99B). *Social Work in Health Care,* 32 (1): 9-23.

Baker, Marjorie E. (2000). Knowledge and attitudes of health care social workers regarding advance directives. *Social Work in Health Care,* 32 (2): 61-74.

Bartlett, Maria, C., and Baum, Bernard H. (1995). What happens to patients after nursing home placement? *Social Work in Health Care,* 22 (1): 69-79.

Becker, Nancy E., and Becker, Fred W. (1986). Early identification of high social risk. *Health and Social Work,* 11 (1): 26-35.

Beckerman, Nancy, and Rock, Marjorie (1996). Themes from the frontlines: Hospital social work with people with AIDS. *Social Work in Health Care,* 23 (4): 75-89.

Bennett, Claire, Legon, Julianne, and Zilberfein, Felice (1989). The significance of empathy in current hospital based practice. *Social Work in Health Care,* 14 (2): 27-40.

Ben-Zur, Hasida, Rappaport, Batya, Ammar, Ronny, and Uretzky, Gideon (2000). Coping strategies, life style changes, and pessimism after open-heart surgery. *Health and Social Work,* 25 (3): 201-209.

Berger, Candyce S., Cayner, Jay, Mizrahi, Terry, Scesny, Alice, and Trachtenberg, Judith (1996). The changing scene of social work in hospitals. *Health and Social Work,* 21 (3): 167-177.

Berger, Candyce S., and Mizrahi, Terry (2001). An evolving paradigm of supervision within a changing health care environment. *Social Work in Health Care,* 32 (4): 1-17.

Berkman, Barbara, Millar, Sally, Holmes, William, and Bonander, Evelyn (1991). Predicting elderly cardiac patients at risk for readmission. *Social Work in Health Care,* 16 (1): 21-38.

Bloch, Linda von (1996). Breaking the bad news when sudden death occurs. *Social Work in Health Care,* 23 (4): 91-97.

Cannon, Ida M. (1923). *Social work in hospitals.* New York: Russell Sage.

Caputi, Marie A. (1978). Social work in health care: Past and future. *Health and Social Work,* 3 (1): 9-29.

Clemens, Elizabeth (1995). Multiple perceptions of discharge planning in one urban hospital. *Health and Social Work,* 20 (4): 254-261.

Congress, Elaine P., and Lyons, Beverly P. (1992). Cultural differences in health beliefs: Implications for social work practice in health care settings. *Social Work in Health Care,* 17 (3): 81-97.

Coulton, Claudia J. (1988). Evaluating screening and early intervention: A puzzle with many pieces. *Social Work in Health Care,* 13 (3): 65-72.

Coulton, Claudia J. (1990). Research in patient and family decision making regarding life sustaining and long term care. *Social Work in Health Care,* 15 (1): 63-78.

Coulton, Claudia J., Dunkle, Ruth E., Haug, Marie, Chow, Julian, and Vielhaber, David P. (1989). Locus of control and decision making for posthospital care. *The Gerontologist,* 29 (5): 627-632.

Cowles, Lois A., and Lefcowitz, Myron J. (1992). Interdisciplinary expectations of the medical social worker in the hospital setting. *Health and Social Work,* 17 (1): 57-65.

Cowles, Lois A., and Lefcowitz, Myron J. (1995). Interdisciplinary expectations of the medical social worker in the hospital setting: Part 2. *Health and Social Work,* 20 (4): 279-286.

Csikai, Ellen L., and Bass, Kelli (2000). Health care social workers' views on ethnical issues, practice, and policy in end-of-life care. *Social Work in Health Care,* 32 (2): 1-22.

Cummings, Sherry M. (1999). Adequacy of discharge plans and rehospitalization among hospitalized dementia patients. *Health and Social Work,* 24 (4): 249-259.

Cuzzi, Lawrence, Holden, Gary, Rutter, Steve, Rosenberg, Gary, and Chernack, Peter (1996). A pilot study of fieldwork rotations vs. year long placements for social work students in a public hospital. *Social Work in Health Care,* 24 (1/2): 73-91.

DeCoster, Vaughn A., and Egan, Marcia (2001). Physician's perceptions and responses to patient emotion: Implications for social work practice in healthcare. *Social Work in Health Care,* 32 (3): 21-40.

Dobrof, Judith (1991). DRG's and the social worker's role in discharge planning. *Social Work in Health Care,* 16 (2): 37-54.

Donnelly, James P. (1992). A frame for defining social work in a hospital setting. *Social Work in Health Care,* 18 (1): 107-119.

Dubowitz, Howard, Black, Maureen, and Harrington, Donna (1992). The diagnosis of child sexual abuse. *American Journal of Diseases of Children,* 146 (June): 688-693.

Egan, Marcia, and Kadushin, Goldie (1995). Competitive allies: Rural nurses' and social workers' perceptions of the social work role in the hospital setting. *Social Work in Health Care,* 20 (3): 1-23.

Epstein, Janet, Kaplan, Giora, Lavi, Bruno, Noy, Shlomo, Shahaf, Poriya, Stanger, Varda, and Rotstein, Zeev (2001). A description of inappropriate hospital stays in selected in-patient services: A study of cases receiving social work services. *Social Work in Health Care,* 32 (4): 43-65.

Evans, Ron L., and Connis, Richard T. (1996). Risk screening for adverse outcomes in subacute care. *Psychological Reports,* 78: 1043-1048.

Evans, Ron L., Hendricks, Robert D., Lawrence-Umlauf, Kaye V., and Bishop, Duane S. (1989). Timing of social work intervention and medical patients' length of hospital stay. *Health and Social Work,* 14 (4): 277-282.

Fahs, Marianne C., and Wade, Kathleen (1996). An economic analysis of two models of hospital care for AIDS patients: Implications for hospital discharge planning. *Social Work in Health Care,* 22 (4): 21-34.

Feather, John (1993). Factors in perceived hospital discharge planning effectiveness. *Social Work in Health Care,* 19 (1): 1-14.

Fillit, Howard, Howe, Judith L., Sachs, Charles, Sell, Laura, Siegel, Patricia, Miller, Myron, and Butler, Robert N. (1992). Studies of hospital social stays in the frail elderly and their relationship to the intensity of social work intervention. *Social Work in Health Care,* 18 (1): 1-22.

Foster, Larry W., Sharp, John, Scesny, Alice, McLellan, Linda, and Cotman, Kathy (1993). Bioethics: Social work's response and training needs. *Social Work in Health Care,* 19 (1): 15-38.

Gentry, Linda R. (1993). Practice forum: The special caretakers program—A hospital's solution to the boarder baby problem. *Health and Social Work,* 18 (1): 75-77.

Germain, Carel B. (1980). Social work identity, competence, and autonomy: The ecological perspective. *Social Work in Health Care,* 6 (1): 1-10.

Ginsberg, Leon (1995). *The social work almanac* (Second edition). Washington, DC: NASW Press.

Glassman, Uania (1991). The social work group and its distinct healing qualities in the health care setting. *Health and Social Work,* 16 (3): 203-212.

Globerman, Judith, and Bogo, Marion (1995). Social work in the new integrative hospital. *Social Work in Health Care,* 21 (3): 1-21.

Globerman, Judith, Davies, Joan MacKenzie, and Walsh, Susan (1996). Social work in restructuring hospitals: Meeting the challenge. *Health and Social Work,* 21 (2): 178-188.

Greenlick, Merwyn R., and Brody, Kathleen K. (1997). Home health services in a managed care system: Policy recommendations from a program of research. In Fox, Daniel M. and Raphael, Carol (Eds.), *Home-based care for a new century.* Malden, MA: Blackwell Publishers, 99-119.

Hall, James A., Jensen, Greg V., Fortney, Mark A., Sutter, Joy, Locher, Jan, and Cayner, Jay J. (1996). Education of staff and students in health care settings: Integrating practice and research. *Social Work in Health Care,* 24 (1/2): 93-113.

Hanson, James G., and Rapp, Charles A. (1992). Families' perceptions of community mental health programs for their relatives with a severe mental illness. *Community Mental Health Journal,* 28 (3): 181-197.

Hanson, Meridith, Foreman, Lewis, Tomlin, Willie, and Bright, Yvonne (1994). Facilitating problem drinking clients' transition from inpatient to outpatient care. *Health and Social Work,* 19 (1): 23-28.

Hazard, William R. (1995). Elder abuse: Definitions and implications for medical education. *Academic Medicine,* 70 (11): 979-981.

Herbert, Margot, and Levin, Ron (1996). The advocacy role in hospital social work. *Social Work in Health Care,* 22 (3): 71-83.

Holliman, Diane C., Dziegielewski, Sophia, Datta, Priyadarshi (2001). Discharge planning and social work practice. *Social Work in Health Care,* 32 (3): 1-19.

James, Catherine D., and Studs, Dip Soc (1987). An ecological approach to defining discharge planning. *Social Work in Health Care,* 12 (4): 47-59.

Julia, Maria C. (1996). *Multicultural awareness in the health care professions.* Boston, MA: Allyn and Bacon.

Kadushin, Goldie, and Kulys, Regina (1995). Job satisfaction among social work discharge planners. *Health and Social Work,* 20 (3): 174-186.

Keehn, Debra S., Roglitz, Cathy, and Bowden, M. Leora (1994). Impact of social work on recidivism and non-medical complaints in the emergency department. *Social Work in Health Care,* 20 (1): 65-75.

Landau, Ruth (2000a). Ethical dilemmas in general hospitals: Differential perceptions of direct practitioners and directors of social services. *Social Work in Health Care,* 30 (4): 25-44.

Landau, Ruth (2000b). Ethical dilemmas in general hospitals: Social worker's contribution to ethical decision-making. *Social Work in Health Care,* 32 (2): 75-92.

Lauria, Marie M., Hockenberry-Eaton, Marilyn, Pawletko, Terese M., and Mauer, Alvin M. (1996). Psychosocial protocol for childhood cancer. *Cancer,* 78 (6): 1345-1356.

Marcus, Leonard (1990). Research on organizational issues in health care social work. *Social Work in Health Care,* 15 (1): 79-95.

Mayer, Jane B. (1995). The effective healthcare social work director: Managing the social work department at Beth Israel Hospital. *Social Work in Health Care,* 20 (4): 61-72.

McCoy, H. Virginia, Kipp, C. William, and Ahern, Melissa (1992). Reducing older patients' reliance on the emergency department. *Social Work in Health Care,* 17 (1): 23-37.

Mizrahi, Terry, and Abramson, Julie S. (2000). Collaboration between social workers and physicians: Perspectives on a shared case. *Social Work in Health Care,* 31 (3): 1-24.

Mizrahi, Terry, and Berger, Candyce S. (2001). Effect of a changing health care environment on social work leaders: Obstacles and opportunities in hospital social work. *Social Work,* 46 (2): 170-182.

Morrow-Howell, Nancy, and Proctor, Enola (1994). Discharge destinations of Medicare patients receiving discharge planning: Who goes where? *Medical Care,* 32 (5): 486-497.

Nacman, Martin (1977). Social work in health settings: A historical review. *Social Work in Health Care,* 2 (4): 407-418.

Naleppa, Matthias J., and Reid, William J. (2000). Integrating case managment and brief-treatment stretegies: A hospital-based geriatric program. *Social Work in Health Care,* 31 (4): 1-23.

National Association of Social Workers (1987). *NASW standards for social work in health care settings.* Washington, DC: NASW Press, 3-30.

National Association of Social Workers (1990). *NASW clinical indicators for social work and psychosocial services in the acute care medical hospital.* Washington, DC: NASW Press, 1-8.

National Association of Social Workers (1997). Government relations alert: Large volume of letters needed to convince HCFA to retain definition of qualified social workers in Medicare's home health program. <http://www.nasw.org>.

Oktay, Julianne S., Steinwachs, Donald M., Manon, Joyce, Bone, Lee R., and Fahey, Maureen (1992). Evaluating social work discharge planning services for elderly people: Access, complexity, and outcome. *Health and Social Work,* 17 (4): 290-298.

Ortiz, Elizabeth Thompson, and Bassoff, Betty Z. (1988). Proprietary hospital social work. *Health and Social Work,* 13 (2): 114-121.

Ponto, Jade M., and Berg, William (1992). Social work services in the emergency department: A cost-benefit analysis of an extended coverage program. *Health and Social Work,* 17 (1): 66-73.

Posen, Jennie, Moore, Orna, Tassa, Dafna Sadeh, Ginsberg, Karni, Drory, Margalit, and Giladi, Nir (2000). Young women with P.D. *Social Work in Health Care,* 32 (1): 77-91.

Pray, Jackie E. (1991). Responding to psychosocial needs: Physician perceptions of their referral practices for hospitalized patients. *Health and Social Work,* 16 (3): 184-192.

Proctor, Enola K., Morrow-Howell, Nancy, Kitchen, Alice, and Wang, Yeong-Tsyr (1995). Pediatric discharge planning: Complications, efficiency, and adequacy. *Social Work in Health Care,* 22 (1): 1-18.

Proctor, Enola, K., Morrow-Howell, Nancy, Li, Hong, and Dore, Peter (2000). Adequacy of home care and hospital readmission for elderly congestive heart failure patients. *Health and Social Work,* 25 (2): 87-96.

Rauch, Julia B., and Schreiber, Hanita (1985). Discharge planning as a teaching mechanism. *Health and Social Work,* 10 (3): 208-216.

Resnick, Cheryl, and Dziegielewski, Sophia F. (1996). The relationship between therapeutic termination and job satisfaction among medical social workers. *Social Work in Health Care,* 23 (3): 17-32.

Robinson, James C. (1994). The changing boundaries of the American hospital. *The Milbank Quarterly,* 72 (2): 259-275. (Quoted material reprinted with permission of Blackwell Publishers, Malden, MA.)

Rosen, George (1958). *A history of public health: MD monographs on medical history.* New York: MD Publications.

Ross, Judith W. (1993). Editorial: Redefining hospital social work: An embattled professional domain. *Health and Social Work,* 18 (4): 243-246.

Ross, Judith W. (1995). Hospital social work. In Edwards, Richard L. (Ed.), *The encyclopedia of social work* (Nineteenth edition). Washington, DC: NASW Press, 1365-1377.

Ruster, Pamela L. (1995). The evolution of social work in a community hospital. *Social Work in Health Care,* 20 (4): 73-88.

Showers, Nancy (1992). How satisfaction with hospital field work affects social work students' willingness to accept employment in hospital settings. *Social Work in Health Care,* 16 (4): 19-35.

Smith, David R., and Anderson, Ron J. (1995). Feudal vs. futile medicine: Can we have cost containment without prevention? In Eve, Susan Brown, Havens, Betty, and Ingman, Stanley E. (Eds.), *The Canadian health care system: Lessons for the United States.* Lanham, MD: University Press of America, 247-255.

Soskolne, Varda, and Auslander, Gail K. (1993). Follow-up evaluation of discharge planning by social workers in an acute-care medical center in Israel. *Social Work in Health Care,* 18 (2): 22-48.

Spitzer, William, and Burke, Laurie (1993). Practice forum: A critical incident stress debriefing program for hospital-based health care personnel. *Health and Social Work,* 18 (2): 149-156.

Spitzer, William, and Neely, Keith (1992). Critical incident stress: The role of hospital-based social work in developing a statewide intervention system for first-responders delivering emergency services. *Social Work in Health Care,* 18 (1): 39-58.

Stuen, Cynthia, and Monk, Abraham (1990). Discharge planning: The impact of Medicare's prospective payment on elderly patients. In A. Monk (Ed.), *Health care of the aged: Needs, policies and services.* Binghamton, NY: The Haworth Press, Inc., 149-164.

Task Force on Adolescent Assault Victim Needs (1996). Adolescent assault victim needs: A review of issues and a model protocol. *Pediatrics,* 98 (5): 991-1001.

Trattner, Walter I. (1989). *From poor law to welfare state: A history of social welfare in America* (Fourth edition). New York: The Free Press.

Travis, Shirley S., Moore, Suzanne R., and McAuley, William J. (1991). A comparison of hospitalization experiences for demented and non-demented elders: Findings of a retrospective chart review. *Journal of Gerontological Social Work,* 17 (1/2): 35-46.

U.S. Census Bureau (1999). *Current population survey.* Washington, DC: Author. March.

U.S. Government Printing Office (2000a). *Health, United States.* Washington, DC: Author.

U.S. Government Printing Office (2000b). *Statistical abstracts of the United States.* Washington, D.C.: Author.

Walsh, Susan (1985). The psychiatric emergency service as a setting for social work training. *Social Work in Health Care,* 11 (1): 21-31.

Wolock, Isabel, Schlesinger, Elfriede, Dinerman, Miriam, and Seaton, Richard (1987). The posthospital needs and care of patients: Implications for discharge planning. *Social Work in Health Care,* 12 (4): 6176.

Chapter 5

Applewhite, Steven Lozano (1995). Curanderismo: Demystifying the health beliefs and practices of elderly Mexican-Americans. *Health and Social Work,* 20 (4): 247-253.

Aranda, Maria P. (1996). *Implications of diversity for practice.* Presented at the California Geriatric Education Center, Cultural Diversity in Aging, Faculty Development Program, UCLA, June 18.

Balinsky, Warren (1994). *Home care.* San Francisco, CA: Jossey-Bass Publishers.

Barnes, Carla L., Given, Barbara A., and Given, Charles W. (1992). Caregivers of elderly relatives: Spouses and adult children. *Health and Social Work,* 17 (4): 282-289.

Berg-Weger, Marla, Rubio, Doris McGartland, and Tebb, Susan Steigner (2000). The caregiver well-being scale revisited. *Health and Social Work,* 25 (4): 255-269.

Berkman, Barbara (1996). The emerging health care world: Implications for social work practice and education. *Social Work,* 41 (5): 541-555.

Binney, Elizabeth A., Estes, Carroll L., and Ingman, Stanley R. (1990). Medicalization, public policy and the elderly: Social services in jeopardy? *Social Science in Medicine,* 30 (7): 761-771.

Blazer, Dan (1988). Home health care: House calls revisited. *American Journal of Public Health,* 78 (3): 238-239.

Braus, Patricia (1994). When mom needs help. *American Demographics,* 16 (March): 38-47.

Brody, Elaine M. (1981). Women in the middle and family help to older people. *The Gerontologist,* 21 (5): 471-480.

California's Caregiver Resource Center (2001). Who are the caregivers? <http://www.caregiver.org>.

Cannon, Ida M. (1923). *Social work in hospitals.* New York: Russell Sage.

Center for the Advanced Study of Aging Services, School of Social Welfare, University of California, Berkeley (2001). Newsletter (Fall): 4.

Chadiha, Letha A., Proctor, Enola K., Morrow-Howell, Nancy, Darkwa, Osei K., and Dore, Peter (1995). Post-hospital home care for African-American and white elderly. *The Gerontologist,* 35 (2): 233-239.

Clemen-Stone, Susan H., Eigsti, Diane G., and McGuire, Sandra L. (1987). *Comprehensive family and community health nursing* (Second edition). New York: McGraw-Hill.

Concoran, Kevin, and Fischer, Joel (2000). *Measures for clinical practice: A sourcebook* (Third edition). Volume 2: *Adults*. New York: The Free Press.

Corin, Ellen E. (1994). The social and cultural matrix of health and disease. In Evans, Robert G., Barer, Morris L., and Marmor, Theodore R. (Eds.), *Why are some people healthy and others not? The determinants of health of populations*. New York: Aldine de Gruyter, 93-132.

Cox, Carole (1992). Expanding social work's role in home care: An ecological perspective. *Social Work*, 37 (2): 179-183.

Damon-Rodriguez, JoAnn, Wallace, Steven, and Kington, Raynard (1994). Service utilization and minority elderly: Appropriateness, accessibility, and acceptability. In Wieland, Daryl, Benton, Donna, Kramer, B. Josea, and Dawson, Grace D. (Eds.), *Cultural diversity and geriatric care: Challenges to the health professions*. Binghamton, NY: The Haworth Press, Inc., 45-63.

Davitt, Joan K., and Kaye, Lenard W. (1996). Supporting patient autonomy in home health care. *Social Work*, 41 (1): 41-50.

Duke University Center for the Study of Aging and Human Development (1978). *The OARS methodology* (Second edition). Durham, NC: Duke University Press.

Egan, Marcia, and Kadushin, Goldie (1999). The social worker in the emerging field of home care: Professional activities and ethical concerns. *Health and Social Work*, 24 (1): 43-55.

Ell, Kathleen (1996). Social work and health care practice and policy: A psycho-social research agenda. *Social Work*, 41 (6): 583-592.

Erikson, Erik (1950). The problem of ego identity. *Psychological Issues*, 101-164.

Erikson, Erik (1956). The problems of ego identity. *The Journal of the American Psychoanalytic Association*, 4: 56-121.

Erikson, Erik (1959). Identity and the life cycle. In Klein, George S. (Ed.), *Psychological Issues*. Independence, MD: International Universities Press, 56-121.

Ettner, Susan L. (1994). The effect of the Medicaid home care benefit on long-term care choices of the elderly. *Economic Inquiry*, XXXII (January): 103-127.

Evans, Robert G., Barer, Morris L., Marmor, Theodore R. (Eds.) (1994). *Why are some people healthy and others not? The determinants of health of populations*. New York: Aldine de Gruyter.

Fandetti, Donald V., and Goldmeier, John (1988). Social workers as culture mediators in health care settings. *Health and Social Work*, 13 (3): 171-179.

Fashimpar, Gary (1983). A management tool for evaluating the adequacy and quality of homemaker-home health aide programs. *The Gerontologist*, 23 (2): 127-131.

Fashimpar, Gary (1991). Evaluating homemaker-home health aide programs: Practical applications of the homemaker-home health aide program evaluation questionnaire. *Journal of Gerontological Social Work*, 18 (1/2): 3-16.

Fessler, Susan R., and Adams, Catherine G. (1985). Nurse/social worker role conflict in home health care. *Journal of Gerontological Social Work*, 9 (1): 113-123.

Fredman, Lisa, Droge, Janet, and Rabin, David (1992). Functional limitations among home health care users in the national health interview survey supplement on aging. *The Gerontologist*, 32 (5): 641-646.

Garner, Dianne J. (1995). Long-term care. In Edwards, Richard L. (Ed.), *The ency-clopedia of social work* (Nineteenth edition). Washington, DC: NASW Press, 1625-1634.

Ginsberg, Leon (1995). *The social work almanac* (Second edition). Washington, DC: NASW Press.

Giordano, Joseph (1992). Ethnicity and aging. In Mellor, M. Joanna and Solomon, Renee (Eds.), *Geriatric social work education*. Binghamton, NY: The Haworth Press, Inc., 23-37.

Goldberg, Allen J. (1994). Book reviews: Home health care—An annotated bibli-ography. *Journal of the American Geriatric Society*, 42 (8): 910-911.

Hamama, Rachel, Ronen, Tammie, and Feigin, Rena (2000). Self-control, anxiety, and loneliness in siblings of children with cancer. *Social Work in Health Care*, 31 (1): 63-83.

Horowitz, A. (1984). Family caregiving to the frail elderly. In Eisdorfer, Carl (Ed.), *The annual review of gerontology and geriatrics*. New York: Springer, 194-246.

Jacobs, Phillip E., and Lurie, Abraham (1984). A new look at home care and the hospital social worker. In Dobrof, Rose (Ed.), *Gerontological social work in home health care*. Binghamton, NY: The Haworth Press, Inc., 89-90.

Jette, Alan M., Smith, Kevin W., and McDermott, Susan M. (1996). Quality of Medicare-reimbursed home health care. *The Gerontologist*, 36 (4): 492-501.

Kadushin, Goldie, and Egan, Marcia (2001). Ethical dilemmas in home health care: A social work perspective. *Health and Social Work*, 26 (3): 136-147.

Kane, Robert L., Finch, Michael, Blewett, Lynn, Chen, Qing, Burns, Risa, and Moskowitz, Mark (1996). Use of post-hospital care by Medicare patients. *Jour-nal of the American Geriatric Society*, 44 (3): 242-250.

Kane, Robert L., Kane, Rosalie A., Finch, Michael, Harrington, Charlene, New-comer, Robert, Miller, Nancy, and Hulbert, Melissa (1997). S/HMO's, the sec-ond generation: Building on the experience of the first social health maintenance organization demonstrations. *Journal of the American Geriatric Society*, 45 (1): 101-107.

Karger, Howard Jacob, and Stoesz, David (1994). *American social welfare policy: A pluralistic approach* (Second edition). New York: Longman.

Kaye, Lenard W., and Davitt, Joan K. (1995). Provider and consumer profiles of tra-ditional and high-tech home health care. *Health and Social Work*, 20 (4): 262-271.

Kenney, Genevieve M. (1993). Is access to home health care a problem in rural ar-eas? *American Journal of Public Health*, 83 (3): 412-414.

Kerson, Toba Schwaber, and Michelson, Renee W. (1995). Counseling home-bound clients and their families. *Journal of Gerontological Social Work*, 24 (3/4): 159-190.

Kramer, Andrew M., Shaughnessy, Peter W., Bauman, Marjorie K., and Crisler, Kathryn S. (1990). Assessing and assuring the quality of home health care: A conceptual framework. *The Milbank Quarterly*, 68 (3): 413-443.

Lawlor, Edward F., and Raube, Kristiana (1995). Social interventions and outcomes in medical effectiveness research. *Social Service Review*, 69 (3): 383-404. (Quoted material reprinted with permission of University of Chicago Press, Chi-cago, IL.)

Linsk, Nathan, Keigher, Sharon M., and Osterbusch, Suzanne E. (1988). States' policies regarding paid family caregiving. *The Gerontologist,* 28 (2): 204-212.

Loewenberg, F. M., and Dolgoff, R. (1996). *Ethical decisions for social work practice* (Fifth edition). Itasca, IL: F.E. Peacock Co.

Mailick, Mildred D., and Jordon, Pearl (1977). A multimodal approach to collaborative practice in health settings. *Social Work in Health Care,* 2 (4): 445-455.

Marder, Reggi, and Linsk, Nathan L. (1995). Addressing AIDS long-term care issues through education and advocacy. *Health and Social Work,* 20 (1): 75-80.

McCormick, Wayne C., Uomoto, Jay, Young, Heather, Graves, Amy B., Vitaliano, Peter, Mortimer, James A., Edland, Steven D., and Larson, Eric B. (1996). Attitudes toward use of nursing homes and home care in older Japanese-Americans. *Journal of the American Geriatric Society,* 44 (7): 769-777.

McDowell, Ian, and Newell, Claire (1996). *Measuring health: A guide to rating scales and questionnaires* (Second edition). New York: Oxford University Press.

Mindel, Charles, and Wright, Roosevelt (1982). Satisfaction in multigenerational households. *Journal of Gerontology,* 37 (4): 483-489.

Moody, Harry (1982). Ethical dilemmas in long-term care. *Journal of Gerontological Social Work,* 5 (1/2): 97-111.

Morrow-Howell, Nancy, Chadiha, Letha A., Proctor, Enola K., Hourd-Bryant, Maggie, and Dore, Peter (1996). Racial differences in discharge planning. *Health and Social Work,* 21 (2): 131-139.

Mullen, Edward J., and Magnabosco, Jennifer L. (Eds.) (1997). *Outcomes measurement in the human services: Cross-cutting issues and methods.* Washington, DC: NASW Press.

National Association for Home Care (1996). *Basic statistics about home care.* Washington, DC: Author.

National Association for Home Care (2000). *Basic statistics about home care.* <http://www.nahc.org/Consumer/hcstats.html>.

National Association of Social Workers (1987). *NASW standards for social work in health care settings.* Washington, DC: NASW Press, 1-31.

National Association of Social Workers (1995). *NASW clinical indicators for social work and psychosocial services in home health care.* Washington, DC: NASW Press, 1-9.

Olson, Laura Katz (1994). Public policy and privatization: Long-term care in the United States. In Olson, Laura Katz (Ed.), *The graying of the world: Who will care for the frail elderly?* Binghamton, NY: The Haworth Press, Inc., 25-58.

Proctor, Enola K., Morrow-Howell, Nancy, and Kaplan, Sally J. (1996). Implementation of discharge plans for chronically ill elders discharged home. *Health and Social Work,* 21 (1): 30-39.

Reamer, Frederic G., and Abramson, Marcia (1982). *The teaching of social work ethics.* Hastings on Hudson, NY: Institute of Society, Ethics, and the Life Sciences.

Robbins, Dennis, A. (1996). *Ethical and legal issues in home health and long-term care: Challenges and solutions.* Gaithersburg, MD: Aspen Publishers.

Silverstone, Barbara, and Burack-Weiss, Ann (1983). The social work function in nursing homes and home care. *The Journal of Gerontological Social Work,* 5 (1/2): 7-33.

Simmons, June (1994). Community based care: The new health social work paradigm. *Social Work in Health Care,* 20 (1): 35-46.

Tanjasiri, Sora P., Wallace, Steven P., and Shibata, Kazue (1995). Picture imperfect: Hidden problems among Asian Pacific Islander elderly. *The Gerontologist,* 35 (6): 753-760.

Tebb, S. S. (1995). An aid to empowerment: A caregiver wellbeing scale. *Health and Social Work,* 20: 87-92.

U.S. Department of Health and Human Services, National Institute of Health, National Institute on Aging (1993). *Profiles of America's Elderly: Racial and Ethnic Diversity of America's Elderly Population.* Number 3, November, POP/93-1-8.

U.S. Government Printing Office (1990). *The Pepper Commission final report: A call for action.* Washington, DC: Author, 101-114.

U. S. Government Printing Office (2000a). *Health, United States.* Washington, DC: Author.

U.S. Government Printing Office (2000b). *Statistical Abstracts of the United States.* Washington, DC: Author.

Wallace, Steven P. (1990). The political economy of health care for elderly blacks. *International Journal of Health Services,* 20 (4): 665-680.

Wallace, Steven P. (1996). *Stratification, ethnicity, and aging public policy.* Presented at the California Geriatric Education Center, Cultural Diversity in Aging, Faculty Development Program, UCLA, June 18.

Ware, John E., and Sherbourne, Cathy D. (1992). The MOS 36-item short-form health survey (SF-36). *Medical Care,* 30 (6): 473-483.

Welch, H. Gilbert, Wennberg, David E., and Welch, W. Pete (1996). The use of Medicare home health care services. *The New England Journal of Medicine,* 335 (5): 324-329.

White-Means, Shelly I., and Thornton, Michael C. (1990a). Ethnic differences in the production of informal home health care. *The Gerontologist,* 30 (6): 758-768.

White-Means, Shelly I., and Thornton, Michael C. (1990b). Labor market choices and home health care provision among employed ethnic caregivers. *The Gerontologist,* 30 (6): 769-775.

Wilcox, Julie A., and Taber, Merlin A. (1991). Informal helpers of elderly home care clients. *Health and Social Work,* 16 (4): 258-265.

Zimmer, James G., Groth-Juncker, Annemarie, and McCusker, Jane (1985). A randomized controlled study of a home health care team. *The American Journal of Public Health,* 75 (2): 134-141.

Chapter 6

Barber, Clinton E., and Iwai, Mieko (1996). Role conflict and role ambiguity as predictors of burnout among staff caring for elderly dementia patients. *Journal of Gerontological Social Work,* 26 (1/2): 101-117.

Beirne, Nancy F., Patterson, Margery N., Galie, Michelle, and Goodman, Patricia (1995). Effects of a fast-tract closing on a nursing facility population. *Health and Social Work,* 20 (2): 117-123.

Bogo, Marion (1987). Social work practice with family systems in admission to homes for the aged. *Journal of Gerontological Social Work,* 10 (1/2): 5-19.

Boondas, Jennifer (1991). Nursing home resident assessment classification and focused care. *Nursing and Health Care,* 12 (6): 308-312.

Brannon, Diane (1992). Toward second-generation nursing home research. *The Gerontologist,* 32 (3): 293-294. (Quoted material reprinted with permission of The Gerontological Society of America, Washington, DC.)

Brown, Lil (1989). Is there sexual freedom for our aging population in long-term care institutions? *Journal of Gerontological Social Work,* 13 (3/4): 75-93.

Bruno, Ronald (1994). Policy for the people: One facility's introduction to restraint reduction. *Journal of Gerontological Social Work,* 22 (3/4): 129-142.

Bullard-Poe, Laura, Powell, Cicely, and Mulligan, Thomas (1994). The importance of intimacy to men living in a nursing home. *Archives of Sexual Behavior,* 23 (2): 231-236.

Caplan, Arthur L. (1990). The morality of the mundane: Ethical issues arising in the daily lives of nursing home residents. In Kane, Rosalie A. and Caplan, Arthur L. (Eds.), *Everyday ethics: Resolving dilemmas in nursing home life.* New York: Springer, 37-50.

Cohen-Mansfield, Jiska, Rabinovich, Beth A., Marx, Marcia S., Braun, Judith, and Fleshner, Edith (1991). Nurses' and social workers' perceptions of elderly nursing home residents' well-being. *Journal of Gerontological Social Work,* 16 (3/4): 135-147.

Cox, Carole (1993). Dealing with the aggressive nursing home resident. *Journal of Gerontological Social Work,* 19 (3/4): 179-192.

Dane, B. O., and Simon, B. L. (1991). Resident guests: Social workers in host settings. *Social Work,* 36: 208-213.

Dempsey, Norah P., and Pruchno, Rachel A. (1993). The family's role in the nursing home: Predictors of technical and non-technical assistance. *Journal of Gerontological Social Work,* 21 (1/2): 127-145.

Dhooper, Surjit S., Green, Sharon M., Huff, Marlene B., and Austin-Murphy, Judy (1993). Efficacy of a group approach to reducing depression in nursing home residents. *Journal of Gerontological Social Work,* 20 (3/4): 87-100.

Dieckmann, Janna L. (1993). From almshouse to city nursing home: Philadelphia's Riverview home for the aged, 1945-1965. *Nursing History Review,* 1: 217-228.

Evans, L., and Strumpf, F. (1989). Tying down the elderly: A review of the literature on physical restraint. *Journal of the American Geriatrics Society,* 37 (1): 65-74.

Fairchild, Susan, Carrino, Gerard E., and Ramirez, Mildred (1996). Social workers' perceptions of staff attitudes toward resident sexuality in a random sample of New York State nursing homes. *Journal of Gerontological Social Work,* 26 (1/2): 153-169.

Flaherty, Ellen (2001). Nursing home staff. *Aging Research and Training News,* 24 (5): 49.

Foldes, Steven S. (1990). Life in an institution: A sociological and anthropological view. In Kane, Rosalie A. and Caplan, Arthur L. (Eds.), *Everyday ethics: Resolving dilemmas in nursing home life.* New York: Springer, 21-36.

Freed, Anne O. (1990). How Japanese families cope with fragile elderly. *Journal of Gerontological Social Work,* 15 (1/2): 39-56.

Freeman, Iris C. (1988). "Weighing the costs of care," in Point/Counterpoint: Caring for persons with aids in geriatric nursing homes. *Health and Social Work,* 13 (2): 156-158.

Gale Publishing Company (1997). *Wards Business Directory of U.S. Private and Public Companies.* Volume 5. Detroit, MI: Author.

Getzel, Jessica (1983). Resident councils and social action. In Getzel, George S. and Mellor, M. Joanna (Eds.), *Gerontological social work practice in long-term care.* Binghamton, NY: The Haworth Press, Inc., 179-185.

Greene, Roberta, Vourlekis, Betsy S., Gelfand, Donald, and Lewis, Judith S. (1992). Current realities: Practice and education needs of social workers in nursing homes. *Journal of Gerontological Social Work,* 18 (3/4): 39-54.

Gutheil, Irene (1991). Intimacy in nursing home friendships. *Journal of Gerontological Social Work,* 17 (1/2): 59-73.

Hancock, Tina U. (1992). Field placements in for-profit organizations: Policies and practices of graduate programs. *Journal of Social Work Education,* 28 (3): 330-340.

Harrington, Charlene, Woolhandler, Steffie, Mullan, Joseph, Carrillo, Helen, and Himmelstein, David (2001). Does investor ownership of nursing homes compromise the quality of care? *American Journal of Public Health,* 91 (9): 1452-1455. Also available online: <http://www.ajph.org/cgi/content/full/91/9/1452>.

Health Care Financing Administration (1989). *Medicare and Medicaid data book 1988.* HCFA publication number 03270. Baltimore, MD: Office of Research and Demonstrations.

Health Care Financing Administration (2000). *HCFA's National Restraint Newsletter.* VIII(1) (Summer). <http://www.hcfa.gov/pubforms/rrnews>.

Hoffman, Rosemary G. (1991). Companion animals: A therapeutic measure for elderly patients. *Journal of Gerontological Social Work,* 18 (1/2): 195-204.

Horejsi, Gloria (1987). Nursing home consultation. *Health and Social Work,* 12 (2): 155-156.

Institute of Medicine (1981). *Health care in a context of civil rights.* Washington, DC: National Academy Press.

Joint Commission on the Accreditation of Healthcare Organizations (1993). *Accreditation Manual for Long Term Care: 1994.* Volume 1, *Organization Standards.* Oak Brook Terrace, IL: JCAHO.

Kaas, M. J. (1978). Sexual expression of the elderly in nursing homes. *The Gerontologist,* 18 (4): 372-378.

Kane, Rosalie A., and Caplan, Arthur L. (Eds.) (1990). *Everyday ethics: Resolving dilemmas in nursing home life.* New York: Springer.

Karger, Howard Jacob, and Stoesz, David (1994). *American social welfare policy: A pluralistic approach* (Second edition). New York: Longman.

Kramer, Betty J. (2000). Husbands caring for wives with dementia: A longitudinal study of continuity and change. *Health and Social Work,* 25 (2): 97-107.

Kruzich, Jean M. (1995). Empowering organizational contexts: Patterns and predictors of perceived decision-making influence among staff in nursing homes. *The Gerontologist,* 35 (2): 207-216.

Kruzich, Jean M., and Powell, William E. (1995). Decision-making influence: An empirical study of social workers in nursing homes. *Health and Social Work,* 20 (3): 215-222.

Lerer, Gertie (1995). Helping the irascible patient in long term care: Toward a theoretical and practice design. *Journal of Gerontological Social Work,* 24 (1/2): 169-184.

Linsk, Nathan L., and Marder, Reggi E. (1992). Medical social work long term care referrals for people with HIV infection. *Health and Social Work,* 17 (2): 105-115.

Margolis, Richard J. (1990). *Risking old age in America.* Boulder, CO: Westview Press.

Mead, Nelson B. (1991). Some nursing home experiences. *Journal of Gerontological Social Work,* 16 (3/4): 3-15.

Mercer, Susan O. (1994). Navajo elders in a reservation nursing home: Health status profile. *Journal of Gerontological Social Work,* 23 (1/2): 3-29.

Mercer, Susan O. (1996). Navajo elderly people in a reservation nursing home: Admission predictors and culture care practices. *Social Work,* 41 (2): 181-189.

Monahan, Deborah J. (1995). Informal caregivers of institutionalized demential residents: Predictors of burden. *Journal of Gerontological Social Work,* 23 (3/4): 65-82.

Montgomery, Rhonda J. V., and Kosloski, Karl (1994). A longitudinal analysis of nursing home placement for dependent elders care by spouses vs. adult children. *Journal of Gerontology,* 49 (2): S62-S74.

Morrison, Barbara Jones (1995). A research and policy agenda on predictors of institutional placement among minority elderly. *Journal of Gerontological Social Work,* 24 (1/2): 17-28.

Morrow-Howell, Nancy, Chadiha, Letha A., Proctor, Enola K., Hourd-Bryant, Maggie, and Dore, Peter (1996). Racial differences in discharge planning. *Health and Social Work,* 21 (2): 131-139.

Mosher-Ashley, Pearl M., Turner, Barbara F., and O'Neill, Darcy (1991). Attitudes of nursing and rest home administrators toward deinstitutionalized elders with psychiatric disorders. *Community Mental Health Journal,* 27 (4): 241-253.

Nasr, S., and Osterweil, D. (1999). The nonpharmacologic management of agitation in the nursing home: A concensus approach. *Annals of Long-Term Care,* 7 (5): 171-180.

National Association for Home Care (2000). *Basic statistics about home care,* <http://www.nahc.org/Consumer/hcstats.html>.

National Association of Social Workers (1981). *NASW standards for social work services in long-term care facilities.* Washington, DC: NASW Press, 1-11.

National Association of Social Workers (1993). *NASW clinical indicators for social work and psychosocial services in nursing homes.* Washington, DC: NASW Press, 1-12.

Nelson, Wayne H. (1995). Long-term care volunteer roles on trial: Ombudsman effectiveness revisited. *Journal of Gerontological Social Work,* 23 (3/4): 25-46.

Olson, Laura Katz (1994). Public policy and privatization: Long-term care in the United States. In Olson, Laura Katz (Ed.), *The graying of the world: Who will care for the frail elderly?* Binghamton, NY: The Haworth Press, Inc., 25-58.

Ouslander, J., Osterweil, D., and Morley, J. (Eds.) (1997). *Medical care in the nursing home* (Second edition). Whitehouse Station, NJ: McGraw-Hill.

Palmer, Diane S. (1991). Co-leading a family council in a long-term care facility. *Journal of Gerontological Social Work,* 16 (3/4): 121-134.

Pepper Commission (1990). *A call for action: Final report.* Washington, DC: U.S. Government Printing Office.

Quam, Jean K., and Whitford, Gary S. (1992). Educational needs of nursing home social workers at the baccalaureate level. *Journal of Gerontological Social Work,* 18 (3/4): 143-156.

Reinardy, James R. (1995). Relocation to a new environment: Decisional control and the move to a nursing home. *Health and Social Work,* 20 (1): 31-38.

Riddick, Carol Cutler, Cohen-Mansfield, Jiska, Fleshner, Edith, and Kraft, Gladys (1992). Caregiver adaptations to having a relative with dementia admitted to a nursing home. *Journal of Gerontological Social Work,* 19 (1): 51-75.

Sahyoun, Nadine R., Pratt, Laura A., Lentzner, Harold, Dey, Achintya, and Robinson, Kristen (2001). The changing profile of nursing home residents: 1985-1997. *Aging Trends,* 4 (March). Hyattsville, MD: National Center for Health Statistics, 1-8.

Salive, Marcel E., Collins, Karen S., Foley, Daniel J., and George, Linda K. (1993). Predictors of nursing home admission in a biracial population. *American Journal of Public Health,* 83 (12): 1765-1767.

Scharlach, Andrew (1988). Peer counselor training for nursing home residents. *The Gerontologist,* 28 (4): 500-502.

Silverstone, Barbara, and Burack-Weiss, Ann (1982). The social work function in nursing homes and home care. *The Journal of Gerontological Social Work,* 5 (1/2): 7-33.

Smith, David Barton (1990). Population ecology and the racial integration of hospitals and nursing homes in the United States. *The Milbank Quarterly,* 68 (4): 561-596.

Society for Social Work Leadership in Health Care (2000). Friends or foes: Redefining hospital/nursing home relationships. *Social Work Leader,* 26 (5): 1.

Solovy, Alden (2000). Pain management: Tools for inplementing JCAHO's new standards. *Hospitals and Health Networks,* 74 (11): 51-63.

Spears, Renee, Drinka, Paul J., and Voeks, Susan K. (1993). Obtaining a durable power of attorney for health care from nursing home residents. *The Journal of Family Practice,* 36 (4): 409-413.

Tennstedt, Sharon L., Skinner, Katherine M., Sullivan, Lisa M., and McKinlay, John B. (1992). Response comparability of family and staff proxies for nursing home residents. *American Journal of Public Health,* 82 (5): 747-749.

Teno, Joan (2001). Inadequate pain treatment in nursing homes. *Aging Research and Training News,* 24 (5): 50.

Teno, J. M., Weitzen, S., Wetle, T., and Mor, V. (2001). Persistent pain in nursing home residents (letter to the editor). *JAMA,* 285 (16): 2081.

U.S. Civil Rights Commission (1963). *Civil rights: Report of the United States Civil Rights Commission.* Washington, DC: U.S. Government Printing Office.

U.S. Government Printing Office (1999). Annual statistical supplement to the *Social Security Bulletin.* Washington, DC: Social Security Administration, December.

U.S. Government Printing Office (2000a). *Health, United States.* Washington, DC: Author.

U.S. Government Printing Office (2000b). *Statistical abstracts of the United States.* Washington, DC: Author.

U.S. Senate Special Committee on Aging (1990). *Developments in aging: 1990,* Volume 1. Washington, DC: U.S. Government Printing Office.

Vinton, Linda, and Mazza, Nicholas (1994). Aggressive behavior directed at nursing home personnel by residents' family members. *The Gerontologist,* 34 (4): 528-533.

Vogel, William (1991). A personal memoir of the state hospitals of the 1950's. *Hospital and Community Psychiatry,* 42 (6): 593-597.

Vourlekis, Betsy S., Gelfand, Donald E., and Greene, Roberta R. (1992). Psychosocial needs and care in nursing homes: Comparison of views of social workers and home administrators. *The Gerontologist,* 32 (1): 113-119. (Copyright The Gerontological Society of America. Reproduced by permission of the publisher.)

Wasow, Mona, and Loeb, Martin (1979). Sexuality in nursing homes. *Journal of the American Geriatrics Society,* 27: 73-79.

Weisberg, Judith (1991). Social worker as client: My education as a family member in a nursing home. *Journal of Gerontological Social Work,* 16 (1/2): 195-203.

Williams, Ann (1997). American Healthcare Association spokesperson. Phone conversation with author, July 23.

Williams, Carter C. (1989). Liberation: Alternative to physical restraints. *The Gerontologist,* 29 (5): 385-386.

Wullschleger, Karla Scroggin, Lund, Dale A., Caserta, Michael S., and Wright, Scott D. (1996). Anxiety about aging: A neglected dimension of caregivers' experience. *Journal of Gerontological Social Work,* 26 (3/4): 3-18.

Chapter 7

Abrahm, Janet (2001). Optimal pain management in older patients: Achieving effective assesment and treatment. *Healthcare and Aging,* 8 (2) <http://www.asaging.org/han>. Reprinted with permission of Janet L. Abrahm, MD.

Allison, Helen, Gripton, James, and Rodway, Margaret (1990). Social work services as a component of palliative care with terminal cancer patients. In Davidson, Kay W. and Clarke, Sylvia S. (Eds.), *Social work in health care: A handbook for practice,* Part I. Binghamton, NY: The Haworth Press, Inc., 205-223.

Amar, Deborah F. (1994). The role of the hospice social worker in the nursing home setting. *The American Journal of Hospice and Palliative Care,* 11 (3): 18-22.

American Society on Aging (2001). Hospice needs and Medicare rules. *Aging Today,* 22 (4): 15.

Bern-Klug, Mercedes, Gessert, Charles, and Forbes, Sarah (2001). The need to revise assumptions about the end of life: Implications for social work practice. *Health and Social Work,* 26 (1): 38-48.

Buckingham, Robert W. (1996). *The handbook of hospice care.* New York: Prometheus Books.

Cassell, Eric (1982). The nature of suffering and the goals of medicine. *The New England Journal of Medicine,* 306: 639-645.

Corbett, Terry L., and Hai, Dorothy M. (1979). Searching for euthanatos: The hospice alternative. *Hospital Progress,* 60 (3): 38-41.

Corr, Charles, and Corr, Donna (1985). Situations involving children: A challenge for the hospice movement. *The Hospice Journal,* 1 (2): 63-77.

Donovan, Jenny A. (1984). Team nurse and social worker: Avoiding role conflict. *American Journal of Hospice Care,* 1 (1): 21-23.

Doyle, Derek (1994). *Domiciliary palliative care: A guide for the primary care team.* Oxford, New York, Tokyo: Oxford University Press.

Dush, David M. (1988a). Psychosocial research in hospice care: Toward a specificity of therapeutic mechanisms. *The Hospice Journal,* 4 (2): 9-36.

Dush, David M. (1988b). Trends in hospice research and psychosocial palliative care. *The Hospice Journal,* 4 (3): 13-28.

Fish, Nina Millet (1994). Social work practice in hospice care. In Holosko, M.J. and Taylor, P.A. (Eds.), *Social work practice in health care settings* (Second edition). Toronto, Canada: Canadian Scholar's Press, 403-418.

Freund, Peter E. S., and McGuire, Meridith B. (1991). *Health, illness and the social body: A critical sociology.* Englewood Cliffs, NJ: Prentice-Hall.

Germain, Carel Bailey (1984). *Social work practice in health care: An ecological perspective.* New York: The Free Press.

Gummer, Burton (1988). The hospice in transition: organizational and administrative perspectives. In F. D. Perlmutter (Ed.), *Alternative social agencies: Administrative strategies.* Binghamton, NY: The Haworth Press, 31-43.

Hayslip, Bert, and Leon, Joel (1992). *Hospice care.* Newbury Park, CA: Sage Publications.

Kaye, Lenard W., and Davitt, Joan K. (1995). Provider and consumer profiles of traditional and high-tech home health care. *Health and Social Work,* 20 (4): 262-271.

Kerr, Derek (1993). Mother Mary Aikenhead, the Irish Sisters of Charity and Our Lady's Hospice for the Dying. *The American Journal of Hospice and Palliative Care,* 10 (3): 13-20.

Kovacs, Pamela J., and Bronstein, Laura R. (1999). Preparation for oncology settings: What hospice workers say they need. *Health and Social Work,* 24 (1): 57-64.

Kron, Joan (1978). Designing a better place to die. In Schwartz, Howard D. and Kart, Cary S. (Eds.), *Dominant issues in medical sociology.* Reading, MA: Addison-Wesley, 548-554.

Kübler-Ross, Elisabeth (1969). *On death and dying.* New York: Macmillan.

Kulys, R., and Davis, M. (1986). An analysis of social services in hospice. *Social Work,* 31 (6): 448-456.

Lusk, Mark (1983). The psychosocial evaluation of the hospice patient. *Health and Social Work,* 8 (3): 210-218.

McDonald, Douglas (1991). Hospice social work: A search for identity. *Health and Social Work,* 16 (4): 274-280.

McNulty, Elizabeth G., and Holderby, Robert A. (1983). *Hospice: A caring challenge.* Springfield, IL: Charles C Thomas.

Moore, Kathleen (1984). Training social workers to work with the terminally ill. *Health and Social Work,* 19 (4): 268-273.

Mount, Balfour (1993). Whole person care: Beyond psychosocial and physical needs. *The American Journal of Hospice and Palliative Care* (January/February): 28-37.

Naierman, Naomi (2001). The Medicare hospice benefit: Learning about a well-kept secret. *Healthcare and Aging,* 8 (2): 1-8.

National Association for Home Care (1996). *Basic statistics about home care.* Washington, DC: Author.

National Association for Home Care (2001). *Basic statistics about hospice* (1999 statistics, updated July 2001). Washington, DC: Author.

National Association of Social Workers (1997). *Social work speaks* (Fourth edition). Washington, DC: Author.

National Hospice and Palliative Care Organization (2001). NHPCO facts and figures. Phone: 703-837-3137. Alexandria, VA: Author.

Paradis, Lenora Finn (1985). *Hospice handbook: A guide for managers and planners.* Rockford, MD: Aspen Systems.

Parry, Joan K., and Ryan, Angela Shen (Eds.) (1995). *A cross-cultural look at death, dying, and religion.* Chicago, IL: Nelson Hall.

Phipps, E. E. (1988). The origin of hospices/hospitals. *Death Studies,* 12 (2): 91-99.

Pilsecker, C. (1979). Terminal cancer: A challenge for social work. *Social Work in Health Care,* 4 (4): 369-379.

Preston, Robert (1979). *The dilemmas of care.* New York: Elsevier Press.

Proffitt, Linda J. (1987). Hospice. In Minahan, Anne (Ed.), *The encyclopedia of social work* (Eighteenth edition). Washington, DC: NASW Press, 812-816.

Quig, L. (1989). The role of the hospice social worker. *American Journal of Hospice Care,* 6 (4): 22-23.

Reece, Dona, and Sontag, Mary-Ann (2001). Successful interprofessional collaboration on the hospice team. *Health and Social Work,* 26 (3): 167-175.

Richman, Jack M. (1995). Hospice. In Edwards, Richard L. (Ed.), *The encyclopedia of social work* (Nineteenth edition). Washington, DC: NASW Press, 1358-1364.

Rodway, Margaret R., and Blythe, Judith (1994). Social work practice in palliative care. In Holosko, M.J. and Taylor, P.A. (Eds.), *Social work practice in health care settings* (Second edition). Toronto, Canada: Canadian Scholar's Press, 419-437.

Rusnack, Betty, Schaefer, Sarajane McNulty, and Moxley, David (1988). "Safe passage": Social work roles and functions in hospice care. *Social Work in Health Care,* 13 (3): 3-18.

Saunders, Cicely (1982). Hospice care. In Ajemian, Ina and Mount, Balfour (Eds.), *The R.V.H. manual on pallative hospice care: A resource manual.* Salem, NH: Ayer, 21-26.

Smith, Wade (1994). Building a hospice: A personal viewpoint. In Kornblum, William and Smith, Carolyn D. (Eds.), *The healing experience: Readings on the social context of health care.* Englewood Cliffs, NJ: Prentice-Hall, 203-208.

Sontag, Mary-Ann (1996). A comparison of hospice programs based on Medicare certification status. *The American Journal of Hospice and Palliative Care,* 13 (2): 32-41.

Sontag, Mary-Ann, Nadig, Jennifer, and Henry, Lisa (1994). The children's grief workshop: Social work practice in hospice. *The American Journal of Hospice and Palliative Care,* 11 (3): 23-29.

Stark, Doretta E., and Johnson, Edith M. (1983). Implications of hospice concepts for social work practice with oncology patients and their families in an acute care teaching hospital. *Social Work in Health Care,* 9 (1): 63-70.

Storey, Porter (1993). Hospice settings around the world. *The American Journal of Hospice and Palliative Care,* 10 (4) (July/August): 4-5.

Strang, P. (1992). Emotional and social aspects of cancer pain. *Acta Oncologica,* 31 (3): 323-326.

Stubblefield, Kristine S. (1990). A preventive program for bereaved families. In Davidson, Kay W. and Clarke, Sylvia S. (Eds.), *Social work in health care: A handbook for practice,* Part I. Binghamton, NY: The Haworth Press, Inc., 385-400.

U.S. Government Printing Office (1994). *State operations manual: Provider certification.* Health Care Financing Administration. Transmittal number 265. (Interpretative Guidelines-Hospice; regulation 418.68, tag number 265).

U.S. Government Printing Office (2000). *Statistical abstracts of the United States.* Washington, DC: Author.

Van Loon, Ruth Anne (1999). Desire to die in terminally ill people: A framework for assessment and intervention. *Health and Social Work,* 24 (4): 260-268.

Weiner, Herbert (1984). An integrative model of health, illness, and disease. *Health and Social Work,* 9 (4): 253-260.

Weisman, Avery D. (1972). *On death and dying—A psychiatric study of the terminally ill.* New York: Behavioral Publications.

Chapter 8

Ball, Robert M. (1996). Medicare's roots: What Medicare's architects had in mind. *Generations,* 20 (2): 13-19.

Belcher, John R. (1993). The trade-offs of developing a case management model for chronically mentally ill people. *Health and Social Work,* 18 (1): 20-31.

Billings, John (1999). Access to health care services. In Kovner, Anthony R. and Jonas, Steven (Eds.), *Health care delivery in the United States*. New York: Springer, 401-438.

Chambliss, Catherine, Pinto, Debra, and McGuigan, Joan (1997). Reactions to managed care among psychologists and social workers. *Psychological Reports*, 80 (1): 147-154.

Cornelius, Donald S. (1994). Managed care and social work: Constructing a context and a response. *Social Work in Health Care*, 20 (1): 47-63.

Davidson, Jeanette R., and Davidson, Tim (1996). Confidentiality and managed care: Ethical and legal concerns. *Health and Social Work*, 21 (3): 208-215.

Freeman, Michael A., and Trabin, Tom (1994). *Managed behavioral health care: History, models, key issues, and future course*. Rockville, MD: U.S. Center for Mental Health Services.

Friedland, Robert B. (1996). Managed care and all of us: The role of managed care in the future. *Generations*, 20 (2): 37-41.

Friedman, Emily (1996). Capitation, integration, and managed care. *JAMA*, 275 (12): 957-962.

Grayson, Mary (1998). An interview with Dick Davidson. *Hospitals and Health Networks*, 73 (July 5): 12-16.

Hodge, Melville H. (1996). Health care and America's rolling depression. *Health Care Management Review*, 21 (3): 7-12.

Kane, Robert L. (1995). Canadian lessons in health care reform: Reading between the lines. In Eve, Susan Brown, Havens, Betty, and Ingman, Stanley R. (Eds.), *The Canadian health care system: Lessons for the United States*. Lanham, MD: University Press, 7-18.

Karger, Howard Jacob, and Stoesz, Howard (1998). *American social welfare policy: A pluralistic approach* (Third edition). New York: Longman.

Kirkman-Liff, Bradford L. (1996). Health care reform in the Netherlands, Israel, Germany, England, and Sweden. *Generations*, 20 (2): 65-69.

Kovner, Anthony R. (1999). Health maintenance organizations and managed care. In Kovner, Anthony R. and Jonas, Steven (Eds.), *Health care delivery in the United States*. New York: Springer, 279-302.

Lave, Judith R. (1996). Rethinking Medicare. *Generations*, 20 (2): 19-23.

Limbacher, P.B. (1998). A taste of profit. *Modern Healthcare*, 28(6).

Lyons, Barbara, Rowland, Diane, and Hanson, Kristina (1996). Another look at Medicaid. *Generations*, 20 (2): 24-29.

Manderscheid, Rondals W., and Henderson, Marilyn J. (1998). Federal and state legislative program directions for managed care. In Mullen, Edward J. and Magnabosco, Jennifer L. (Eds.), *Outcomes measurement in the human services: Cross-cutting issues and methods*. Washington, DC: NASW Press, 113-123.

Mechanic, David (1999). *Mental health and social policy: The emergence of managed care* (Fourth edition). Boston: Allyn and Bacon.

Mizrahi, Terry (1993). Managed care and managed competition: A primer for social work. *Health and Social Work*, 18 (2): 86-91.

Moore, C.W. (1986). *The mediation process: Practical strategies for resolving conflict*. San Francisco: Jossey-Bass.

Munson, Carlton E. (1997). The future of clinical social work and managed cost organizations. *Psychiatric Services,* 48 (4): 479-482.

Newhouse, Joseph P. (1996). An iconoclastic view of health care cost containment.
Generations, 20 (2): 61-63.

Rachlis, Michael M. (1995). The Canadian experience with public health insurance.
In Eve, Susan Brown, Havens, Betty, and Ingman, Stanley R. (Eds.), *The Cana-
dian health care system: Lessons for the United States.* Lanham, MD: University
Press, 143-154.

Rovner, Julie (1998). Brace yourself: Expect an explosion of data about Medicare's
new options. *AARP Bulletin,* 39 (8): 2, 18.

Sarudi, Dagmara (2001a). Keeping patients safe. *Hospitals and Health Networks,*
75 (4): 42-46.

Sarudi, Dagmara (2001b). The leapfrog effect. *Hospitals and Health Networks,* 75 (5):
32-36.

Schuster, James M., Kern, Edward E., Kane, Vince, and Nettleman, Leslie (1994).
Changing roles of mental health clinicians in multidisciplinary teams. *Hospital
and Community Psychiatry,* 45 (12): 1187-1189.

Shi, Leiyu (2000). Type of health insurance and quality of primary care experience.
American Journal of Public Health, 90 (12): 1848-1855.

Shindul-Rothschild, Judith (2001). The macroeconomic impact of managed care. In
Veeder, Nancy W. and Peebles-Wilkins, Wilma (Eds.), *Managed care services:
Policy, programs, and research.* London: Oxford University Press, 15-30.

Simmons, Henry E. (1996). The nation's least understood health care problem—
The quality of medical care. *Generations,* 20 (2): 57-61.

Strom-Gottfried, Kimberly (1998a). Applying a conflict resolution framework to
disputes in managed care. *Social Work,* 43 (5): 393-401.

Strom-Gottfried, Kimberly (1998b). Informed consent meets managed care. *Health
and Social Work,* 23 (1): 25-33.

U.S. Government Printing Office (1997a). *Health, United States, 1996-1997.* Washington, DC: Author.

U.S. Government Printing Office (1997b). *Statistical abstracts of the United States.*
Washington, DC: Author.

U.S. Government Printing Office (2000a). *Health, United States.* Washington, DC:
Author.

U.S. Government Printing Office (2000b). *Statistical abstracts of the United States.*
Washington, DC: Author.

Woolhandler, Steffie, and Himmelstein, David U. (1997). Costs of care and administration at for-profit and other hospitals in the United States. *New England Journal of Medicine,* 336 (11): 769-799.

Zis, Michael, Jacobs, Lawrence R., and Shapiro, Robert Y. (1996). The elusive
common ground: The politics of public opinion and health care reform. *Generations,* 20 (2): 7-11.

Chapter 9

Armstrong, Pat, and Armstrong, Hugh, with Fedan, Claudia (1998). *Universal healthcare: What the United States can learn from the Canadian experience.* New York: The New Press.

Auslander, Gail K. (2000). Outcomes of social work intervention in health care settings. *Social Work in Health Care,* 31 (2): 31-46.

Berkman, Barbara (1998). Outcomes measurement for social work research and practice in health care. In Mullen, Edward J. and Magnabosco, Jennifer L. (Eds.), *Outcomes measurement in the human services: Cross-cutting issues and methods.* Washington, DC: NASW Press, 218-223.

Berman, William H., and Hurt, Stephen W. (1997). Developing clinical outcomes systems: Conceptual and practical issues. In Mullen, Edward J. and Magnabosco, Jennifer L. (Eds.), *Outcomes measurement in the human services: Cross-cutting issues and methods.* Washington, DC: NASW Press, 81-97.

Bloom, Samuel W. (2000). Social work and the behavioral sciences: Past history, future prospects. *Social Work in Health Care,* 31 (3): 25-37.

Bracht, Neil (Ed.) (1999). *Health promotion at the community level: New advances* (Second edition). Thousand Oaks, CA: Sage Publications.

Brown Eve, Susan, Havens, Betty, and Ingman, Stanley R. (1995). *The Canadian health care system: Lessons for the United States.* New York: University Press of America.

Concoran, Kevin, and Fischer, Joel (2000). *Measures for clinical practice: A sourcebook* (Third edition), Volume 2: Adults. New York: The Free Press.

Davidson, Kay (1998). Educating students for social work in health care today. In Schamess, Gerald and Lightburn, Anita (Eds.), *Humane managed care.* Washington, DC: NASW Press, 425-429.

Davis, King (1998). Managed health care: Forcing social work to make choices and changes. In Schamess, Gerald and Lightburn, Anita (Eds.), *Humane managed care.* Washington, DC: NASW Press, 409-424.

Ell, Kathleen (1996). Social work and health care practice and policy: A psychosocial research agenda. *Social Work,* 41 (6): 583-592.

Evans, Robert G., Barer, Morris L., and Marmor, Theodore R. (Eds.) (1994). *Why are some people healthy and others not? The determinants of health of populations.* New York: Aldine De Gruyter.

Kawachi, Ichiro, Kennedy, Bruce, and Wilkinson, Richard (1999). *The society and population health reader.* New York. The New Press.

Keigher, Sharon M. (1997). What role for social work in the new health care practice paradigm? *Health and Social Work,* 22 (2): 149-155.

Kelner, M. (1985). Community support networks: Current issues. *Canadian Journal of Public Health,* 76 (Supplement 1): 69-70.

Lee,W., Eng, C., Fox, N., and Etienne M. (1998). PACE: A model for integrated care of frail older patients. *Geriatrics,* 53 (June): 62-73.

McDowell, Ian, and Newell, Claire (1987). *Measuring health: A guide to rating scales and questionnaires.* New York: Oxford University Press.

McDowell, Ian, and Newell, Claire (1996). *Measuring health: A guide to rating scales and questionnaires* (Second edition). New York: Oxford University Press.

McKay, Mary McKernan, Stoewe, Judith, McCadam, Kathleen, and Gonzales, Jude (1998). Increasing access to child mental health services for urban children and their caregivers. *Health and Social Work,* 23 (1): 9-23.

Mechanic, David (1978). *Medical sociology.* New York: The Free Press.

Miringoff, Marc, and Miringoff, Marque-Luisa (1999). *The social health of the nation: How America is really doing.* New York: Oxford University Press.

Monkman, Marjorie McQueen (1991). Outcome objectives in social work practice: Persons and environment. *Social Work,* 36 (3): 253-258.

Mullen, Edward J., and Magnabosco, Jennifer L. (Eds.) (1997). *Outcomes measurement in the human services: Cross-cutting issues and methods.* Washington, DC: National Association of Social Workers Press.

Munson, Carlton E. (1998). Evolution and trends in the relationship between clinical social work practice and managed cost organizations. In Schamess, Gerald and Lightburn, Anita (Eds.), *Humane managed care.* Washington, DC: NASW Press, 308-324.

O'Neill, John (2001). Social interventions in health care pushed. *NASW NEWS,* 16 (5): 3.

Payne, Malcolm (2000). *Teamwork in multiprofessional care.* Chicago: Lyceum Books, Inc.

Poland, Blake, D., Green, Lawrence, and Rootman, Irving (Eds.) (2000). *Settings for health promotion: Linking theory and practice.* Thousand Oaks: Sage Publications.

Raczynski, James M., and DiClemente, Ralph J. (1999). Future directions in research and practice. In Raczynski, James M. and DiClemente, Ralph J. (Eds.), *Handbook of health promotion and disease prevention.* New York: Kluwer Academic/Plenum Publishers, 661.

Robbins, Susan P., Chatterjee, Pranab, and Canda, Edward R. (1998). *Contemporary human behavior theory: A critical perspective for social work.* Boston: Allyn and Bacon.

Rosenberg, Gary (1998). Social work in a health and mental health managed care environment. In Schamess, Gerald and Lightburn, Anita (Eds.), *Humane managed care.* Washington, DC: NASW Press, 3-22.

Schamess, Gerald, and Lightburn, Anita (Eds.) (1998). *Humane managed care.* Washington, DC: NASW Press.

Vaghy, Andrea (1998). Report identifies health care issues affecting social work education. *Social Work Education Reporter,* 46 (3): 8, 36.

Van Hook, Mary P., Berkman, Barbara, and Dunkle, Ruth (1996). Assessment tools for general health settings: PRIME MD, OARS, and SF-36. *Health and Social Work,* 21 (3): 230-234.

Veeder, Nancy W., and Peebles-Wilkins, Wilma (1998). Research needs in managed behavioral health care. In Schamess, Gerald and Lightburn, Anita (Eds.), *Humane managed care.* Washington, DC: NASW Press, 483-504.

Volland, Patricia J. (1996). Social work practice in health care: Looking to the future with a different lens. *Social Work in Health Care,* 24 (1/2): 35-51.

Volland, Patricia J., Berkman, Barbara, Stein, Gary, and Vaghy, Andrea (2000). *Social work education for practice in health care: Final report* (Second edition). New York: The New York Academy of Medicine. <http://www.nyam.org>.

Wernet, Stephen (Ed.) (1999). *Managed care in human services.* Chicago: Lyceum Books, Inc.

World Health Organization (1986). Ottawa Charter for Health Promotion. <http://www.who.dk/policy/ottawa.htm>.

Index

SOCIAL WORK IN THE HEALTH FIELD
A Care Perspective, Second Edition

_____in hardbound at $52.46 (regularly $69.95) (ISBN: 0-7890-2118-8)

_____in softbound at $29.96 (regularly $39.95) (ISBN: 0-7890-2119-6)

Or order online and use Code HEC25 in the shopping cart.

COST OF BOOKS_____

OUTSIDE US/CANADA/
MEXICO: ADD 20%_____

POSTAGE & HANDLING_____
(US: $5.00 for first book & $2.00
for each additional book)
Outside US: $6.00 for first book
& $2.00 for each additional book)

SUBTOTAL_____

IN CANADA: ADD 7% GST_____

STATE TAX_____
(NY, OH & MN residents, please
add appropriate local sales tax)

FINAL TOTAL_____
(If paying in Canadian funds,
convert using the current
exchange rate, UNESCO
coupons welcome)

☐ **BILL ME LATER:** ($5 service charge will be added)

(Bill-me option is good on US/Canada/Mexico orders only;
not good to jobbers, wholesalers, or subscription agencies.)

☐ Check here if billing address is different from
shipping address and attach purchase order and
billing address information.

Signature_____

☐ **PAYMENT ENCLOSED: $**_____

☐ **PLEASE CHARGE TO MY CREDIT CARD.**

☐ Visa ☐ MasterCard ☐ AmEx ☐ Discover
☐ Diner's Club ☐ Eurocard ☐ JCB

Account # _____

Exp. Date_____

Signature_____

Prices in US dollars and subject to change without notice.

NAME_____

INSTITUTION_____

ADDRESS_____

CITY_____

STATE/ZIP_____

COUNTRY_____ COUNTY (NY residents only)_____

TEL_____ FAX_____

E-MAIL_____

May we use your e-mail address for confirmations and other types of information? ☐ Yes ☐ No
We appreciate receiving your e-mail address and fax number. Haworth would like to e-mail or fax special
discount offers to you, as a preferred customer. **We will never share, rent, or exchange your e-mail address
or fax number.** We regard such actions as an invasion of your privacy.